Infectious Disease Threats

Editor

DOUGLAS S. PAAUW

MEDICAL CLINICS
OF NORTH AMERICA

www.medical.theclinics.com

July 2013 • Volume 97 • Number 4

ELSEVIER

1600 John F. Kennedy Boulevard • Suite 1800 • Philadelphia, Pennsylvania, 19103-2899

http://www.theclinics.com

MEDICAL CLINICS OF NORTH AMERICA Volume 97, Number 4
July 2013 ISSN 0025-7125, ISBN-13: 978-1-4557-5584-4

Editor: Pamela Hetherington

Medical Clinics of North America (ISSN 0025-7125) is published bimonthly by Elsevier Inc., 360 Park Avenue South, New York, NY 10010-1710. Months of issue are January, March, May, July, September, and November. Periodicals postage paid at New York, NY, and additional mailing offices. Subscription prices are USD 241 per year for US individuals, USD 441 per year for US institutions, USD 121 per year for US students, USD 307 per year for Canadian individuals, USD 572 per year for Canadian institutions, USD 190 per year for Canadian students, USD 372 per year for international individuals, USD 572 per year for international institutions and USD 190 per year for international students. To receive student/resident rate, orders must be accompanied by name of affiliated institution, date of term, and the *signature* of program/residency coordinator on institution letterhead. Orders will be billed at individual rate until proof of status is received. Foreign air speed delivery is included in all *Clinics* subscription prices. All prices are subject to change without notice. **POSTMASTER:** Send address changes to *Medical Clinics of North America*, Elsevier Health Sciences Division, Subscription Customer Service, 3251 Riverport Lane, Maryland Heights, MO 63043. **Customer Service: Telephone: 1-800-654-2452** (U.S. and Canada); **1-314-447-8871** (outside U.S. and Canada). **Fax: 1-314-447-8029. E-mail: journalscustomerservice-usa@elsevier.com** (for print support); **journalsonlinesupport-usa@elsevier.com** (for online support).

Reprints. For copies of 100 or more of articles in this publication, please contact the Commercial Reprints Department, Elsevier Inc., 360 Park Avenue South, New York, NY 10010-1710. Tel.: 212-633-3812; Fax: 212-462-1935; E-mail: reprints@elsevier.com.

Medical Clinics of North America is also published in Spanish by McGraw-Hill Interamericana Editores S. A., P.O. Box 5-237, 06500 Mexico, D.F., Mexico.

Medical Clinics of North America is covered in *MEDLINE/PubMed (Index Medicus), Current Contents, ASCA, Excerpta Medica, Science Citation Index, and ISI/BIOMED.*

Printed in the United States of America.

PROGRAM OBJECTIVE
The goal of the *Medical Clinics of North America* is to keep practicing physicians up to date with current clinical practice by providing timely articles reviewing the state of the art in patient care.

TARGET AUDIENCE
All practicing physicians and other healthcare professionals.

LEARNING OBJECTIVES
Upon completion of this activity, participants will be able to:
1. Review enterohemorrhagic E. coli infections and the hemolytic-uremic syndrome.
2. Discuss the management of urinary tract infections in the era of rising antimicrobial resistance.
3. Describe clostridium difficile infections, methicillin-resistant staphylococcus aureus infections, and serious group A streptococcal infections.

ACCREDITATION
The Elsevier Office of Continuing Medical Education (EOCME) is accredited by the Accreditation Council for Continuing Medical Education (ACCME) to provide continuing medical education for physicians.

The EOCME designates this enduring material for a maximum of 15 *AMA PRA Category 1 Credit*(s)™. Physicians should claim only the credit commensurate with the extent of their participation in the activity.

All other health care professionals requesting continuing education credit for this activity will be issued a certificate of participation.

DISCLOSURE OF CONFLICTS OF INTEREST
The EOCME assesses conflict of interest with its instructors, faculty, planners, and other individuals who are in a position to control the content of CME activities. All relevant conflicts of interest that are identified are thoroughly vetted by EOCME for fair balance, scientific objectivity, and patient care recommendations. EOCME is committed to providing its learners with CME activities that promote improvements or quality in healthcare and not a specific proprietary business or a commercial interest.

The planning committee, staff, authors and editors listed below have identified no financial relationships or relationships to products or devices they or their spouse/life partner have with commercial interest related to the content of this CME activity:

Richard W. Arnold, MD; Samuel Y. Ash, MD; Mayan Bomstzyk, MD; Pamela Hetherington; Christopher L. Knight, MD; Angelena M. Labella, MD; Sandy Lavery; Conrad Liles, MD, PhD; Ajit P. Limaye, MD; John B. Lynch, MD, MPH; Eileen K. Maziarz, MD; Jill McNair; Susan E. Merel, MD; Kim O'Connor, MD; Douglas S. Paauw, MD, MACP; Genevieve L. Pagalilauan, MD; Andrea V. Page, MD, MSc; Lindsay Parnell; Paul S. Pottinger, MD; Santha Priya; John V.L. Sheffield, MD; Amanda Kay Shepherd, MD; Tara B. Spector, MD; Dennis L. Stevens, PhD, MD; Christina M. Surawicz, MD; Christopher J. Wong, MD; Jenny Wright, MD.

The planning committee, staff, authors and editors listed below have identified financial relationships or relationships to products or devices they or their spouse/life partner have with commercial interest related to the content of this CME activity:

UNAPPROVED/OFF-LABEL USE DISCLOSURE
The EOCME requires CME faculty to disclose to the participants:
1. When products or procedures being discussed are off-label, unlabelled, experimental, and/or investigational (not US Food and Drug Administration (FDA) approved); and
2. Any limitations on the information presented, such as data that are preliminary or that represent ongoing research, interim analyses, and/or unsupported opinions. Faculty may discuss information about pharmaceutical agents that is outside of FDA-approved labelling. This information is intended solely for CME and is not intended to promote off-label use of these medications. If you have any questions, contact the medical affairs department of the manufacturer for the most recent prescribing information.

TO ENROLL
To enroll in the *Medical Clinics of North America* Continuing Medical Education program, call customer service at 1-800-654-2452 or sign up online at http://www.theclinics.com/home/cme. The CME program is available to subscribers for an additional annual fee of USD $267.

METHOD OF PARTICIPATION
In order to claim credit, participants must complete the following:
1. Complete enrolment as indicated above.
2. Read the activity.
3. Complete the CME Test and Evaluation. Participants must achieve a score of 70% on the test. All CME Tests and Evaluations must be completed online.

CME INQUIRIES/SPECIAL NEEDS
For all CME inquiries or special needs, please contact elsevierCME@elsevier.com.

MEDICAL CLINICS OF NORTH AMERICA

FORTHCOMING ISSUES

September 2013
The Diabetic Foot
Andrew J. Boulton, *Editor*

November 2013
Pre-Operative Management of the Patient with Chronic Disease
Jeffrey Kirsch, and Ansgar Brambrink, *Editors*

January 2014
Diagnosis and Management of Chronic Liver Diseases
Anne Larson, *Editor*

RECENT ISSUES

May 2013
Early Diagnosis and Intervention in Predementia Alzheimer's Disease
José L. Molinuevo, MD, PhD,
Jeffrey L. Cummings, MD, ScD,
Bruno Dubois, MD, and
Philip Scheltens, MD, *Editors*

March 2013
Management of Acute and Chronic Headache Pain
Steven D. Waldman, MD, JD, *Editor*

January 2013
Diabetic Chronic Kidney Disease
Mark E. Williams, MD, FACP, FASN, *Editor*

RELATED INTEREST

Infectious Disease Clinics of North America Volume 27, Issue 1 (March 2013)
Community-Acquired Pneumonia: Controversies and Questions
Thomas M. File Jr, MD, MSc, *Editor*

DOWNLOAD
Free App!

Review Articles
THE CLINICS

NOW AVAILABLE FOR YOUR iPhone and iPad

Contributors

EDITOR

DOUGLAS S. PAAUW, MD, MACP
Professor of Medicine, Division of General Internal Medicine, Rathmann Family
Foundation Endowed Chair for Patient-Centered Clinical Education; Medicine Student
Programs, Rathmann Family Foundation Endowed Chair for Patient-Centered Clinical
Education, Professor of Medicine, University of Washington School of Medicine, Seattle,
Washington

AUTHORS

RICHARD W. ARNOLD, MD, FACP
Clinical Professor of Medicine, Department of Medicine, University of Washington, Seattle,
Washington

SAMUEL Y. ASH, MD
Chief Resident, Department of Medicine, University of Washington Medical Center,
Seattle, Washington

MAYAN BOMSZTYK, MD
Acting Instructor, Department of Medicine, University of Washington, Seattle, Washington

CHRISTOPHER L. KNIGHT, MD
Associate Professor of Medicine, Division of General Internal Medicine, Department of
Medicine, University of Washington School of Medicine, Seattle, Washington

ANGELENA M. LABELLA, MD
Assistant Professor, Section of Hospital Medicine, Division of General Medicine,
Department of Medicine, New York Presbyterian, Columbia University Medical Center,
New York, New York

W. CONRAD LILES, MD, PhD
Affiliate Professor of Medicine, Division of Infectious Diseases, Department of Medicine,
Mount Sinai Hospital-University Health Network, University of Toronto, Toronto, Ontario,
Canada; Associate Chair and Professor of Medicine, Division of Allergy and Infectious
Diseases, Department of Medicine, University of Washington School of Medicine, Seattle,
Washington

AJIT P. LIMAYE, MD
Professor, Division of Allergy and Infectious Disease, University of Washington School of
Medicine, University of Washington, Seattle, Washington

JOHN B. LYNCH, MD, MPH
Assistant Professor, Department of Medicine, Division of Allergy and Infectious Diseases,
University of Washington School of Medicine, Seattle, Washington

EILEEN K. MAZIARZ, MD
Fellow, Division of Infectious Diseases and International Health, Department of Internal Medicine, Duke University Medical Center, Durham, North Carolina

SUSAN E. MEREL, MD
Assistant Professor, Hospital Medicine Program, Division of General Internal Medicine, Department of Medicine, University of Washington Medical Center, Seattle, Washington

KIM M. O'CONNOR, MD, FACP
Assistant Professor of Medicine, Division of General Internal Medicine, University of Washington School of Medicine, Seattle, Washington

DOUGLAS S. PAAUW, MD, MACP
Professor of Medicine, Division of General Internal Medicine, Rathmann Family Foundation Endowed Chair for Patient-Centered Clinical Education; Medicine Student Programs, Rathmann Family Foundation Endowed Chair for Patient-Centered Clinical Education, Professor of Medicine, University of Washington School of Medicine, Seattle, Washington

GENEVIEVE L. PAGALILAUAN, MD, FACP
Assistant Professor, Division of General Internal Medicine, University of Washington School of Medicine, Seattle, Washington

ANDREA V. PAGE, MD, MSc
Assistant Professor, Division of Infectious Diseases, Department of Medicine, Mount Sinai Hospital-University Health Network, University of Toronto, Toronto, Ontario, Canada

PAUL S. POTTINGER, MD
Associate Professor of Medicine, Division of Allergy and Infectious Diseases; Associate Director, Infectious Diseases Fellowship Training Program, University of Washington, Seattle, Washington

JOHN V.L. SHEFFIELD, MD
Professor, Division of General Internal Medicine, Department of Medicine, Harborview Medical Center, University of Washington, Seattle, Washington

AMANDA KAY SHEPHERD, MD
Acting Instructor, Department of Medicine, University of Washington, Seattle, Washington

TARA B. SPECTOR, MD
Acting Instructor of Medicine, Division of General Internal Medicine, University of Washington Medical Center, Seattle, Washington

DENNIS L. STEVENS, PhD, MD
Chief, Infectious Diseases Section, Veterans Administration Medical Center, Boise, Idaho; Professor of Medicine, University of Washington School of Medicine, Seattle, Washington

CHRISTINA M. SURAWICZ, MD
Professor of Medicine, Division of Gastroenterology, Department of Medicine, University of Washington School of Medicine, Seattle, Washington

CHRISTOPHER J. WONG, MD
Assistant Professor, Division of General Internal Medicine, Department of Medicine, University of Washington, Seattle, Washington

JENNY WRIGHT, MD
Acting Instructor of Medicine, University of Washington School of Medicine; General Internal Medicine Center, University of Washington Medical Center, Seattle, Washington

Contents

Preface: Infectious Disease Threats: What Are We to Do?   **xiii**

Douglas S. Paauw

Herpes Zoster   **503**

Kim M. O'Connor and Douglas S. Paauw

> Herpes zoster is a common condition that significantly affects health-related quality of life. Most cases occur in immunocompetent individuals older than 60 years; however, immunosuppressed patients are at particularly high risk. Post-herpetic neuralgia is the most common serious complication of herpes zoster, and is much more common in the very elderly. Vaccination with the zoster vaccine is recommended for most people older than 60, and reduces the incidence of herpes zoster and the occurrence of post-herpetic neuralgia.

Clostridium difficile Infection   **523**

Christopher L. Knight and Christina M. Surawicz

> _Clostridium difficile_ is emerging as a common cause of infectious diarrhea. Incidence has increased dramatically since 2000, associated with a new strain that features both increased toxin production and increased resistance to antibiotics. For patients with mild to moderate disease, oral metronidazole is usually the first choice of treatment, and those with severe disease should be treated with vancomycin, with additional intravenous metronidazole in some cases. Fecal microbiota transplantation is a potentially promising therapy for patients with multiple recurrences of _C difficile_ infection. Prevention of nosocomial transmission is crucial to reducing disease outbreaks in health care settings.

Pertussis   **537**

Tara B. Spector and Eileen K. Maziarz

> Pertussis, or whopping cough, is an upper respiratory tract infection caused by _Bordetella pertussis_. It has long been a concern in pediatric populations, leading to aggressive vaccination strategies to help decrease pediatric disease. In recent years, recognition of pertussis infection in adult populations has increased, leading to more frequent diagnosis and recommendations for booster immunizations in the adult population. Early recognition and treatment as well as vaccination will help reduce the current increase in this disease.

Multidrug-resistant Tuberculosis   **553**

John B. Lynch

> Multidrug-resistant tuberculosis (MDR-TB) threatens to become the dominant form of tuberculosis in many parts of the world because of decades of inappropriate treatment on a global scale. Infection with MDR-TB is

associated with poor outcomes because of delays in treatment and the need for complex, toxic, and long medication regimens. Most cases are undetected because of technological and economic barriers to diagnosing tuberculosis and the availability of assays to test for drug resistance. Experience in treating MDR-TB is scarce. Tuberculosis was once curable, but could become a potentially untreatable infectious disease unless efforts are made to control it.

Infections in Transplant Patients   581

Genevieve L. Pagalilauan and Ajit P. Limaye

Recipients of solid organ transplants (SOT) need primary care providers (PCPs) who are familiar with their unique needs and understand the lifelong infectious risks faced by SOT patients because of their need for lifelong immunosuppressive medications. SOT recipients can present with atypical and muted manifestations of infections, for which the knowledgable PCP will initiate a comprehensive evaluation. The goal of this article is to familiarize PCPs with the infectious challenges facing SOT patients. General concepts are reviewed, and a series of patient cases described that illustrate the specific learning points based on common presenting clinical symptoms.

Methicillin-Resistant *Staphylococcus aureus* Infections   601

Paul S. Pottinger

Methicillin-resistant *Staphylococcus aureus* (MRSA) is an important pathogen that has exploded into clinical prominence in a short period. New medications are available for the treatment of MRSA infections, each with its own pitfalls and caveats. However, the resistance profile of the bacteria is becoming more complex. Recent guidelines from the Infectious Diseases Society of America provide an evidence-based framework for the management of MRSA infections. This article provides additional practical advice on approaches to MRSA, including the detection, prevention, and management of a variety of its common presentations.

Influenza   621

Angelena M. Labella and Susan E. Merel

Influenza is a common virus whose ability to change its genetic makeup allows for disease of pandemic proportion. This article summarizes the different strains of influenza circulating in the United States for the past century, the diagnosis and treatment of influenza, as well as the different ways to prevent disease. This information will be of value to clinicians caring for patients both in the hospital and in the community.

Pneumococcus   647

Samuel Y. Ash and John V.L. Sheffield

Pneumococcus is one of the most common bacterial pathogens encountered in medicine. This article summarizes the risk factors, pathogenesis, treatment, and prevention of the spectrum of disease caused by pneumococcus with particular emphasis on antibiotic resistance as well as immunization. This information is useful for physicians caring for patients both as inpatients and outpatients as well as for those concerned with public health and disease prevention.

Complications of Antibiotic Therapy   667

Jenny Wright and Douglas S. Paauw

Antibiotics have greatly changed the practice of medicine for the better. Many infections commonly treated in the outpatient setting with antibiotics (eg, urinary tract infections, streptococcal pharyngitis), which previously caused significant morbidity and mortality, are now typically benign. However, with antibiotic therapy come side effects, ranging in severity from mild nausea to life-threatening cytopenias. This article highlights important complications of antibiotic therapy that may be encountered by outpatient providers. Side effects by system are discussed, and a few important drug-specific complications and important drug-drug interactions highlighted.

Enterohemorrhagic *Escherichia coli* Infections and the Hemolytic-Uremic Syndrome   681

Andrea V. Page and W. Conrad Liles

Enterohemorrhagic Escherichia coli (EHEC; Shiga toxin/verotoxin-producing E. coli) can cause bloody diarrhea and the hemolytic-uremic syndrome (HUS), typically following consumption of contaminated food (including ground beef, leafy greens, and sprouts) and water. Often associated with foodborne outbreaks, EHEC possess unique virulence factors that facilitate effective colonization of the human gastrointestinal tract and subsequent release of Shiga toxin. This article reviews the epidemiology, pathogenesis, clinical presentation, treatment, and prevention of EHEC infections, focusing on E. coli O157:H7, the serotype most common in North America, and E. coli O104:H4, the serotype responsible for the EHEC outbreak in Germany in 2011.

Infections in Travelers   697

Mayan Bomsztyk and Richard W. Arnold

Travel medicine continues to grow as international tourism and patient medical complexity increases. This article reflects the state of the current field, but new recommendations on immunizations, resistance patterns, and treatment modalities constantly change. The US Centers for Disease Control and the World Health Organization maintain helpful Web sites for both patient and physician. With thoughtful preparation and prevention, risks can be minimized and travel can continue as safely as possible.

Serious Group A Streptococcal Infections   721

Christopher J. Wong and Dennis L. Stevens

The spectrum of illnesses caused by group A streptococcus (GAS) includes invasive infections, noninvasive infections, and noninfectious complications. Increasingly virulent infections associated with high morbidity and mortality have been observed since the late 1980s and continue to be prevalent in North America and worldwide. Penicillin remains the therapy of choice, with the addition of clindamycin recommended in high risk cases. Early recognition of GAS as the cause of these serious clinical syndromes is critical for timely administration of appropriate therapy. In this review, the pathophysiology, clinical manifestations, and treatment of invasive GAS infections are discussed.

Management of Urinary Tract Infections in the Era of Increasing Antimicrobial Resistance   737

Amanda Kay Shepherd and Paul S. Pottinger

Antimicrobial resistance of urinary pathogens is increasing. Most urinary tract infections (UTIs) should still be treated empirically. However, patients with recurrence or other risk factors for resistance may benefit from urine culture. Patients with recurrent UTI often resort to antibiotic prevention, a risky proposition in terms of resistance. Non-antimicrobial preventative methods should be considered first. If preventative antibiotics must be used, postcoital patient-initiated protocols are effective and reduce overall antibiotic exposure compared with continuous prophylaxis. Consider referring patients for urologic evaluation when at risk for complicated UTIs or when recurrence continues despite conservative interventions.

Index   759

Preface

Infectious Disease Threats: What Are We to Do?

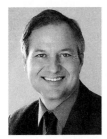

Douglas S. Paauw, MD, MACP
Editor

Over the past fifty years there has been a dramatic change in many of the infectious diseases that we diagnose and treat. A half century ago, we were just beginning to be armed with therapies that were effective for such common diseases as tuberculosis, *Staphylococcus aureus* infection, community-acquired pneumonia, and urinary tract infections. Therapies became widely available and it appeared that we had conquered many of the infectious disease problems that had plagued patients for centuries. Expectations arose that physicians should be able to treat and cure all infectious diseases. Antibiotics were the new miracle, and the public began to believe that all you needed was an antibiotic to feel better when you got sick.

The example of *S aureus* is a good one for us to learn from. In the 1940s, penicillin was discovered and became an extremely effective treatment for *S aureus*. Within a few years, resistance to penicillin began to arise, but by the late 1950s the antibiotic methicillin was developed that effectively treated penicillin-resistant *S aureus* infections. It didn't take long for resistance to form to methicillin, occurring within a few years. By the late 1960s, MRSA was present in the United States, but was found only rarely as a hospital-acquired infection, and then over the next decade, as an infection seen in injection drug users. By the late 1990s MRSA began appearing as an infection in the community, not confined to patients with hospital exposure or injection drug use. Now community-acquired MRSA is common, and the assumption is that all *S aureus* infections are MRSA until proven otherwise. Vancomycin has been the gold-standard drug for the treatment of MRSA but now a strain of vancomycin-resistant *S aureus* has emerged.

Another example of the times we live in is the emergence and dominance of *Clostridium difficile* infection. Clinical infection with *C difficile* was first recognized in the late 1970s. It was almost always seen in the setting of antibiotic use and was considered a hospital-acquired organism. We have learned over the past 2 decades that there are many more risk factors for *C difficile* beyond antibiotics, including advanced age,

Med Clin N Am 97 (2013) xiii–xiv
http://dx.doi.org/10.1016/j.mcna.2013.04.006
0025-7125/13/$ – see front matter © 2013 Published by Elsevier Inc.

medical.theclinics.com

proton pump inhibitors, inflammatory bowel disease, chemotherapy, and tube feedings. In the early 2000s a new strain that was more severe, leading to worse disease and more frequent recurrences, was described. One major risk factor for this strain was past floroquinolone use. In addition, more patients without risk factors began developing *C difficile*. Since 2005, the incidence of *C difficile* infections has more than doubled.

Antibiotics are needed and crucial to the treatment of some infectious diseases. Unfortunately, the use of antibiotics is a double-edged sword, with the risk of development of resistance and the increase in antibiotic-related disease such as *C difficile*. Antibiotics also have direct side effects that can be severe and dangerous. The expectation of the public is that we can treat all infectious diseases with antibiotics. This public pressure in the form of patient expectations pushes the inappropriate use of antibiotics. It is only through our careful antibiotic stewardship and increased public education that we can move forward in the treatment of our patients safely and wisely.

Douglas S. Paauw, MD, MACP
Professor of Medicine
University of Washington School of Medicine
Seattle, WA, USA

E-mail address:
DPaauw@medicine.washington.edu

Herpes Zoster

Kim M. O'Connor, MD*, Douglas S. Paauw, MD, MACP

KEYWORDS

- Herpes zoster • Shingles • Varicella zoster virus • Immunosuppression

KEY POINTS

- The condition known as shingles is due to a reactivation of the varicella zoster virus.
- More than 90% of cases occur in immunocompetent individuals; however, immunosuppression increases the risk by 20- to 100-fold.
- The prodrome of shingles may last up to several weeks before the development of a vesicular rash.
- The zoster vaccine reduces the incidence of herpes zoster by approximately 50% and the occurrence of post-herpetic neuralgia by two-thirds, with vaccinated individuals experiencing attenuated or shortened symptoms.
- The zoster vaccine should be offered to most individuals older than 60 years.

EPIDEMIOLOGY

Varicella zoster virus (VZV) causes 2 distinct clinical entities. Primary infection with the varicella virus results in a diffuse vesicular rash commonly called chicken pox. The reactivation of latent varicella infection manifests as a painful blistering rash called herpes zoster or shingles, and tends to present in adulthood as cellular immunity declines. Ninety percent of the United States population has serologic evidence of varicella infection and is at risk for the development of herpes zoster.[1] Around 1 in 3 people will develop zoster during their lifetime, resulting in approximately 1 million episodes in the United States annually.[2] In an average general medicine practice of 1500 patients, a provider will see 3 to 5 patients per year with zoster.[3] Considering these statistics, familiarity with this condition is important.

Herpes zoster adversely affects health-related quality of life, and is an economic burden for individuals and the health care system. Based on a prospective study of 261 adult patients recruited from general and subspecialty medicine clinics in Canada, a diagnosis of zoster interfered with all health-related quality of life measures, with more than 50% of the patients identifying interference with sleep, enjoyment of life, and daily activities.[4] Based on a retrospective, population-based study of adult

Conflict of Interest: None.
Division of General Internal Medicine, University of Washington School of Medicine, WA, USA
* Corresponding author.
E-mail address: koconnor@u.washington.edu

patients in Minnesota, extrapolated estimates of the annual medical care cost of treating incident herpes zoster cases in the United States was $1.1 billion.[5]

More than 90% of cases of herpes zoster occur in immunocompetent people.[5] The greatest risk factor for herpes zoster is age, owing to a decrease in cellular immunity. In one study, the incidence of zoster increased 10-fold in adults aged 80 to 89 years compared with children younger than 10 years.[6] The most dramatic increases in disease rates begin after age 50 years.[6] The risk of post-herpetic neuralgia (PHN) also increases with age, with one study demonstrating a 27-fold increase in PHN in patients older than 50 in comparison with those younger than 50 years.[7]

Immunosuppressed patients have a 20 to 100 times greater risk of herpes zoster than immunocompetent individuals of the same age.[8] Immunosuppressive conditions associated with increased rates of zoster include human immunodeficiency virus (HIV) infection, organ transplant recipients, patients on immunomodulating therapies (including corticosteroids), and malignancies (especially lymphoproliferative disorders).[1] Despite the increased risk of shingles in patients with malignancies, the development of shingles in otherwise healthy patients should not automatically trigger a search for cancer.[9] Because shingles occurs at much higher rates in HIV-seropositive patients, it may be prudent to screen for HIV in otherwise young healthy patients who develop herpes zoster if risk factors for HIV are present.[10] Before the highly active antiretroviral (HAART) era, about 8% of HIV-infected patients developed herpes zoster, with an average CD4 count of 315.[10] More recent data, in the era of HAART, show a lower incidence of herpes zoster (9.3 per 1000 person-years) than in the pre-HAART era.[11] Risk factors associated with increased risk of herpes zoster include recent start of antiretroviral therapy, a viral load of more than 400 copies/mL, and a CD4 count of less than 350.[11]

The rate of herpes zoster in solid organ transplant recipients ranges from 3% to 25%, with incidence varying depending on the organ transplanted, type of immunosuppression, and type of antiviral prophylaxis.[12] Based on a retrospective study of transplant patients between 1994 and 1999, the overall incidence of herpes zoster was 8.6% (liver 5.7%, renal 7.4%, lung 15.1%, and heart 16.8%).[13] The immunosuppressants included in the study were azathioprine, cyclosporine, steroids, mycophenolate mofetil, tacrolimus, and antithymocyte globulin. Independent organ-specific risk factors for development of herpes zoster included female gender, mycophenolate mofetil therapy for liver transplantation, and antiviral therapies other than prolonged cytomegalovirus (CMV) prophylaxis in renal and heart transplant patients.[13] Independent predictors of herpes zoster for all organs combined included a history of induction therapy and antiviral treatments other than prolonged CMV prophylaxis. The median time of onset of herpes zoster was 9 months.[13] Considering these risks, pre-transplant immunization against varicella zoster, regardless of immune status, may be preventive.

Patients with rheumatic and immune-mediated diseases such as inflammatory bowel disease are 1.5 to 2 times more likely to develop herpes zoster. Both the underlying disease process and the use of immunosuppressive therapies and disease-modifying antirheumatic drugs (DMARDs) contribute to this increased risk. Recommendations regarding herpes zoster vaccine in this patient population are discussed later in this article.

Concerns were raised about whether widespread immunization with varicella vaccine in childhood would lead to an increased risk of vaccine-associated herpes zoster or increase the incidence of herpes zoster in the general population, owing to the decreased circulation of wild-type virus and a decline in T-cell immunity. To date these concerns have not materialized.[14] In a study of 548 children with acute lymphocytic leukemia, the incidence of zoster was lower in the group who received the Oka live attenuated VZV vaccine compared with those who had prior natural varicella infection.[15] An 11-year study by Juman and colleagues[16] demonstrated that the incidence of varicella decreased from 2.63 cases to 0.92 cases/1000 person-years after the introduction of the varicella vaccine without an increase in incidence of herpes zoster.

PATHOGENESIS

VZV is a DNA herpesvirus, which infects susceptible individuals through airborne transmission. The virus enters the body through contact with mucous membranes, where it replicates and disseminates via the blood and lymphatics. The virus incubates and replicates for approximately 2 weeks, at which time it overwhelms the host immune response, and the disseminated vesicular rash of chicken pox develops.[8] During the course of varicella, the VZV infects the sensory nerve endings and travels along the axons, eventually establishing lifetime latency in the dorsal root ganglia. Reactivation occurs when varicella zoster–specific cellular immunity declines and can no longer contain the virus, and replication begins. This process is followed by severe inflammation and hemorrhagic necrosis of nerve cells. The varicella virus travels down the sensory nerve, usually causing intense neuritis, and eventually reaches the skin where it produces a vesicular rash. The rash of herpes zoster occurs most often in the first (ophthalmic) division (V1) of the trigeminal nerve and from T1 to L2, because these are the dermatomes in which the rash of varicella achieves the highest density.[8]

PRESENTATION

The rash of herpes zoster starts with erythematous macules or papules developing into grouped vesicular lesions or bullae in a dermatomal distribution. Over the course of 7 to 10 days, the lesions develop into pustules and eventually crust over. If a patient continues to develop new lesions after about 1 week, the possibility of immunodeficiency should be explored.[17] Zoster involving mucous membranes is often overlooked because the fragile epidermis in these areas may not allow for the development of vesicles but rather, shallow ulcerations. Once a lesion is crusted over, it is no longer considered infectious. Complete healing may take up to 4 weeks, and postinflammatory hypopigmentation or hyperpigmentation may persist for months to years.

In most cases shingles is unilateral in location, and does not cross the midline. Lesions that develop on the back may cross the midline and still involve only one dermatome, owing to the anatomy of the spinal nerves. A small medial branch arising from the posterior primary ramus of each spinal nerve crosses a few centimeters past the midline (**Fig. 1**).[18] Zoster generally involves a single dermatome of a single sensory ganglion; however, in 20% of cases adjacent dermatomes may be involved.[19] Some patients will experience a few scattered vesicles located at some distance from the involved dermatome. The most common sites for shingles are the thoracic nerves and the ophthalmic division (V1) of the trigeminal nerve.[8] Fewer than 20% of patients have significant systemic symptoms, such as fever, headache, malaise, or fatigue.[17]

Immunocompromised patients are at risk of developing disseminated zoster, which often presents with a generalized distribution of vesicular lesions affecting several distinct dermatomes and frequently crossing the midline. Evaluation for visceral involvement including hepatitis, pneumonitis, and cerebritis is important. Often these visceral manifestations can occur in the absence of skin lesions or with late development of blisters, which can lead to delayed diagnosis and treatment. Recognizing disseminated zoster is important because the mortality is 5% to 15% in these patients, with most deaths attributable to pneumonia.[19]

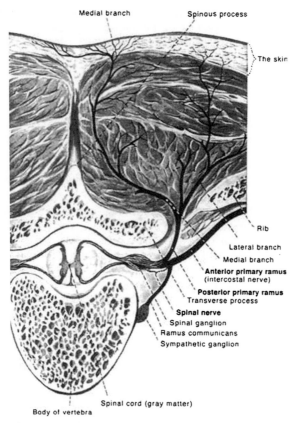

Fig. 1. Anatomy of the spinal nerves. (*From* Usatine RP, Clemente C. Is herpes zoster unilateral? West J Med 1999;170(5):263; with permission.)

In more than 75% of patients, the rash of zoster is generally preceded by a period of pain in the dermatome where the rash subsequently appears.[17] The pain has been described as deep "burning," "throbbing," "stabbing," or "shock-like."[20] Pain may be constant or only present when touched. Sensitivity to touch (paresthesia), exaggerated response to stimuli (hyperesthesia), or pain provoked by otherwise trivial stimuli (allodynia) have all been described. Repeated stimulation leading to escalating pain (windup pain) can also occur.[20] Some people only describe unbearable pruritus at the site.

Classic textbooks state that the herpes zoster prodrome generally lasts 48 to 72 hours; however, the prodrome of zoster has not been well documented in the literature and may be prolonged in some patients.[21] Goh and Khoo[22] reported a series of 164 patients with herpes zoster presenting to a dermatology clinic in Singapore, representing the largest such documentation of herpes zoster prodromal duration to date. The investigators reported prodromal symptoms of pain, itching, and hyperesthesia occurring on average 4.4, 4.7, and 3.4 days before skin eruptions, respectively. In some subsets, for example itching in men, prodromal symptoms predated skin eruption by an average of 6.2 days. A recent case report by Zerngast and colleagues[23] identified 7 patients with herpes zoster prodromes ranging from 6 to 18 days.

The concept of "zoster sine herpete," which is defined as dermatomal distribution of pain without antecedent rash, has also been raised.[24] Evaluations of a few patients with dermatomal pain without rash have demonstrated rising titers of VZV-specific antibody in cerebrospinal fluid (CSF) and serum along with DNA in CSF and mononuclear cells in peripheral blood detectable by polymerase chain reaction (PCR). Whether zoster sine herpete is a true clinical entity is still up for debate, and anecdotal reports of response to antiviral therapy are inconsistent.[25]

A prolonged prodrome or the absence of rash in the setting of pain is subject to a wide array of misdiagnoses, including, for example, myocardial infarction, pleurisy, cholecystitis, appendicitis, duodenal ulcer, ovarian cyst, herniated intervertebral disc, and renal colic, depending on the dermatome involved.[23] The longer the duration of pain before the development of rash, the more likely other causes will be explored, not only leading to delays in treatment but often resulting in the implementation of unnecessary and costly medical expenses.

Until recently it was believed that recurrent episodes of zoster generally occurred in immunocompromised patients only. An article by Yawn and colleagues[26] demonstrated higher rates of zoster recurrence in immunocompetent and immunocompromised patients than was previously expected. In this cohort study of 1669 patients with a previous history of herpes zoster, the recurrence rate of 6.2% at 8 years was equal to the incidence of a first episode. Eighty-five percent of recurrences occurred in immunocompetent patients; however, immunocompromised patients, women older than 50 years at the time of first infection, and pain lasting longer than 30 days at first infection predicted a higher likelihood for recurrence. This information is important because practitioners often remove herpes zoster from their differential diagnosis in healthy patients with unilateral pain complaints if they report a previous history of shingles. These new data constitute a reminder to consider recurrent zoster regardless of immune status.

WHAT ARE THE MOST IMPORTANT COMPLICATIONS OF HERPES ZOSTER?

PHN is the most common complication of herpes zoster. Risk factors for PHN include advanced age, and severity of rash and pain at the time of initial infection.[27,28] There is no consensus on the actual definition of PHN.[26] Definitions range from pain persisting beyond 30 days from the initial onset of rash to pain persisting beyond 3 months from initial rash. The actual prevalence of PHN varies greatly depending on the definition used. In one study, PHN incidence was as high as 30% in people younger than 40 and up to 74% in those older than 60 years when using the definition of 30 days of pain.[29] In a different study, when using the definition of pain lasting longer than 90 days, incidence rates were 6% in those younger than 40 and 12% in those 60 years and older.[30] In either case rates of PHN are high and symptoms are debilitating, so focus on prevention and treatment is important. PHN symptoms may include pain, numbness, dysesthesias (abnormal sensation), and allodynia (pain triggered by nonnoxious stimuli).

Additional complications from herpes zoster are associated with location of the rash.

Herpes zoster ophthalmicus (HZO) is a sight-threatening condition that occurs in 10% to 20% of all zoster cases.[31] Prodromal symptoms include malaise, low-grade fever, photophobia, and pain or itching on the forehead. These symptoms generally precede by about a week the onset of a vesicular rash in the V1 distribution of the trigeminal nerve. The V1 distribution includes the scalp, forehead, upper eyelid, conjunctiva, cornea, tip, side or root of the nose (Hutchinson sign), and nasal mucosa.

Clinicians should pay particular attention to the presence of any vesicles in the distribution of the nasociliary nerve (Hutchinson sign) (**Fig. 2**), because this predicts a higher likelihood of ocular involvement (80%).[32] The nasociliary nerve innervates the skin at the inner corner of the eye, and the tip and the side of the nose. Ocular complications may include lid edema, lid droop, conjunctivitis, episcleritis, scleritis, uveitis, and keratitis. More than 60% of patients will develop corneal involvement (keratitis) and 40% will develop iritis. Prompt initiation of antiviral therapy and referral to ophthalmology in patients with visual complaints, red eye, or involvement of the nasociliary nerve are critical in preventing loss of vision. Late complications such as acute retinal necrosis can occur at any time, therefore HZO should be included on a patient's problem list in the medical file.

If a patient with a history of recent herpes zoster complains of visual changes and eye pain weeks to months after the resolution of a shingles infection, one must consider the development of acute retinal necrosis (ARN). The initial infection could have occurred in any dermatome, not just the trigeminal nerve, hence suggesting that the retinal infection was caused by hematogenous spread of the virus. This condition may occur in immunocompetent patients, but is rare and is usually less severe.[1] Patients with advanced HIV and AIDS are at higher risk for ARN and tend to have a rapidly progressive course, resulting in blindness within months in 75% to 85% of involved eyes.[25] ARN may affect both eyes in 33% to 82% of patients, with the higher rates occurring in HIV patients.[33,34] Fundoscopic examination demonstrates multifocal nonhemorrhagic necrotizing lesions initially involving the peripheral retina, eventually extending and coalescing.[25] Retinal detachment is a common complication. Rapid initiation of intravenous acyclovir therapy, possibly combined with systemic steroids, often preserves vision in immunocompetent patients. In patients with HIV, the involved eye is rarely salvageable, so treatment with intravenous and intravitreal antivirals aims to prevent disease progression to the other eye.

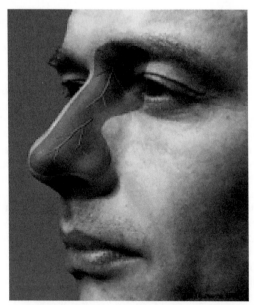

Fig. 2. Visual representation of the nasociliary dermatome. (*From* Opstelten W, Zaal MJ. Managing ophthalmic herpes zoster in primary care. BMJ 2005;331(7509):147–51; with permission.)

Despite these interventions, results are often disappointing, and many HIV patients will suffer vision loss.[1,25,33]

A triad of ipsilateral facial paralysis, ear pain, and vesicles in the auditory canal and auricle is known as herpes zoster oticus or the Ramsay Hunt syndrome. Because of the close proximity of cranial nerve (CN) VII to CN V and CN VIII, patients may complain of problems with hearing (tinnitus, hyperacusis), lacrimation, taste perception, or vertigo. Facial paralysis associated with VZV reactivation is generally more severe than that seen in Bell palsy, and is associated with a higher likelihood of permanent sequelae and multiple CN involvement. Prompt initiation of antiviral therapy and steroids may improve outcomes.[35]

Neurologic complication of herpes zoster include aseptic meningitis, peripheral motor neuropathy, transverse myelitis, acute or chronic encephalitis, Guillain-Barré syndrome, and stroke symptoms secondary to VZV infection of the cerebral arteries. These complications may occur coincident to or days to months after initial herpes zoster infection.[25]

After PHN, the most common complication of herpes zoster is the development of secondary bacterial infections. Most common pathogens are *Staphylococcus aureus* and *Streptococcus pyogenes*. Treatment with oral antibiotics for cellulitis are recommended, and may decrease the development of postinflammatory scarring, which is more likely to occur when zoster lesions become superinfected.[25]

WHAT IS THE DIFFERENTIAL DIAGNOSIS FOR HERPES ZOSTER?

There are numerous conditions that mimic the presentation of disseminated zoster. The focus here is on the more common causes of localized rashes in adults that may present similarly to dermatomal zoster. Herpes simplex virus generally affects the lips, genitalia, and buttocks. The initial infection is often severe with associated lymphadenopathy, fever, and flu-like symptoms. Recurrence is common and usually occurs in the same location. When herpes simplex virus presents in less typical locations, it can be misdiagnosed as herpes zoster. Several studies demonstrated that as many as 10% of specimens submitted to the laboratory from patients with presumed herpes zoster actually have herpes simplex virus infections.[17] A sample of the lesion sent for PCR or DFA testing will help in determining the type of infection.

Vesicular rashes that are intensely pruritic should make one think of contact dermatitis, palmoplantar dishydrotic eczema, dermatophytosis, and dermatitis herpetiformis. Contact dermatitis develops at sites that come in contact with the inciting substance. It most often affects the face, dorsum of hands, and finger webs. Common irritants include detergents, surfactants, solvents, water and wet work, metal tools, wood, fiberglass, and poison ivy. An occupational and recreational history should be obtained to look for a trigger.

Patients with palmoplantar dishydrotic eczema will report a history of recurrent severely pruritic vesicles, most often symmetrically involving the palms, lateral aspect of the fingers, or soles of the feet.

Acute dermatophytosis or tinea pedis is usually self-limited, intermittent, and recurrent, often occurring after activities that make the feet sweat. Unilateral or bilateral development of intensely pruritic, sometimes painful erythematous vesicles develop between the toes and on the soles, often extending up the instep. Evaluation of blister fluid with potassium hydroxide aids in diagnosis.

The cutaneous manifestation of gluten sensitivity is called dermatitis herpetiformis. These pruritic vesicular lesions tend to develop on extensor surfaces of the extremities, scalp, and buttocks. Diagnosis is confirmed by biopsy showing deposits of granular immunoglobulin A along the nonaffected subepidermal basement membrane. This condition should be considered in patients with other potential manifestations of celiac disease such as diarrhea or iron-deficiency anemia.

Cellulitis may develop blisters; however, this is usually secondary to edema at the site of infection, and the vesicles present focally rather than as a cluster as with herpes zoster. The presence of warmth, tenderness, erythema, fever, and leukocytosis with a left shift also support the diagnosis of cellulitis.[36]

Fixed drug eruptions manifest as single or multiple dusky erythematous to violaceous round plaques with central bullae. Commonly implicated drugs include phenolphthalein (laxatives), tetracyclines, barbiturates, sulfonamides, nonsteroidal anti-inflammatories, and salicylates. Pronounced postinflammatory hyperpigmentation is common, and recurrent episodes occur in exactly the same location with drug reexposure. The lips, genitalia, face, and acral areas are affected most often.

Phytophotodermatitis develops after skin exposure to certain plant-derived substances such as celery, wild parsnip, parsley, lemons, and limes, and usually develops 24 hours after sun exposure. The erythematous, edematous, nonpruritic, painful, blistering lesions usually present in a bizarre or linear pattern on sun-exposed skin, reflecting the manner in which the individual came into contact with the fruit or plant. Hyperpigmentation that may take months to years to resolve is common. Bartenders, gardeners, and workers in the food industry would be at highest risk for this condition.

HOW IS HERPES ZOSTER DIAGNOSED?

Most often the diagnosis of herpes zoster is made clinically. However, on occasion confirmation of infection may be necessary; this becomes more important in patients with atypical rash, especially in an immunocompromised host or if there is concern for disseminated disease with or without skin lesions. Key elements of the history used to diagnose herpes zoster clinically include: (1) painful or abnormal sensory prodrome (not always present); (2) dermatomal distribution; (3) grouped vesicles or papules; (4) multiple sites filling the dermatome (especially where divisions of the sensory nerve are represented); (5) lack of history of similar recurrent rash in the same distribution (suggestive of herpes simplex virus); and (6) pain and allodynia in the area of the rash.[17] Despite these criteria, in several studies from clinical diagnostic laboratories it has be shown that up to 10% of specimens submitted from patients with presumed herpes zoster in fact contained herpes simplex virus.[17]

The most sensitive and specific test for diagnosis is PCR testing for viral DNA, which takes approximately 1 day to receive results but can be costly. PCR testing is particularly helpful in the evaluation of "old" lesions that have crusted over, because the DNA is amplified through the testing process.[17] PCR testing can be done on fluid from skin lesions, blood, plasma, CSF, and bronchoalveolar lavage fluid. Direct florescent antibody (DFA) testing can be done on scrapings from active vesicular skin lesions that have not yet crusted. Turnaround time for DFA results is within a few hours. DFA tends to be inexpensive, and can simultaneously detect herpes simplex virus and VZV. DFA sensitivity is approximately 90% and the specificity is 95%; however, this decreases as the lesions progress past the vesicular stage.[17] Viral culture is not recommend because of poor sensitivity (approximately 65%–75%) when compared with PCR testing, and typically requires several weeks' turnaround time for results.[17] Sensitivity of culture also declines as lesions progress past the vesicular stage. Serologic testing is not helpful for the diagnosis of acute infection but may be helpful for a retrospective diagnosis. Most often it is used for screening health care workers to determine if varicella vaccination is needed.

HOW CONTAGIOUS ARE PATIENTS WITH HERPES ZOSTER?

Although less contagious than primary varicella, it is important to counsel patients with herpes zoster about the risk of transmitting the infection to others. Susceptible individuals such as those without a history of varicella infection or varicella vaccination are at risk of developing primary varicella infection. Contagiousness begins when the rash develops, and lasts until the lesions crust over.[19] Transmission can occur either by direct contact or via airborne spread from respiratory secretions, or aerosolization of virus from skin lesions. Small case studies have demonstrated airborne transmission from localized herpes zoster. The presence of VZV in the saliva of patients with herpes zoster has been documented in several small case series.[37] Whether saliva is a vehicle of transmission, however, is still not known. Patients with localized zoster should be advised to cover the lesions with bandages or clothing to reduce transmission. If viral spread via saliva is proved in the future, these recommendations may include respiratory precautions as well. Because airborne transmission is more likely to occur in patients with disseminated zoster, hospitalized patients with disseminated disease or immunocompromised patients with localized zoster who are at high risk of developing dissemination should be placed in strict isolation.

TREATMENT OF HERPES ZOSTER
Does Treatment with Antivirals Shorten Infection and Change Clinical Course in Immunocompetent Patients?

The goal of treatment for herpes zoster is to shorten and lessen the clinical course and possibly decrease complications from the disease. There is evidence that treatment with the antiretrovirals acyclovir, famciclovir, and valacyclovir lessens acute neuritis and hastens healing of the rash.[38–41] Optimal duration of treatment is 7 days; there appears to be no benefit for prolonged courses of treatment.[42] One head-to-head trial of valacyclovir and acyclovir showed quicker healing in the valacyclovir-treated arm.[41] Therapy should be initiated within 72 hours of the onset of lesions. The dosing regimen for acyclovir makes it a difficult drug to use clinically. It must be given 5 times a day to achieve adequate drug levels in order to achieve the high minimum inhibitory concentration needed to treat varicella zoster infection; this is especially difficult in the elderly population who are more commonly afflicted with zoster. Acyclovir has the advantage of being cheaper (about $20 for a 1-week course) compared with $60 for generic famciclovir and $80 for generic valacyclovir. With a dosing schedule of 3 times a day, famciclovir or valacyclovir are preferable from the standpoint of compliance and, probably, real-life efficacy.

Does Treatment with Antivirals Prevent PHN?

This topic has long been one of considerable debate. It is difficult to make strong statements based on the literature, because the definition of PHN has differed in different studies. Studies of all available antiviral drugs for herpes zoster show that the duration of pain suffered by patients is lessened with antiviral treatment.[38,41,43] What is not known for sure is whether long-term severe, permanent PHN is changed by treatment with antiviral drugs. The risk of PHN is less than 2% for patients younger than 60[44] and much higher for patients older than 70 years, in whom the risk is almost 19%.[30] The benefit of treatment for herpes zoster is likely greatest in elderly patients, for whom resolution of pain is less likely to happen quickly in comparison with younger patients.

In the Acute Setting, Does the Addition of Other Treatments Affect Pain from Herpes Zoster?

Historically, corticosteroids were commonly used at the time of clinical onset of herpes zoster. Early studies suggested a possible benefit in reducing pain in patients who took corticosteroids.[45] No studies have shown an effect on the development of PHN.[46] There is some evidence that pain relief might occur slightly more quickly and that quality-of-life scores may be improved in patients who use corticosteroids.[42,45,47] The use of gabapentin for the acute pain of herpes zoster is not helpful.[48] Narcotics are probably the best option for pain relief for patients with painful zoster in the acute setting.

What Treatments Are Effective for PHN?

Pain lasting beyond the resolution of the zoster rash is common. The definition of PHN is clouded by different time courses having been used in different studies. Studies on therapy have used time frames of pain persisting from 1 to 6 months for inclusion. Tricyclic antidepressants (TCA) have long been the mainstay for the treatment of PHN. Amitriptyline, nortriptyline, and desipramine are TCAs that have shown effectiveness for PHN,[49–53] but these agents are greatly limited by their side-effect profile. Most of the patients who develop PHN are elderly, and more prone to the serious side effects of tricyclic antidepressants. Urinary retention in men, orthostatic hypotension, and the risk for arrhythmia in patients with coronary artery disease markedly limit TCA use in the elderly. Gabapentin is a commonly used drug for PHN. A meta-analysis of studies of gabapentin for the treatment of neuropathic pain showed efficacy with a number needed to treat (NNT) of 6.8 for substantial benefit. When the studies evaluating PHN were teased out, there was an NNT of 5.5 for "much improved" for PHN pain.[54] The side effects for gabapentin were predominately dizziness (21%), somnolence (16%), gait disturbance (9%), and edema (8%), with 12% of patients stopping therapy because of side effects.[54] In a study comparing gabapentin, nortriptyline, or both for the treatment of PHN, there was a statistically significant benefit to the combination of both drugs over either drug alone.[55]

Pregabalin is efficacious in the treatment of PHN.[56] On a dose-equivalent basis, it does not appear to be more effective than gabapentin.[57] Side effects are similar to those of gabapentin, with slightly more patients developing edema. In a small (50 patients) comparative open-label randomized trial of amitriptyline and pregabalin, improvement in pain perception at the end of 8 weeks was greater in the pregabalin group ($P<.05$).[58] In a very small trial comparing amitriptyline, pregabalin, or both in the treatment of PHN, the combination of amitriptyline plus pregabalin was superior to either drug alone for pain relief.[59]

Topical capsaicin has some benefit in the treatment of PHN. In a study of topical 0.075% capsaicin applied for up to 2 years, it was helpful in reducing pain from PHN.[60] The only side effect was some stinging with application of the cream. More recently, an 8% capsaicin patch has been developed and tested for the treatment of PHN. Compared with a 0.04% control capsaicin patch, the 8% capsaicin patch applied for 60 minutes showed efficacy over a 4- to 8-week study period.[61,62] The only significant side effect was transient pain at the application site.

Topical lidocaine has been shown to be effective in a small number of studies. In a meta-analysis of treatment of PHN therapies, 5% topical lidocaine was as good as gabapentin, but with the caveat that there was limited study of 5% topical lidocaine.[63] In a large observational study (625 participants) of patients receiving 5% lidocaine patches through a compassionate-use program for the treatment of PHN, there was a significant decrease in the use of other pain medications in patients receiving lidocaine patches.[64]

Opioids have long been a mainstay in the treatment of PHN, and are effective.[53] The side effects of opioids do limit their use somewhat, especially because most of the patients are elderly. Constipation and drowsiness are the most common limiting side effects. Cognitive impairment and falls are also concerns. Opioids appear to be at least as effective as tricyclic antidepressants for the treatment of PHN.[65,66] Tramadol appears to be effective, based on limited evidence (one randomized controlled trial).[67]

How Should Immunocompromised Patients be Treated when they Develop Herpes Zoster?

Patients who have disorders of cell-mediated immunity are at greater risk for developing herpes zoster, and those with the most profound immunosuppression are at highest risk for disseminated zoster and involvement of visceral organs. Patients who should be considered at high risk are organ transplant recipients, patients receiving chronic corticosteroids (especially at higher doses), patients with advanced HIV disease and low CD4 counts, and patients with lymphoproliferative malignancies. Use of intravenous acyclovir for the treatment of herpes zoster in bone marrow transplant patients is very effective at preventing dissemination of herpes zoster. In 2 studies, none of the 51 transplant patients had dissemination after starting on acyclovir.[68,69] Severely immunocompromised patients should receive intravenous acyclovir for the initial treatment of herpes zoster. The patient populations that should definitely be treated with intravenous acyclovir include allogenic stem cell transplant patients within 4 months of transplant, hematopoietic stem cell transplant patients with moderate to severe graft-versus-host disease, and any transplant recipients receiving aggressive antirejection therapy.[17] Once the infection is controlled, patients can complete their course with oral antiviral medications. The use of oral antiviral therapy for uncomplicated zoster in immunocompromised patients appears to be effective.[70,71] Patients with HIV disease can be safely managed with oral antiviral drugs.

How Should Herpes Zoster be Managed During Pregnancy?

Chicken pox can be very dangerous in a pregnant adult, and the virus can be transmitted to the fetus, leading to congenital varicella infection. Herpes zoster infection in the mother does not pose a risk to the fetus. There have not been any documented cases of congenital varicella occurring because of maternal herpes zoster.[17] Acyclovir and valacyclovir appear to be safe for the fetus when given to pregnant women, including in the first trimester.[72] Because of the infrequency of PHN in young adults, treatment should be reserved for women with HZO or who have extremely painful and/or extensive rash. Acyclovir is excreted in breast milk. Its safety in neonates is not fully known, so avoiding treatment with antivirals for mild cases makes sense.

What is the Treatment for Herpes Zoster Ophthalmicus?

HZO is a sight-threatening condition caused by the reactivation of the herpes zoster virus within the trigeminal ganglion. Early recognition and treatment is critical in preventing progressive corneal involvement and possible visual loss. Patients with herpetic lesions in the V1 distribution of the trigeminal nerve are at risk for ocular involvement, and may require ophthalmologic evaluation. The V1 distribution includes the scalp, forehead, upper eyelid, inner corner of the eye, conjunctiva, cornea, tip, side or root of the nose (Hutchinson sign), and nasal mucosa. The presence of a Hutchinson sign predicts an 80% likelihood of ocular involvement. The presence of a red eye, reduced visual acuity, Hutchinson sign, and/or oculomotor palsy should trigger a referral to ophthalmology. An ophthalmologist should see any patient with a red eye and reduced vision on the same day. A red eye alone without visual complaints can be evaluated within 24 to 48 hours. Patients with a Hutchinson sign but no red eye or visual complaints should be seen within 1 to 2 weeks.[32]

Oral antiviral therapy reduces the frequency of late ocular complications from 50% down to 20% to 30%, and lessens acute pain.[1] Seven to 10 days of oral antiviral therapy with acyclovir, valacyclovir, or famciclovir should be started as soon as possible, even if patients present after 72 hours. Efficacy is equal between all antivirals, but in general valacyclovir or famciclovir are recommended owing to their ease of use with thrice-daily dosing.[73] The ophthalmologist may recommend the use of topical ocular steroid drops for corneal immune disease, episcleritis, scleritis, or iritis. Topical antivirals do not appear to be effective. Oral steroids may be added in the presence of moderate to severe pain or rash, or significant orbital edema.[17] Intravenous acyclovir is recommended for patients with retinitis, immunocompromised patients, or persons requiring hospitalization for sight-threatening disease. A history of ophthalmic zoster should be included in a patient's problem list because once an eye has been affected by herpes zoster, it is vulnerable to future complications even months to years later.[31]

HOW EFFECTIVE IS ZOSTER VACCINE AND WHO SHOULD RECEIVE IT?

More than 95% of adults aged 50 years and older have had chicken pox, putting them at risk for developing shingles. The risk of developing shingles increases significantly after age 50 as cell-mediated immunity wanes. A boost in VZV-specific T-cell immune response likely explains the mechanism behind zoster vaccine efficacy in preventing and attenuating disease.[74] In 2006, the Food and Drug Administration (FDA) approved a zoster vaccine for the prevention of shingles in individuals aged 60 and older. The zoster vaccine (trade name Zostavax) is a live, attenuated vaccine that contains the same strain of virus as the varicella vaccines, but at a much higher potency. FDA approval was based on the double-blind, placebo-controlled Shingles Prevention Study (SPS) of more than 38,000 adults aged 60 years and older. In this study, zoster vaccine reduced the incidence of herpes zoster by approximately 50% and the occurrence of PHN by two-thirds, with vaccinated individuals experiencing attenuated or shortened symptoms.[30,75]

In 2011, the FDA also approved the use of the vaccine in patients aged 50 to 59 years, based on the Zostavax Efficacy and Safety Trial (ZEST). In this multicenter, multinational study, approximately 22,000 individuals aged 50 to 59 were randomized to receive either Zostavax or placebo. At 1 year of follow-up, the risk of developing shingles was reduced by 70% in patients who received the vaccine.[76] Because individuals younger than 60 are at lower risk of contracting shingles and because there have been shortages of the shingles vaccine in the past, the Advisory Committee on Immunization Practices (ACIP) is not recommending routine vaccination for patients aged 50 to 59 years at this time.[77] Consideration should be given to offering the vaccine to patients aged 50 to 59 who would poorly tolerate zoster infection or PHN. This population may include patients with preexisting issues of chronic pain, severe depression, comorbid medical conditions, intolerances to medications used to treat PHN, or employment responsibilities that may be compromised by zoster infection.[77]

Regarding duration of protection provided by the vaccine, the SPS demonstrated protective efficacy 4.5 years beyond vaccination. A subpopulation of participants from the SPS were followed for up to 7 years after vaccination as part of the Short-Term Persistence Study, and showed persistent efficacy.[78] The Long-Term Persistence Study will assess efficacy for 7 to 10 years after vaccination; however, results are still pending.[79] At present, no additional booster shot is recommended.

There are only limited data examining zoster vaccination in patients who report a previous history of zoster. Although an episode of herpes zoster has an immunizing effect, some studies suggest that recurrence rates of zoster may be comparable with those in persons without a history of zoster.[26,77] This risk, coupled with the lack of a laboratory test to evaluate for previous occurrence of zoster and the fact that self-reports of herpes zoster may be inaccurate, led to the ACIP recommendation for zoster vaccine in all individuals aged 60 years and older, regardless of zoster status.

What if your Patient Reports No Prior History of Chicken Pox or Varicella Vaccination, Should we be Serologically Screening Individuals Before Administering the Zoster Vaccine?

In the United States the varicella vaccine was licensed in 1995, therefore in most cases patients born and raised in the United States before 1980 can be considered immune. Individuals with diminished immune systems and those who are at high risk for exposure and transmission of varicella such as health care personnel and pregnant women may need to be screened. If they are not immune and not immunosuppressed or pregnant then they should receive 2 doses of varicella vaccine administered at least 4 weeks apart in place of the zoster vaccine.[80] Nonimmune pregnant women should receive their first dose immediately post-partum. At this time, there are no recommendations to administer zoster vaccine to individuals who report a history of varicella vaccination.[2]

The zoster vaccine can be administered concurrently with other live and inactivated vaccines including pneumococcal, influenza and tetanus. Side effects are uncommon, with the most common being injection site reactions such as redness, pain, swelling, pruritus, warmth, hematoma and headache. In the SPS, these injection site reactions occurred in 48% of people who received the vaccine versus 17% in the placebo arm.[75] Headaches were reported in 9.4% of vaccine recipients and 8.2% of placebo.[81]

Patients may be concerned about developing a shingles or chicken pox like rash after receiving the zoster vaccine. In the SPS, only 53 patients out of 38,000 developed zoster or varicella-like rashes (17 in vaccinated group, 36 in placebo group). In the 41 specimens that were available for PCR testing, wild-type virus was detected in 5 of the specimens from the vaccinated group and 20 from the placebo group. The Oka/Merck strain, which is the virus strain present in Zostavax, was not detected in any of the specimens. In clinical trials of zoster vaccine completed before the SPS, only 17 patients in the vaccination and placebo groups developed noninjection site zoster–like and varicella-like rashes. Of the 10 specimens available for PCR testing, only 2 demonstrated the Oka/Merck strain in patients who reported varicella-like rashes.[81]

If your Patient is Currently on an Antiviral Medication, Should He or She Receive the Shingles Vaccine?

Antivirals with efficacy against the herpes virus family include acyclovir, famciclovir, and valacyclovir. These antivirals may interfere with replication of the live, VZV-based zoster vaccine. Consequently, patients should be advised to discontinue these medications 24 hours before administration of the zoster vaccine and to not restart these medications for at least 14 days after vaccination.[2]

Should we Immunize Patients who are Anticipating Upcoming Immunosuppression?

Providers should encourage their patients older than 60 to receive the zoster vaccine if they anticipate future treatment with immunosuppressives because severe morbidity and mortality is much greater in immunocompromised individuals. The zoster vaccine should be administered at least 14 days before initiation of immunosuppressive therapy; however, some experts recommend waiting at least 1 month If possible.[2]

What if your Patient is Already Immunosuppressed?

According to recommendations by the ACIP updated in 2008, the following conditions are considered contraindications: patients with AIDS or HIV with clinical manifestations including CD4$^+$ T-lymphocyte values 200 per mm^3 or less, or 15% or less of total lymphocytes; persons with leukemia, lymphoma, or malignant neoplasms affecting the bone marrow or lymphatic system; patients with unspecified cellular immunodeficiency; and patients undergoing hematopoietic stem cell transplantation (HSCT). However, data supporting this recommendation were limited, and providers may consider the vaccine in HSCT patients on a case-by-case basis.

Patients on the following immunosuppressive regimens should also avoid the vaccine: high-dose corticosteroids ($\geq$20 mg/d of prednisone or equivalent) lasting 2 or more weeks; and human immune mediators and immune modulators such as the antitumor necrosis factor agents adalimumab, infliximab, and etanercept. However, data supporting this recommendation in patients on immune modulators and mediators were also limited, and providers may again consider the vaccine in these patients on a case-by-case basis.[2] Patients should wait at least 2 weeks after stopping long-term high-dose steroids, or 1 month after discontinuing immune mediators and modulators, before receiving the zoster vaccine.[2]

Because patients with rheumatic and immune-mediated disease are 1.5 to 2 times more likely to develop zoster because of either their underlying disease process or the treatments used for these conditions, data supporting the use of herpes zoster vaccine in these patient populations would be useful. In 2012, a retrospective cohort analysis of 463,541 Medicare beneficiaries diagnosed with autoimmune disease (ankylosing spondylitis, inflammatory bowel disease, psoriatic arthritis/psoriasis, or rheumatoid arthritis) was published.[82] The aim of the study was to examine the possible association between the receipt of the zoster vaccine and the incidence of herpes zoster in the short term (<42 days after vaccination) and long term (median of 2 years of follow-up). Only 4% of the patients received the herpes zoster vaccine. The overall crude herpes zoster incidence rate was 7.8 cases per 1000 person-years (95% confidence interval [CI] 3.7–16.5) within 42 days after vaccination. The rate among the unvaccinated was 11.6 cases per 1000 person-years (95% CI 11.4–11.9).

Of the 633 patients on immunosuppressives (tumor necrosis factor [TNF]-α blockers, non-TNF biologics, DMARDS, and oral/or glucocorticoids) who received the zoster vaccine, there were no cases of herpes zoster, varicella, or meningitis/encephalitis within 42 days of vaccination. The adjusted hazard ratio for the vaccine was 0.61 at a median of 2 years of follow-up. These results suggest that the live zoster vaccination may not increase the risk of herpes zoster in the short term in patients with certain autoimmune diseases, including those exposed to immunomodulating medications. The investigators acknowledge that there were several limitations to their study and that further studies should be conducted to determine the safety of using zoster vaccine in this patient population.[82]

Which Patients with Potentially Immunocompromising Conditions can Receive the Zoster Vaccine?

Zoster vaccine may be administered to patients with leukemia who are in remission and who have not received chemotherapy or radiation for at least 3 months; patients with impaired humoral immunity, for example, hypogammaglobulinemia or

Table 1
Treatment of post-herpetic neuralgia

Therapy	Quality of Evidence	Side Effects
Tricyclic antidepressants (amitriptyline, nortriptyline, desipramine)	Class 1 and class 2	Dry mouth, orthostatic hypotension, constipation, urinary retention, arrhythmia
Gabapentin, pregabalin	Class 1	Drowsiness, dizziness, edema
Opioids (controlled-release oxycodone and morphine, methadone)	Class 1	Drowsiness, confusion, nausea, constipation, risk of fall, urinary retention, respiratory depression
Tramadol	Class 2	Seizures, suicidal ideation, dizziness, drowsiness, constipation, risk of serotonergic syndrome
Topical lidocaine	Class 1	Local skin reactions
Topical capsaicin	Class 1 (weak effect)	Skin burning

dysgammaglobulinemia; patients on high-dose steroids for less than 2 weeks, low-to-moderate steroid doses (<20 mg/d of prednisone or equivalent), topical, intranasal, or intra-articular steroids; and patients being treated with low doses of methotrexate (≤0.4 mg/kg/wk), azathioprine (≤3.0 mg/kg/d), or 6-mercaptopurine (≤1.5 mg/kg/d) for treatment of rheumatoid arthritis, psoriasis, polymyositis, sarcoidosis, inflammatory bowel disease, and other conditions.

Other contraindications include pregnancy or a history of anaphylactic/anaphylactoid reactions to any component of the vaccine, including gelatin and neomycin. A history of contact dermatitis to neomycin does not constitute a contraindication, because contact dermatitis represents a delayed-type immune response.[2]

Can Patients who are in Close Contact with Immunocompromised Individuals Still Receive the Zoster Vaccine?

Person-to-person transmission of the vaccine virus was not reported in the herpes zoster vaccine clinical trials. Person-to-person transmission has occurred after the varicella vaccine; however, these events were rare and only occurred when recipients of the varicella vaccine developed a varicella-like rash after vaccination. If a recipient of herpes zoster vaccine develops a varicella-like rash, recommendations for contact precautions should be initiated to prevent possible spread to susceptible individuals **(Table 1)**.[2,75,81]

SUMMARY

Herpes zoster is a common condition that significantly affects health-related quality of life. The majority of cases occur in immunocompetent individuals older than 60 years; however, immunosuppressed patients are at particularly high risk. Diagnosis is most often made clinically. If the diagnosis is unclear, the results of a DFA test can be obtained within a few hours, allowing for early initiation of treatment. PHN is the most common complication of herpes zoster, and can be debilitating. The prevention of herpes zoster through the administration of the zoster vaccine is the best way to avoid the development or lessen the severity of PHN. Early treatment with antivirals in patients with shingles may reduce the severity of PHN pain over the long term, but data supporting this are still limited. The herpes zoster vaccine should be offered to all patients older than 60, regardless of whether they report a history of shingles in the past, deny ever having chicken pox, or report a history of receiving the varicella vaccine. Certain conditions or medications associated with immunosuppression are still considered contraindications to vaccination with this live virus vaccine. Further studies are needed to determine whether the vaccine is safe in immunosuppressed individuals.

REFERENCES

1. Gnann JW Jr, Whitley RJ. Clinical practice. Herpes zoster. N Engl J Med 2002; 347(5):340–6.
2. Harpaz R, Ortega-Sanchez IR, Seward JF, et al. Prevention of herpes zoster: recommendations of the Advisory Committee on Immunization Practices (ACIP). MMWR Recomm Rep 2008;57(RR-5):1–30 [quiz: CE2–4].
3. Wareham DW, Breuer J. Herpes zoster. BMJ 2007;334(7605):1211–5.
4. Drolet M, Brisson M, Schmader KE, et al. The impact of herpes zoster and post-herpetic neuralgia on health-related quality of life: a prospective study. CMAJ 2010;182(16):1731–6.
5. Yawn BP, Itzler RF, Wollan PC, et al. Health care utilization and cost burden of herpes zoster in a community population. Mayo Clin Proc 2009;84(9):787–94.
6. Hope-Simpson RE. Postherpetic neuralgia. J R Coll Gen Pract 1975;25(157): 571–5.
7. Choo PW, Galil K, Donahue JG, et al. Risk factors for postherpetic neuralgia. Arch Intern Med 1997;157(11):1217–24.
8. Schmader KE, Oxman MN. Chapter 194. Varicella and Herpes Zoster. In: Goldsmith LA, Katz SI, Gilchrest BA, et al, editors. Fitzpatrick's Dermatology in General Medicine. New York: McGraw-Hill; 2012. http://www.accessmedicine. com/content.aspx?aID=56088542. Accessed on March 29, 2013.
9. Ragozzino MW, Melton LJ 3rd, Kurland LT, et al. Risk of cancer after herpes zoster: a population-based study. N Engl J Med 1982;307(7):393–7.
10. Buchbinder SP, Katz MH, Hessol NA, et al. Herpes zoster and human immuno-deficiency virus infection. J Infect Dis 1992;166(5):1153–6.
11. Blank LJ, Polydefkis MJ, Moore RD, et al. Herpes zoster among persons living with HIV in the current antiretroviral therapy era. J Acquir Immune Defic Syndr 2012;61(2):203–7.
12. Manuel O, Kumar D, Singer LG, et al. Incidence and clinical characteristics of herpes zoster after lung transplantation. J Heart Lung Transplant 2008;27(1):11–6.
13. Gourishankar S, McDermid JC, Jhangri GS, et al. Herpes zoster infection following solid organ transplantation: incidence, risk factors and outcomes in the current immunosuppressive era. Am J Transplant 2004;4(1):108–15.
14. Whitley RJ. Changing dynamics of varicella-zoster virus infections in the 21st century: the impact of vaccination. J Infect Dis 2005;191(12):1999–2001.
15. Hardy I, Gershon AA, Steinberg SP, et al. The incidence of zoster after immunization with live attenuated varicella vaccine. A study in children with leukemia. Varicella Vaccine Collaborative Study Group. N Engl J Med 1991;325(22):1545–50.
16. Jumaan AO, Yu O, Jackson LA, et al. Incidence of herpes zoster, before and after varicella-vaccination-associated decreases in the incidence of varicella, 1992-2002. J Infect Dis 2005;191(12):2002–7.
17. Dworkin RH, Johnson RW, Breuer J, et al. Recommendations for the management of herpes zoster. Clin Infect Dis 2007;44(Suppl 1):S1–26.
18. Usatine RP, Clemente C. Is herpes zoster unilateral? West J Med 1999;170(5):263.
19. Sampathkumar P, Drage LA, Martin DP. Herpes zoster (shingles) and postherpetic neuralgia. Mayo Clin Proc 2009;84(3):274–80.

20. Kost RG, Straus SE. Postherpetic neuralgia—pathogenesis, treatment, and prevention. N Engl J Med 1996;335(1):32–42.
21. Whitley R. Chapter 137 Varicella-Zoster Virus. In: Mandell, Douglas, Bennett, editors. Principles and Practice of Infectious Diseases, Seventh Edition. Philadelphia: Churchill Livingstone Elsevier; 2010. p. 1963–9. Accessed on March 29, 2013.
22. Goh CL, Khoo L. A retrospective study of the clinical presentation and outcome of herpes zoster in a tertiary dermatology outpatient referral clinic. Int J Dermatol 1997;36(9):667–72.
23. Zerngast W, O'Connor K, Paauw D. Varicella zoster with extended prodrome: a case series. Am J Med 2013;126(4):359–61.
24. Gilden DH, Kleinschmidt-DeMasters BK, LaGuardia JJ, et al. Neurologic complications of the reactivation of varicella-zoster virus. N Engl J Med 2000;342(9): 635–45.
25. Gnann JW Jr. Varicella-zoster virus: atypical presentations and unusual complications. J Infect Dis 2002;186(Suppl 1):S91–8.
26. Yawn BP, Wollan PC, Kurland MJ, et al. Herpes zoster recurrences more frequent than previously reported. Mayo Clin Proc 2011;86(2):88–93.
27. Nagasako EM, Johnson RW, Griffin DR, et al. Rash severity in herpes zoster: correlates and relationship to postherpetic neuralgia. J Am Acad Dermatol 2002; 46(6):834–9.
28. Dworkin RH, Boon RJ, Griffin DR, et al. Postherpetic neuralgia: impact of famciclovir, age, rash severity, and acute pain in herpes zoster patients. J Infect Dis 1998;178(Suppl 1):S76–80.
29. Klompas M, Kulldorff M, Vilk Y, et al. Herpes zoster and postherpetic neuralgia surveillance using structured electronic data. Mayo Clin Proc 2011;86(12):1146–53.
30. Oxman MN, Levin MJ, Johnson GR, et al. A vaccine to prevent herpes zoster and postherpetic neuralgia in older adults. N Engl J Med 2005;352(22):2271–84.
31. Opstelten W, Zaal MJ. Managing ophthalmic herpes zoster in primary care. BMJ 2005;331(7509):147–51.
32. Lam FC, Law A, Wykes W. Herpes zoster ophthalmicus. BMJ 2009;339:b2624.
33. Ormerod LD, Larkin JA, Margo CA, et al. Rapidly progressive herpetic retinal necrosis: a blinding disease characteristic of advanced AIDS. Clin Infect Dis 1998;26(1):34–45 [discussion: 46–7].
34. Hellinger WC, Bolling JP, Smith TF, et al. Varicella-zoster virus retinitis in a patient with AIDS-related complex: case report and brief review of the acute retinal necrosis syndrome. Clin Infect Dis 1993;16(2):208–12.
35. Angles EM, Nelson SW, Higgins GL 3rd. A woman with facial weakness: a classic case of Ramsay Hunt syndrome. J Emerg Med 2013;44(1):e137–8.
36. Ibrahimi OA, Sakamoto GK, Lee JJ. Acute onset vesicular rash. Herpes zoster. Am Fam Physician 2010;82(7):815–6.
37. Mehta SK, Tyring SK, Gilden DH, et al. Varicella-zoster virus in the saliva of patients with herpes zoster. J Infect Dis 2008;197(5):654–7.
38. Tyring S, Barbarash RA, Nahlik JE, et al. Famciclovir for the treatment of acute herpes zoster: effects on acute disease and postherpetic neuralgia. A randomized, double-blind, placebo-controlled trial. Collaborative Famciclovir Herpes Zoster Study Group. Ann Intern Med 1995;123(2):89–96.
39. Shafran SD, Tyring SK, Ashton R, et al. Once, twice, or three times daily famciclovir compared with aciclovir for the oral treatment of herpes zoster in immunocompetent adults: a randomized, multicenter, double-blind clinical trial. J Clin Virol 2004;29(4):248–53.

40. Tyring SK, Beutner KR, Tucker BA, et al. Antiviral therapy for herpes zoster: randomized, controlled clinical trial of valacyclovir and famciclovir therapy in immunocompetent patients 50 years and older. Arch Fam Med 2000;9(9): 863–9.

41. Beutner KR, Friedman DJ, Forszpaniak C, et al. Valaciclovir compared with acyclovir for improved therapy for herpes zoster in immunocompetent adults. Antimicrobial Agents Chemother 1995;39(7):1546–53.

42. Wood MJ, Johnson RW, McKendrick MW, et al. A randomized trial of acyclovir for 7 days or 21 days with and without prednisolone for treatment of acute herpes zoster. N Engl J Med 1994;330(13):896–900.

43. Jackson JL, Gibbons R, Meyer G, et al. The effect of treating herpes zoster with oral acyclovir in preventing postherpetic neuralgia. A meta-analysis. Arch Intern Med 1997;157(8):909–12.

44. Helgason S, Petursson G, Gudmundsson S, et al. Prevalence of postherpetic neuralgia after a first episode of herpes zoster: prospective study with long term follow up. BMJ 2000;321(7264):794–6.

45. Eaglstein WH, Katz R, Brown JA. The effects of early corticosteroid therapy on the skin eruption and pain of herpes zoster. JAMA 1970;211(10):1681–3.

46. Chen N, Yang M, He L, et al. Corticosteroids for preventing postherpetic neuralgia. Cochrane Database Syst Rev 2010;(12):CD005582.

47. Whitley RJ, Weiss H, Gnann JW Jr, et al. Acyclovir with and without prednisone for the treatment of herpes zoster. A randomized, placebo-controlled trial. The National Institute of Allergy and Infectious Diseases Collaborative Antiviral Study Group. Ann Intern Med 1996;125(5):376–83.

48. Dworkin RH, Barbano RL, Tyring SK, et al. A randomized, placebo-controlled trial of oxycodone and of gabapentin for acute pain in herpes zoster. Pain 2009;142(3):209–17.

49. Kishore-Kumar R, Max MB, Schafer SC, et al. Desipramine relieves postherpetic neuralgia. Clin Pharmacol Ther 1990;47(3):305–12.

50. Watson CP, Evans RJ, Reed K, et al. Amitriptyline versus placebo in postherpetic neuralgia. Neurology 1982;32(6):671–3.

51. Watson CP, Vernich L, Chipman M, et al. Nortriptyline versus amitriptyline in postherpetic neuralgia: a randomized trial. Neurology 1998;51(4):1166–71.

52. Max MB, Schafer SC, Culnane M, et al. Amitriptyline, but not lorazepam, relieves postherpetic neuralgia. Neurology 1988;38(9):1427–32.

53. Dubinsky RM, Kabbani H, El-Chami Z, et al. Practice parameter: treatment of postherpetic neuralgia: an evidence-based report of the Quality Standards Subcommittee of the American Academy of Neurology. Neurology 2004;63(6): 959–65.

54. Moore RA, Wiffen PJ, Derry S, et al. Gabapentin for chronic neuropathic pain and fibromyalgia in adults. Cochrane Database Syst Rev 2011;(3):CD007938.

55. Gilron I, Bailey JM, Tu D, et al. Nortriptyline and gabapentin, alone and in combination for neuropathic pain: a double-blind, randomised controlled crossover trial. Lancet 2009;374(9697):1252–61.

56. McKeage K, Keam SJ. Pregabalin: in the treatment of postherpetic neuralgia. Drugs Aging 2009;26(10):883–92.

57. Ifuku M, Iseki M, Hidaka I, et al. Replacement of gabapentin with pregabalin in postherpetic neuralgia therapy. Pain Med 2011;12(7):1112–6.

58. Achar A, Chakraborty PP, Bisai S, et al. Comparative study of clinical efficacy of amitriptyline and pregabalin in postherpetic neuralgia. Acta Dermatovenerol Croat 2012;20(2):89–94.

59. Achar A, Chatterjee G, Ray TG, et al. Comparative study of clinical efficacy with amitriptyline, pregabalin, and amitriptyline plus pregabalin combination in postherpetic neuralgia. Indian J Dermatol Venereol Leprol 2010; 76(1):63–5.

60. Watson CP, Tyler KL, Bickers DR, et al. A randomized vehicle-controlled trial of topical capsaicin in the treatment of postherpetic neuralgia. Clin Ther 1993; 15(3):510–26.

61. Irving GA, Backonja MM, Dunteman E, et al. A multicenter, randomized, double-blind, controlled study of NGX-4010, a high-concentration capsaicin patch, for the treatment of postherpetic neuralgia. Pain Med 2011;12(1):99–109.

62. Backonja M, Wallace MS, Blonsky ER, et al. NGX-4010, a high-concentration capsaicin patch, for the treatment of postherpetic neuralgia: a randomised, double-blind study. Lancet Neurol 2008;7(12):1106–12.

63. Wolff RF, Bala MM, Westwood M, et al. 5% lidocaine-medicated plaster vs other relevant interventions and placebo for post-herpetic neuralgia (PHN): a systematic review. Acta Neurol Scand 2011;123(5):295–309.

64. Clere F, Delorme-Morin C, George B, et al. 5% lidocaine medicated plaster in elderly patients with postherpetic neuralgia: results of a compassionate use programme in France. Drugs Aging 2011;28(9):693–702.

65. Raja SN, Haythornthwaite JA, Pappagallo M, et al. Opioids versus antidepressants in postherpetic neuralgia: a randomized, placebo-controlled trial. Neurology 2002;59(7):1015–21.

66. Mordarski S, Lysenko L, Gerber H, et al. The effect of treatment with fentanyl patches on pain relief and improvement in overall daily functioning in patients with postherpetic neuralgia. J Physiol Pharmacol 2009;60(Suppl 8):31–5.

67. Boureau F, Legallicier P, Kabir-Ahmadi M. Tramadol in post-herpetic neuralgia: a randomized, double-blind, placebo-controlled trial. Pain 2003;104(1–2):323–31.

68. Meyers JD. Treatment of herpesvirus infections in the immunocompromised host. Scand J Infect Dis Suppl 1985;47:128–36.

69. Shepp DH, Dandliker PS, Meyers JD. Treatment of varicella-zoster virus infection in severely immunocompromised patients. A randomized comparison of acyclovir and vidarabine. N Engl J Med 1986;314(4):208–12.

70. Arora A, Mendoza N, Brantley J, et al. Double-blind study comparing 2 dosages of valacyclovir hydrochloride for the treatment of uncomplicated herpes zoster in immunocompromised patients 18 years of age and older. J Infect Dis 2008; 197(9):1289–95.

71. Ljungman P, Lonnqvist B, Ringden O, et al. A randomized trial of oral versus intravenous acyclovir for treatment of herpes zoster in bone marrow transplant recipients. Nordic Bone Marrow Transplant Group. Bone Marrow Transplant 1989;4(6):613–5.

72. Pasternak B, Hviid A. Use of acyclovir, valacyclovir, and famciclovir in the first trimester of pregnancy and the risk of birth defects. JAMA 2010;304(8):859–66.

73. Shaikh S, Ta CN. Evaluation and management of herpes zoster ophthalmicus. Am Fam Physician 2002;66(9):1723–30.

74. Levin MJ, Oxman MN, Zhang JH, et al. Varicella-zoster virus-specific immune responses in elderly recipients of a herpes zoster vaccine. J Infect Dis 2008; 197(6):825–35.

75. Shapiro M, Kvern B, Watson P, et al. Update on herpes zoster vaccination: a family practitioner's guide. Can Fam Physician 2011;57(10):1127–31.

76. Schmader KE, Levin MJ, Gnann JW Jr, et al. Efficacy, safety, and tolerability of herpes zoster vaccine in persons aged 50-59 years. Clin Infect Dis 2012;54(7):922–8.

77. Centers for Disease Control and Prevention. Vaccines and preventable diseases: herpes zoster vaccination for health care professionals. Available at: http://www.cdc.gov/vaccines/vpd-vac/shingles/hcp-vaccination.htm. Accessed October 19, 2012; December 31, 2012.
78. Sanford M, Keating GM. Zoster vaccine (Zostavax): a review of its use in preventing herpes zoster and postherpetic neuralgia in older adults. Drugs Aging 2010;27(2):159–76.
79. Schmader KE, Oxman MN, Levin MJ, et al. Persistence of the efficacy of zoster vaccine in the shingles prevention study and the short-term persistence substudy. Clin Infect Dis 2012;55(10):1320–8.
80. American Colleges of Physicians. American Colleges of Physicians guide to adult immunizations, 4th edition: team-based manual. Available at: http://immunization.acponline.org/. Accessed on March 29, 2013.
81. Merck Canada. Zostavax [package insert]. Kirkland (Quebec). Available at: http://www.merck.ca/assets/en/pdf/products/ZOSTAVAX-PM_E.pdf. Accessed December 31, 2012.
82. Zhang J, Xie F, Delzell E, et al. Association between vaccination for herpes zoster and risk of herpes zoster infection among older patients with selected immune-mediated diseases. JAMA 2012;308(1):43–9.

Clostridium difficile Infection

Christopher L. Knight, MD[a],*, Christina M. Surawicz, MD[b]

KEYWORDS

- *Clostridium difficile* • Metronidazole • Fecal microbiota transplantation

KEY POINTS

- *Clostridium difficile* infection (CDI) is increasing in prevalence and severity.
- Major risk factors include antibiotic use, age, exposure to the organism in health care settings, and (likely) use of proton-pump inhibitors.
- Prevention of transmission is essential in reducing nosocomial outbreaks.
- Oral metronidazole (500 mg 3 times daily for 10 days) is the therapy of choice for mild to moderate disease.
- Oral vancomycin (125 mg 4 times daily for 10 days) is the therapy of choice for severe disease and pregnant/lactating women.
- High-dose oral vancomycin (250–500 mg 4 times daily for 10 days) and intravenous metronidazole are the therapies of choice for complicated disease.
- Rectal vancomycin enemas can be given in patients with ileus, abdominal distention, and anatomic/surgical abnormalities that prevent oral antibiotics from reaching the colon.
- The first recurrence of CDI should be treated the using the same protocol as for initial infection.
- The second recurrence should be treated with oral vancomycin using an extended "pulsed" course.
- The best treatment for third and subsequent recurrences remains unclear, but fecal microbiota transplantation shows considerable promise.

MICROBIOLOGY

In 1935, microbiologists isolated a new species of gram-positive, spore-forming bacteria from human feces. The difficulty of its isolation, requiring an anaerobic environment, gave it its name: *Bacillus difficilis*. In the 1970s, it was recognized that toxins produced by this organism, renamed *Clostridium difficile*, were a major cause of pseudomembranous colitis.[1,2] The 2 primary toxins, toxin A and toxin B, both cause injury

a Division of General Internal Medicine, Department of Medicine, University of Washington School of Medicine, 4245 Roosevelt Way Northeast, Box 354760, Seattle, WA 98109, USA;
b Division of Gastroenterology, Department of Medicine, University of Washington School of Medicine, 325 9th Avenue, Box 359773, Seattle, WA 98104, USA
* Corresponding author.
E-mail address: cknight@uw.edu

Med Clin N Am 97 (2013) 523–536
http://dx.doi.org/10.1016/j.mcna.2013.02.003
0025-7125/13/$ – see front matter © 2013 Elsevier Inc. All rights reserved.

medical.theclinics.com

to intestinal mucosa, but toxin B is much more potent than toxin A, thought to be the reason why some strains of C difficile remain pathogenic despite producing only toxin B.[3] The ability of C difficile to form spores that resist many common disinfectants and can survive for months on environmental surfaces makes it particularly prone to nosocomial transmission.

In 2002, hospitals in Québec and southern Canada began to report dramatically increased rates of C difficile infection (CDI). This and several subsequent outbreaks were eventually attributed to a newly epidemic strain of C difficile. The strain has been named based on the microbiologic techniques used to identify it: North American pulsed-field gel electrophoresis type 1, restriction endonuclease analysis type BI, and PCR ribotype 027, or NAP1/BI/027. This strain produces dramatically more toxin A and B in vitro than do conventional strains of pathogenic C difficile, causing more severe disease.[4]

EPIDEMIOLOGY AND RISK FACTORS

Both the incidence and the severity of CDI have been rising since 2001. From 2000 to 2005, the rate of hospitalizations reporting CDI doubled from 5.5 per 10,000 to 11.2 per 10,000 population, with a similar increase in age-adjusted case-fatality rate from 1.2% to 2.2%.[5] Much of the increase is seen in older patients with exposure to health care settings such as long-term care facilities and hospitals.[6] However, C difficile is also emerging in a pathogen in populations previously thought to be at low risk, such as pregnant women hospitalized for delivery and patients without prior exposure to health care settings.[7–9]

Antibiotic Exposure

Exposure to antibiotics remains the preeminent risk factor for CDI. Any antibiotic can cause CDI, commonly clindamycin, penicillins, cephalosporins, and fluoroquinolones, and especially multiple antibiotics. CDI has also been reported with exposure to metronidazole and vancomycin, which are used for treatment.[10] The effect of antibiotics is presumed to be disruption of the normal gut microbiota, thus allowing proliferation of C difficile.[11]

Antibiotics are the most significant risk factor, and their effect can persist for weeks to months after they are stopped. A case-control study done in the Netherlands showed a 7- to 10-fold increased risk for CDI during antibiotic therapy that persisted for the first month after stopping antibiotics. The risk gradually declined over the following 2 months, returning to baseline 3 months after stopping antibiotic therapy. There was a trend toward increased risk with longer overall duration of antibiotics, although differences were not statistically significant.[12]

Exposure to Toxigenic C difficile

The other major risk factor for health care–associated CDI is exposure to settings where the organism is prevalent. Risk for CDI has been shown to correlate with length of hospital stay, but recently discharged patients and patients who live in long-term care facilities or other health care settings are also at increased risk.[13] By definition, community-acquired CDI is not associated with exposure to a health care setting.

Age

Older age is a well-established risk factor for health care–associated CDI. From 2000 to 2005, the majority of United States hospitalizations with CDI occurred in a group between 65 and 84 years of age, and patients older than 85 are at even higher risk.

Data are more limited for community-acquired infection, but some studies suggest that younger people are at risk. The median age of patients with community-associated CDI tends to be lower, and a study of community-associated CDI in North Carolina showed a higher incidence in the 45- to 64-year-old age group than in those older than 65.[13,14]

Gastric Acid Suppression

Despite a large number of studies regarding an association between gastric acid suppression and CDI, the subject remains somewhat controversial. Many studies evaluated hospitalized patients but some also studied outpatients. Most, but not all, show an increased risk of CDI associated with the use of proton-pump inhibitors (PPIs). Some studies have shown a lesser increase in risk with the use of H2-receptor antagonists, suggesting a correlation with degree of acid suppression.[15,16] Multiple recent meta-analyses of PPI use in patients with CDI have found pooled estimates of between 1.7- and 2.1-fold increase in risk, favoring an association.[17–19]

Inflammatory Bowel Disease

The generalized increase in the incidence of CDI in recent years has been accompanied by a parallel increase in rates among patients with inflammatory bowel disease (IBD). Patients with ulcerative colitis appear to be at particularly high risk, with a tripling of incidence between 1998 and 2005 in one study.[20] In addition to higher incidence rates, patients with IBD present a clinical challenge because CDI can mimic the symptoms of an IBD flare. Patients with IBD who also have CDI have higher rates of colectomy and a 4-fold increase in mortality. Patients with IBD may also experience unique complications of CDI, including pouchitis in patients status post colectomy with ileoanal reconstruction.[21]

CLINICAL MANIFESTATIONS AND DIAGNOSIS
Clinical Manifestations and Disease Severity

The cardinal symptom of CDI is watery diarrhea, which can be up to 10 to 15 stools per day. Diarrhea of CDI is rarely bloody, although it can be in severe cases. Some patients may lose significant amounts of serum proteins in stool, causing hypoalbuminemia, edema, and ascites.[22] In addition, fever ($\geq 38.0^\circ$C), abdominal distension, and leukocytosis ($\geq$15–20,000 white blood cells/mm^3) are significant indicators of severe disease, likely to cause admission to the intensive care unit, surgery for complications of CDI, or death.[23] Leukocytosis may precede diarrhea. A retrospective review of 60 patients with unexplained leukocytosis reported 35 (58%) with *C difficile* toxin in their stool. Of these patients, 30 (86%) eventually had symptoms consistent with colitis, but for 16 (53%) leukocytosis was noted before any mention of colitis symptoms.[24]

Patients with severe CDI frequently have abdominal pain caused by ileus, colonic dilation, and even toxic megacolon. Marked leukocytosis (sometimes as high as 50,000/μL) and lactic acidosis are worrisome signs and should prompt surgical consultation.

Pseudomembranous Colitis

Patients with CDI frequently have pathognomonic findings on lower endoscopy. *C difficile* colitis can be nonspecific or there may be release of proteins and inflammatory cells, which coalesce to form yellowish pseudomembranes (**Fig. 1**). Although a typical endoscopic appearance is virtually pathognomonic for CDI, endoscopy is rarely needed as a diagnostic test when CDI is suspected, because of the availability of less invasive stool studies and the risk of perforation in patients with severe colitis.

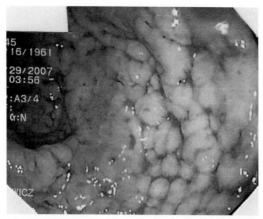

Fig. 1. Confluent pseudomembranes in a patient with *Clostridium difficile* colitis.

Diagnostic Studies

The past gold-standard test for the diagnosis of CDI was the cytotoxin neutralization assay. Culture alone is insufficient because some *C difficile* isolates are nontoxigenic.[25] However, these tests are expensive and time consuming, so they have largely been replaced by more rapid assays.

Enzyme immunoassay (EIA) tests are available for toxins A and B, as well as glutamate dehydrogenase (GDH), an enzyme produced by *Clostridium* species. EIA tests for toxins A and B have a sensitivity of 75% to 95% and a specificity of 83% to 98% in comparison with cytotoxin neutralization assays.[26] GDH may be easier to detect by EIA testing and is sometimes used as an initial screen, but a positive GDH test does not distinguish between toxigenic and nontoxigenic strains. A negative GDH test has good negative predictive value, but a positive GDH test requires additional testing to confirm presence of toxin. GDH testing has been reported to have sensitivities from 75% to more than 90%, with negative predictive values of 95% to 100% in the appropriate clinical setting.[27]

The newest testing methodologies are nucleic acid amplification tests, including polymerase chain reaction (PCR) and loop-mediated isothermal amplification tests. These tests detect genes residing within the pathogenicity locus of the *C difficile* genome such as the toxin A gene (tcdA), toxin B gene (tcdB), and the toxin regulatory gene (tcdC). Overall performance for gene amplification assays shows sensitivities of 90% to 100% with specificities of 94% to 100%.[28] In a head-to-head comparison, gene amplification significantly outperformed EIA-based testing.[29]

Although not needed for diagnosis, computed tomography (CT) imaging of the abdomen can be useful in assessing disease severity. Colon-wall thickening (**Fig. 2**), dilation of the colon, and ascites are all concerning findings. CT can also be helpful in ruling out other pathologic processes, and in determining the presence of perforation.

Surveillance and Repeat Testing

Clinical guidelines issued jointly by the Society for Healthcare Epidemiology of America (SHEA) and the Infectious Disease Society of America (IDSA) recommend evaluating only diarrheal stool from patients thought have symptomatic CDI, unless the patient has ileus, in which case a rectal swab may be used to obtain a specimen for PCR testing.[30] There is no benefit to testing multiple stool specimens. It is not advisable to

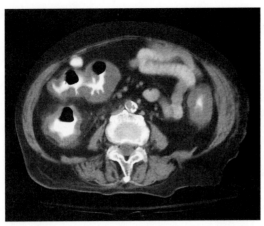

Fig. 2. Colon wall thickening on abdominal computed tomography imaging. Oral contrast fills the lumen of the colon.

retest patients for "clearance" of *C difficile*, because successfully treated patients may continue to have a positive test for CDI for as long as 30 days after starting therapy.[31]

PREVENTION

It is crucial that efforts focus on prevention of initial CDI, especially in health care settings. The cornerstones of these efforts are reduction in the overuse of antimicrobials and efforts to prevent transmission from patient to patient.

Antimicrobial Stewardship

Exposure to antibiotics is the primary risk factor for CDI. Although any antibiotic can cause CDI, the more antibiotics the patient is exposed to and the greater the duration, the higher the risk. There have been multiple studies demonstrating a reduced risk of CDI when institutions initiate programs to limit the use of high-risk antimicrobials.[32–34] In one study an effort to optimize antimicrobial use in response to an epidemic of the NAP1/BI/027 hypervirulent strain reduced nosocomial CDI by 60%.[34] There is also a joint IDSA/SHEA guideline on establishing an institutional program to enhance antimicrobial stewardship.[35]

Reduction of Transmission

C difficile is particularly problematic in health care settings because in its spore form it is resistant to commonly used disinfectants. Alcohol, the active ingredient in many hand gels and cleansers, has been shown to be ineffective against *C difficile* spores.[36] Hand washing with soap and water or chlorhexidine is preferable. Use of gloves when handling body substances was associated with a significant reduction incidence of CDI in one randomized study.[37] Use of surface disinfectants specifically active against *C difficile* has also been shown to be helpful.[38,39]

Probiotics

Probiotics, such as *Lactobacillus* preparations and *Saccharomyces boulardii*, have been shown to reduce overall rates of antibiotic-associated diarrhea. Although most studies focusing specifically on *C difficile* have been small and have not had significant results, a meta-analysis of combining the results of multiple studies showed a statistically significant 66% reduction in CDI. Both *Lactobacillus*-based and *Saccharomyces*-based preparations appeared to be effective.[40]

TREATMENT

Although exposure to antimicrobials is a key part of the pathogenesis of CDI, once the infection is established, antimicrobials are necessary for treatment. Three agents are used for primary treatment of CDI: metronidazole (Flagyl), vancomycin (Vancocin), and fidaxomicin (Dificid). Other drugs have been studied but are not extensively used. Choice of therapy depends on the severity of the patient's illness, and whether one is treating initial infection or recurrent CDI. If possible, antibacterial agents that are not being used to treat CDI should be stopped.

Metronidazole

Metronidazole is a nitroimidazole antibiotic that has broad activity against anaerobic bacteria (including *C difficile*) in vitro. Unlike other agents commonly used to treat CDI, orally administered metronidazole is well absorbed in the proximal gut. However, in patients with colitis, metronidazole and its primary metabolite, hydroxymetronidazole, reach sufficient endoluminal concentrations to have antibacterial activity. In patients without diarrhea, fecal concentrations of metronidazole and metabolites are much lower, suggesting that the infection itself allows metronidazole to reach effective levels in the colon, either by altering the permeability of the colon mucosa or disrupting reabsorption of metronidazole secreted from the biliary tract.[41] Because metronidazole is able to reach the colon via the bloodstream, it can be given intravenously for the treatment of CDI, unlike vancomycin and fidaxomicin.

Metronidazole's primary advantages over other antimicrobials are low cost and lack of concerns about antimicrobial resistance. At the time of writing, a full course of vancomycin costs nearly 100 times as much as a course of metronidazole, and fidaxomicin is even more expensive. Although *C difficile* itself is not typically resistant to vancomycin, other gram-positive organisms are developing vancomycin resistance, providing a compelling reason to avoid its use when other agents might be effective.

Metronidazole's disadvantages relative to other agents relate primarily to adverse effects from systemic absorption, including nausea, a metallic taste in the mouth, and occasionally a disulfiram-like reaction when patients consume alcohol. Metronidazole also readily crosses the placenta and is excreted in breast milk; it has been implicated in facial anomalies when used during the first trimester, making it contraindicated in pregnant and lactating women. Long-term use of metronidazole (2–4 weeks or more) has been associated with a peripheral neuropathy, which is problematic for treating patients with recurrent CDI.[42] There is also limited evidence that metronidazole is less effective than vancomycin in patients with severe CDI (see the section on comparative effectiveness).

Vancomycin

Vancomycin is a glycopeptide antibiotic that is poorly absorbed from the gastrointestinal tract when administered orally. It has broad activity against gram-positive organisms, including *C difficile*. Vancomycin's primary advantage over metronidazole is lack of systemic absorption and the accompanying toxicities. There is also some evidence of greater efficacy in severe CDI (see the section on comparative effectiveness). Its primary disadvantage is cost: the oral form of vancomycin is particularly expensive in the United States. Because of this, some hospitals and compounding pharmacies use the intravenous form administered orally. Anecdotally this appears to be effective, although patients may report a bad taste with this formulation. There is also concern about fostering vancomycin resistance among other organisms, particularly entero-cocci, when using vancomycin to treat CDI. This aspect remains largely theoretical at this point, although one study of 301 patients showed decreased acquisition rates of vancomycin-resistant enterococci with fidaxomicin treatment for CDI when com-pared with vancomycin.[43]

Fidaxomicin

Fidaxomicin is a macrocyclic antibiotic with particularly potent activity against *C difficile*. It is active against some other gram-positive organisms, including enterococci, staph-ylococci, and other clostridial species, but less so than vancomycin. It has little activity against other common bowel flora, particularly gram-negative species.[44] Fidaxomicin has been approved by the United States Food and Drug Administration for the treatment of *C difficile* colitis, based primarily on the results of one randomized controlled trial, which enrolled 629 patients and randomized them to fidaxomicin or vancomycin. Equiv-alent cure rates (88% vs 86%) were found, but some patients receiving fidaxomicin had a somewhat lower recurrence rate than those receiving vancomycin, only apparent in patients without the NAP1/BI/027 hypervirulent strain of *C difficile*.[45] This result gives fidaxomicin an apparent clinical edge over vancomycin. However, the duration of follow-up in the study (4 weeks) may not have been long enough to capture recurrence in all patients. Fidaxomicin is significantly more expensive than oral vancomycin, and dramatically more so than metronidazole. There is also a relative lack of both empirical data and clinical experience, as it is a new therapeutic agent.

Comparative Effectiveness of Antimicrobials

Numerous controlled trials have evaluated the relative effectiveness of various antimi-crobials. Several compare metronidazole and vancomycin, and showed no difference in patients with mild to moderate CDI. In patients with severe CDI, two trials showed a benefit of vancomycin over metronidazole, although one is based on a limited analysis of a small subgroup.[46,47]

A systematic review published in 2011 found that metronidazole, vancomycin, and fidaxomicin were all equally effective for initial therapy. The investigators concur that fidaxomicin appears to have a lower risk of recurrence, but find the evidence supporting superiority of vancomycin in severe CDI to be insufficient, and encourage additional studies.[48]

Antiperistaltic Agents

Antiperistaltic agents (such as loperamide) are generally avoided in the treatment of CDI. The 2010 SHEA/IDSA guidelines recommend against their use "as they may obscure symptoms and precipitate toxic megacolon."[30]

Management of Initial Infection

Assessment of disease severity is a cornerstone of determining treatment for initial CDI. Unfortunately there are no universally accepted or validated criteria for severe disease. The 2010 SHEA/IDSA guidelines propose criteria based on expert opinion, which include as markers of severe disease leukocytosis with a white blood cell count of 15,000 cells/mL or higher, or a serum creatinine level greater than or equal to 1.5 times the patient's baseline level. The guidelines refer to CDI with hypotension, shock, ileus, or megacolon as "complicated" CDI.[30] Other criteria used in research studies in-clude fever or hypothermia, hypoalbuminemia, and advanced age.[47,49] Ultimately, assessment of disease severity relies on the clinical judgment of the treating clinician. The authors suggest criteria to assess severity and a treatment algorithm in **Fig. 3**.

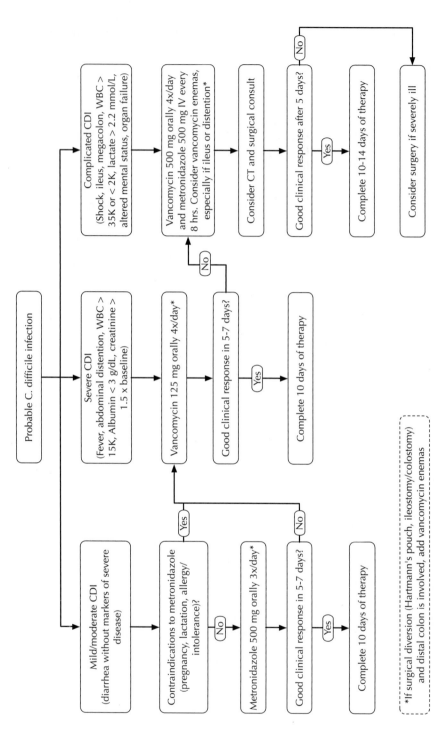

Fig. 3. Algorithm for treatment of initial and first recurrence of *Clostridium difficile* infection. CDI, *C difficile* infection; IV, intravenous; K, thousand; WBC, white blood cells.

Treatment of mild to moderate CDI

Based on evidence showing therapeutic equivalence between metronidazole and vancomycin, the best initial therapy for mild or moderate CDI in patients without contraindications (pregnancy, lactation, allergy/intolerance) is metronidazole, 500 mg 3 times daily for 10 days. Patients who have contraindications or are unable to tolerate metronidazole should be treated with oral vancomycin, 125 mg 4 times daily for 10 days. Most patients will recover within the first week of therapy.[50] For those who fail to respond after 5 to 7 days, the authors recommend switching to oral vancomycin.

Patients with surgical or anatomic abnormalities in whom oral antibiotics cannot reach the colon (eg, Hartmann pouch, ileostomy, or diverting colostomy) should be given vancomycin enemas (500 mg in 500 mL saline) if the distal colon is involved.[51]

Treatment of severe CDI

Although the data supporting the benefit of vancomycin over metronidazole in severe CDI are limited, it is prudent to start initial treatment with oral vancomycin (125 mg 4 times daily) in patients with fever, leukocytosis, hypoalbuminemia, or worsened renal function (see **Fig. 1**). Patients who fail to respond to low-dose vancomycin after 5 to 7 days may benefit from escalation to high-dose (250–500 mg every 6 hours) oral vancomycin plus intravenous metronidazole, 500 mg 3 times a day.[30,31] Patients who develop ileus, abdominal distention, severe colitis, ascites, or other markers of complicated CDI should be treated with oral vancomycin, intravenous metronidazole, and possibly vancomycin enemas.

Treatment of complicated CDI

Patients with complicated CDI (markers include shock, hypotension, ileus, megacolon, severe leukocytosis or leukopenia, elevated serum lactate, altered mental status, and end-organ failure) should be treated with high-dose (500 mg every 6 hours) oral vancomycin plus intravenous metronidazole, 500 mg 3 times a day.[30,31] Patients with ileus, abdominal distention, megacolon, or surgical/anatomic abnormalities in whom oral antibiotics cannot reach the colon (eg, Hartmann pouch, ileostomy, or diverting colostomy) should also be given vancomycin enemas (500 mg in 500 mL saline).[51]

Early surgical consultation is suggested for patients with complicated CDI. Several case series have demonstrated better outcomes with early surgery in patients with fulminant colitis.[52–54] CT of the abdomen may be valuable in assessing disease severity and the need for surgical intervention.

Management of Recurrent Infection

Between 15% and 20% of patients treated for CDI will experience a recurrence of disease within 30 days of initial therapy.[10] Roughly half of recurrent disease is caused by new infection and half by the original organism.[55] Making the distinction clinically is difficult, and does not change management. The most important risk factor for recurrent CDI is intercurrent antibiotic use to treat another infection while completing CDI therapy. Impaired host immune response may be a factor: toxin A is immunogenic, and the presence of antibody to toxin A is associated with a decreased risk of recurrence.[56]

Treatment of first recurrence

Treatment of the first recurrence of CDI follows the same protocol as for initial infection. There is no evidence of increased efficacy of metronidazole or vancomycin, regardless of the drug used for the initial infection.[46] However, patients with severe or complicated recurrent CDI should be treated with vancomycin using the same parameters as for initial infection.

Treatment of second recurrence

Patients with a second recurrence of CDI should be treated with vancomycin rather than metronidazole because of the risk of metronidazole toxicity, especially neurotoxicity, with repeat dosing.[42] Tapering the vancomycin dose or using intermittent "pulsed" dosing may reduce the risk of a subsequent recurrence. One cohort study of patients with recurrent CDI showed that the recurrence rate in the group with pulsed dosing every 2 to 3 days was 14%, compared with 31% with tapered dosing and 40% to 50% with conventional dosing.[57]

Both case series and a randomized trial have shown potential for rifampin and rifaximin to reduce recurrence.[58] However, the randomized study was underpowered to show significant differences, and reports of emerging rifampin resistance suggest that additional study is needed.[59] Rates of recurrence have been shown to be lower with fidaxomicin than with vancomycin when used for initial therapy, but this has never been studied in recurrent CDI.[45]

Treatment of third and subsequent recurrences

Patients with a third or subsequent recurrence of CDI have several therapeutic options, none of which have been definitively studied. Perhaps the most intriguing are efforts to reconstitute the normal fecal microbiota using stool from a healthy donor, a procedure known as fecal microbiota transplantation (FMT).[60] Although reports to date consist largely of case series, a systematic review suggests that resolution is common, occurring a 92% of cases, and adverse events are unusual.[61] One trial, which randomized 43 patients to vancomycin, vancomycin followed by bowel lavage, or a shortened (4 days) course of vancomycin followed by bowel lavage then FMT, found that 81% of patients in the FMT group had no further recurrences after transplant; of the 3 patients who failed to respond, 2 improved with a second transplant, bringing the overall response rate up to 94% 10 weeks after transplant, in comparison with a 23% to 31% response rate in the other 2 groups.[62] Two other randomized trials of FMT are in the recruitment stage at the time of writing.[63,64]

Probiotics, especially *S boulardii*, have also shown some potential as an adjunct to antibiotics for the treatment of recurrent CDI, although studies are small. A meta-analysis concluded that the evidence for *S boulardii* is favorable but weak, and additional trials are needed.[65] Fungemia from *S boulardii* has been reported in patients with central venous catheters, and it should be avoided in critically ill and immunocompromised patients.[66]

REFERENCES

1. Kuipers EJ, Surawicz CM. *Clostridium difficile* infection. Lancet 2008;371(9623): 1486–8.
2. Lessa FC, Gould CV, McDonald LC. Current status of *Clostridium difficile* infection epidemiology. Clin Infect Dis 2012;55(Suppl 2):S65–70.
3. Riegler M, Sedivy R, Pothoulakis C, et al. *Clostridium difficile* toxin B is more potent than toxin A in damaging human colonic epithelium in vitro. J Clin Invest 1995;95(5):2004–11.
4. McDonald LC, Killgore GE, Thompson A, et al. An epidemic, toxin gene-variant strain of *Clostridium difficile*. N Engl J Med 2005;353(23):2433–41.
5. Zilberberg MD, Shorr AF, Kollef MH. Increase in adult *Clostridium difficile*-related hospitalizations and case-fatality rate, United States, 2000-2005. Emerg Infect Dis 2008;14(6):929–31.
6. Diggs NG, Surawicz CM. *Clostridium difficile* infection: still principally a disease of the elderly. Therapy 2010;7(3):295–301.

7. Garey KW, Jiang Z-D, Yadav Y, et al. Peripartum *Clostridium difficile* infection: case series and review of the literature. Am J Obstet Gynecol 2008;199(4): 332–7.

8. Unger JA, Whimbey E, Gravett MG, et al. The emergence of *Clostridium difficile* infection among peripartum women: a case-control study of a *C. difficile* outbreak on an obstetrical service. Infect Dis Obstet Gynecol 2011;2011:267249.

9. Centers for Disease Control and Prevention CDC. Surveillance for community-associated *Clostridium difficile*—Connecticut, 2006. MMWR Morb Mortal Wkly Rep 2008;57(13):340–3.

10. Bartlett JG. Narrative review: the new epidemic of *Clostridium difficile*-associated enteric disease. Ann Intern Med 2006;145(10):758–64.

11. Owens RC, Donskey CJ, Gaynes RP, et al. Antimicrobial-associated risk factors for *Clostridium difficile* infection. Clin Infect Dis 2008;46(Suppl 1):S19–31.

12. Hensgens MP, Goorhuis A, Dekkers OM, et al. Time interval of increased risk for *Clostridium difficile* infection after exposure to antibiotics. J Antimicrob Chemother 2012;67(3):742–8.

13. Vesteinsdottir I, Gudlaugsdottir S, Einarsdottir R, et al. Risk factors for *Clostridium difficile* toxin-positive diarrhea: a population-based prospective case-control study. Eur J Clin Microbiol Infect Dis 2012;31(10):2601–10.

14. Kutty PK, Woods CW, Sena AC, et al. Risk factors for and estimated incidence of community-associated *Clostridium difficile* infection, North Carolina, USA. Emerg Infect Dis 2010;16(2):197–204.

15. Bavishi C, Dupont HL. Systematic review: the use of proton pump inhibitors and increased susceptibility to enteric infection. Aliment Pharmacol Ther 2011; 34(11–12):1269–81.

16. Howell MD, Novack V, Grgurich P, et al. Iatrogenic gastric acid suppression and the risk of nosocomial *Clostridium difficile* infection. Arch Intern Med 2010; 170(9):784–90.

17. Deshpande A, Pant C, Pasupuleti V, et al. Association between proton pump inhibitor therapy and *Clostridium difficile* infection in a meta-analysis. Clin Gastroenterol Hepatol 2012;10(3):225–33.

18. Janarthanan S, Ditah I, Adler DG, et al. *Clostridium difficile*-associated diarrhea and proton pump inhibitor therapy: a meta-analysis. Am J Gastroenterol 2012; 107(7):1001–10.

19. Kwok CS, Arthur AK, Anibueze CI, et al. Risk of *Clostridium difficile* infection with acid suppressing drugs and antibiotics: meta-analysis. Am J Gastroenterol 2012;107(7):1011–9.

20. Rodemann JF, Dubberke ER, Reske KA, et al. Incidence of *Clostridium difficile* infection in inflammatory bowel disease. Clin Gastroenterol Hepatol 2007;5(3): 339–44.

21. Issa M, Ananthakrishnan AN, Binion DG. *Clostridium difficile* and inflammatory bowel disease. Inflamm Bowel Dis 2008;14(10):1432–42.

22. Dansinger ML, Johnson S, Jansen PC, et al. Protein-losing enteropathy is associated with *Clostridium difficile* diarrhea but not with asymptomatic colonization: a prospective, case-control study. Clin Infect Dis 1996;22(6):932–7.

23. Fujitani S, George WL, Murthy AR. Comparison of clinical severity score indices for *Clostridium difficile* infection. Infect Control Hosp Epidemiol 2011;32(3):220–8.

24. Wanahita A, Goldsmith EA, Marino BJ, et al. *Clostridium difficile* infection in patients with unexplained leukocytosis. Am J Med 2003;115(7):543–6.

25. Planche T, Wilcox M. Reference assays for *Clostridium difficile* infection: one or two gold standards? J Clin Pathol 2011;64(1):1–5.

26. Planche T, Aghaizu A, Holliman R, et al. Diagnosis of *Clostridium difficile* infection by toxin detection kits: a systematic review. Lancet Infect Dis 2008;8(12): 777–84.
27. Shetty N, Wren MW, Coen PG. The role of glutamate dehydrogenase for the detection of *Clostridium difficile* in faecal samples: a meta-analysis. J Hosp Infect 2011;77(1):1–6.
28. Deshpande A, Pasupuleti V, Rolston DD, et al. Diagnostic accuracy of real-time polymerase chain reaction in detection of *Clostridium difficile* in the stool samples of patients with suspected *Clostridium difficile* infection: a meta-analysis. Clin Infect Dis 2011;53(7):e81–90.
29. Boyanton BL, Sural P, Loomis CR, et al. Loop-mediated isothermal amplification compared to real-time PCR and enzyme immunoassay for toxigenic *Clostridium difficile* detection. J Clin Microbiol 2012;50(3):640–5.
30. Cohen SH, Gerding DN, Johnson S, et al. Clinical practice guidelines for *Clostridium difficile* infection in adults: 2010 update by the Society for Healthcare Epidemiology of America (SHEA) and the Infectious Diseases Society of America (IDSA). Infect Control Hosp Epidemiol 2010;31(5):431–55.
31. Surawicz CM, McFarland LV, Greenberg RN, et al. The search for a better treatment for recurrent *Clostridium difficile* disease: use of high-dose vancomycin combined with *Saccharomyces boulardii*. Clin Infect Dis 2000;31(4):1012–7.
32. Wilcox MH, Freeman J, Fawley W, et al. Long-term surveillance of cefotaxime and piperacillin-tazobactam prescribing and incidence of *Clostridium difficile* diarrhoea. J Antimicrob Chemother 2004;54(1):168–72.
33. Climo MW, Israel DS, Wong ES, et al. Hospital-wide restriction of clindamycin: effect on the incidence of *Clostridium difficile*-associated diarrhea and cost. Ann Intern Med 1998;128(12 Pt 1):989–95.
34. Valiquette L, Cossette B, Garant M-P, et al. Impact of a reduction in the use of high-risk antibiotics on the course of an epidemic of *Clostridium difficile*-associated disease caused by the hypervirulent NAP1/027 strain. Clin Infect Dis 2007; 45(Suppl 2):S112–21.
35. Dellit TH, Owens RC, McGowan JE, et al. Infectious Diseases Society of America and the Society for Healthcare Epidemiology of America guidelines for developing an institutional program to enhance antimicrobial stewardship. Clin Infect Dis 2007;44(2):159–77.
36. Wullt M, Odenholt I, Walder M. Activity of three disinfectants and acidified nitrite against *Clostridium difficile* spores. Infect Control Hosp Epidemiol 2003;24(10): 765–8.
37. Johnson S, Gerding DN, Olson MM, et al. Prospective, controlled study of vinyl glove use to interrupt *Clostridium difficile* nosocomial transmission. Am J Med 1990;88(2):137–40.
38. Mayfield JL, Leet T, Miller J, et al. Environmental control to reduce transmission of *Clostridium difficile*. Clin Infect Dis 2000;31(4):995–1000.
39. Wilcox MH, Fawley WN, Wigglesworth N, et al. Comparison of the effect of detergent versus hypochlorite cleaning on environmental contamination and incidence of *Clostridium difficile* infection. J Hosp Infect 2003;54(2):109–14.
40. Johnston BC, Ma SS, Goldenberg JZ, et al. Probiotics for the prevention of *Clostridium difficile*-associated diarrhea: a systematic review and meta-analysis. Ann Intern Med 2012;157(12):878–88.
41. Bolton RP, Culshaw MA. Faecal metronidazole concentrations during oral and intravenous therapy for antibiotic associated colitis due to *Clostridium difficile*. Gut 1986;27(10):1169–72.

42. Kapoor K, Chandra M, Nag D, et al. Evaluation of metronidazole toxicity: a prospective study. Int J Clin Pharmacol Res 1999;19(3):83–8.

43. Nerandzic MM, Mullane K, Miller MA, et al. Reduced acquisition and overgrowth of vancomycin-resistant enterococci and Candida species in patients treated with fidaxomicin versus vancomycin for *Clostridium difficile* infection. Clin Infect Dis 2012;55(Suppl 2):S121–6.

44. Finegold SM, Molitoris D, Vaisanen ML, et al. In vitro activities of OPT-80 and comparator drugs against intestinal bacteria. Antimicrobial Agents Chemother 2004;48(12):4898–902.

45. Louie TJ, Miller MA, Mullane KM, et al. Fidaxomicin versus vancomycin for *Clostridium difficile* infection. N Engl J Med 2011;364(5):422–31.

46. Pepin J, Valiquette L, Gagnon S, et al. Outcomes of *Clostridium difficile*-associated disease treated with metronidazole or vancomycin before and after the emergence of NAP1/027. Am J Gastroenterol 2007;102(12):2781–8.

47. Zar FA, Bakkanagari SR, Moorthi KM, et al. A comparison of vancomycin and metronidazole for the treatment of *Clostridium difficile*-associated diarrhea, stratified by disease severity. Clin Infect Dis 2007;45(3):302–7.

48. Drekonja DM, Butler M, MacDonald R, et al. Comparative effectiveness of *Clostridium difficile* treatments: a systematic review. Ann Intern Med 2011;155(12): 839–47.

49. Al-Nassir WN, Sethi AK, Nerandzic MM, et al. Comparison of clinical and microbiological response to treatment of *Clostridium difficile*-associated disease with metronidazole and vancomycin. Clin Infect Dis 2008;47(1):56–62.

50. Musher DM, Aslam S, Logan N, et al. Relatively poor outcome after treatment of *Clostridium difficile* colitis with metronidazole. Clin Infect Dis 2005;40(11): 1586–90.

51. Apisarnthanarak A, Razavi B, Mundy LM. Adjunctive intracolonic vancomycin for severe *Clostridium difficile* colitis: case series and review of the literature. Clin Infect Dis 2002;35(6):690–6.

52. Markelov A, Livert D, Kohli H. Predictors of fatal outcome after colectomy for fulminant *Clostridium difficile* Colitis: a 10-year experience. Am Surg 2011; 77(8):977–80.

53. Ali SO, Welch JP, Dring RJ. Early surgical intervention for fulminant pseudomembranous colitis. Am Surg 2008;74(1):20–6.

54. Butala P, Divino CM. Surgical aspects of fulminant *Clostridium difficile* colitis. Am J Surg 2010;200(1):131–5.

55. Barbut F, Richard A, Hamadi K, et al. Epidemiology of recurrences or reinfections of *Clostridium difficile*-associated diarrhea. J Clin Microbiol 2000;38(6):2386–8.

56. Kyne L, Warny M, Qamar A, et al. Association between antibody response to toxin A and protection against recurrent *Clostridium difficile* diarrhoea. Lancet 2001;357(9251):189–93.

57. McFarland LV, Elmer GW, Surawicz CM. Breaking the cycle: treatment strategies for 163 cases of recurrent *Clostridium difficile* disease. Am J Gastroenterol 2002;97(7):1769–75.

58. Garey KW, Ghantoji SS, Shah DN, et al. A randomized, double-blind, placebo-controlled pilot study to assess the ability of rifaximin to prevent recurrent diarrhoea in patients with *Clostridium difficile* infection. J Antimicrob Chemother 2011;66(12):2850–5.

59. Curry SR, Marsh JW, Shutt KA, et al. High frequency of rifampin resistance identified in an epidemic *Clostridium difficile* clone from a large teaching hospital. Clin Infect Dis 2009;48(4):425–9.

60. Bakken JS, Borody T, Brandt LJ, et al. Treating *Clostridium difficile* infection with fecal microbiota transplantation. Clin Gastroenterol Hepatol 2011;9(12):1044–9.
61. Gough E, Shaikh H, Manges AR. Systematic review of intestinal microbiota transplantation (fecal bacteriotherapy) for recurrent *Clostridium difficile* infection. Clin Infect Dis 2011;53(10):994–1002.
62. van Nood E, Vrieze A, Nieuwdorp M, et al. Duodenal infusion of donor feces for recurrent *Clostridium difficile*. N Engl J Med 2013;368(5):407–15.
63. Oral vancomycin followed by fecal transplant versus tapering oral vancomycin. Available at: ClinicalTrials.gov. Accessed on December 15, 2012.
64. Fecal transplant for relapsing *C. difficile* infection. Available at: ClinicalTrials.gov. Accessed on December 15, 2012.
65. McFarland LV. Systematic review and meta-analysis of *Saccharomyces boulardii* in adult patients. World J Gastroenterol 2010;16(18):2202–22.
66. Enache-Angoulvant A, Hennequin C. Invasive *Saccharomyces* infection: a comprehensive review. Clin Infect Dis 2005;41(11):1559–68.

Pertussis

Tara B. Spector, MD[a],*, Eileen K. Maziarz, MD[b]

KEYWORDS

- Pertussis • *Bordetella pertussis* • Whooping cough • Immunization

KEY POINTS

- The incidence of pertussis has increased in recent years, particularly among adolescents and adults.
- Adolescents and adults serve as important reservoirs of infection, transmitting pertussis to infants and children, who are at greater risk for morbidity and mortality.
- Clinical presentation of pertussis infection is often atypical in adults and adolescents, who often lack classic symptoms and present later in the course of infection; therefore, a high index of suspicion is necessary to diagnose pertussis infection in these populations.
- Treatment is with a macrolide (azithromycin preferred). Treatment is most effective at reducing the severity or duration of cough if administered within the first 7 days of symptoms, often before the onset of coughing paroxysms. Treatment initiated after this period has limited impact on symptom duration, but does lead to faster eradication of the organism from the nasopharynx, thus reducing rates of transmission.
- Recognition of the increased incidence of pertussis infection in these populations has led to the introduction of revised vaccination strategies in many countries to improve disease control and reduce the global burden of disease.

INTRODUCTION

Pertussis, or whooping cough, is an upper respiratory tract infection (URI) caused by *Bordetella pertussis*. The classic clinical syndrome is a prolonged illness characterized by severe coughing paroxysms, inspiratory whooping, and posttussive emesis. Many classic features of pertussis infection are absent or less prominent in previously immunized adolescents and adults.[1]

After the widespread introduction of the pertussis vaccine in the 1940s, the incidence of pertussis declined dramatically.[2] Despite vaccination strategies, however,

Funding Sources: None.
Conflict of Interest: None.
[a] Division of General Internal Medicine, University of Washington Medical Center, Health Science Building, B-503, 1959 Northeast Pacific Street, Seattle, WA 98195, USA; [b] Division of Infectious Diseases and International Health, Department of Internal Medicine, Duke University Medical Center, Hanes House Room 163, Trent Drive, Durham, NC 27710, USA
* Corresponding author.
E-mail address: tbs4@uw.edu

medical.theclinics.com

B pertussis is far from eradicated, even in developed nations, and remains a significant cause of morbidity and mortality worldwide.[3] Unimmunized infants and partially immunized children are at greatest risk for complications and death from pertussis.[4] In the past 2 decades, there has been a resurgence of reported cases of pertussis worldwide, including in the United States.[5] As a result of more sensitive diagnostic techniques, it is increasingly recognized that pertussis immunity (once believed to be lifelong after both natural infection and immunization) wanes over a period 7 to 10 years, resulting in subclinical infection in those previously immunized and subsequent spread of pertussis to unimmunized or partially immunized infants and children.[6]

Diagnosis of pertussis requires a high index of suspicion for the disease and prompt nasopharyngeal sampling for laboratory confirmation. Numerous diagnostic modalities, including traditional culture, polymerase chain reaction (PCR) assays, and serologic-based tests, are available to confirm diagnosis of pertussis.[7] Treatment and postexposure prophylaxis must be initiated early to be effective. Guidelines for pertussis vaccination are updated frequently, with increased attention to provision of booster vaccines to adolescents and adults to prevent transmission of pertussis to at-risk populations.[8]

This article provides clinically relevant information about pertussis and:

- Reviews the microbiology, transmission, pathogenesis, and epidemiology of pertussis
- Describes both classic and atypical clinical presentations of pertussis infection and how these vary based on host factors
- Compares available diagnostic methods and describes appropriate use of these tests and
- Summarizes current treatment, postexposure prophylaxis, and vaccination guidelines.

MICROBIOLOGY

Pertussis or whooping cough is caused by the small gram-negative, strictly aerobic coccobacillus *B pertussis*. *B pertussis* is 1 of 9 known *Bordetella* species, many of which are known for causing illnesses in animal species, including *B bronchoseptica* (the cause of kennel cough in cats and dogs).[9] *B pertussis*, conversely, is a strict human pathogen without an animal reservoir.[1] Most human respiratory infections caused by *Bordetella* species are caused by *B pertussis or B parapertussis,* which causes a clinically similar, although usually less severe respiratory illness.[9] *Bordetella* species are highly fastidious organisms, the growth of which is inhibited by many components of common laboratory media; isolation of the organism, therefore, requires a high index of suspicion and preparation on appropriate media (see section on laboratory diagnosis).

TRANSMISSION

Pertussis is transmitted from person to person via respiratory droplets spread by coughing. The incubation period is approximately 7 to 10 days.[1] Pertussis is highly contagious; on contact with an infected patient, up to 34% of household contacts develop clinical pertussis and as many as 46% of asymptomatic household contacts show laboratory evidence of nasopharyngeal colonization, suggesting that asymptomatic individuals or carriers can serve as a reservoir of disease.[10] Unimmunized infants are particularly at risk for complications from pertussis, and epidemiologic studies have shown that infants most commonly contract pertussis from a household source.[11,12]

PATHOGENESIS

Once droplets of B pertussis are inhaled, infection occurs through a 4-step process, each mediated by specific virulence factors. These steps are attachment, evasion of host defenses, local tissue damage, and systemic manifestations.[1]

B pertussis attaches to ciliated epithelial cells of the upper respiratory tract via at least 8 different adhesion factors. The most important of these adhesins are filamentous hemagglutinin and fimbriae, highly immunogenic proteins required for airway colonization and included in most acellular pertussis vaccines.[1]

Two virulence factors are primarily responsible for evasion of host defenses: adenylate cyclase toxin (ACT) and pertussis toxin (PT). ACT inhibits neutrophil chemotaxis and phagocytosis by catalyzing excessive amounts of cyclic adenosine monophosphate from adenosine triphosphate. PT, the major virulence determinant of B pertussis, comprises 2 interdependent components: the active (A) and binding (B) subunits. The B subunit is responsible for binding to cell membranes, facilitating entry of the A subunit, which acts via G-protein coupled receptor pathways to alter cell function[13] and to inhibit migration of neutrophils, lymphocytes, and macrophages, preventing them from reaching areas of infection.[1] PT, a major component of most pertussis vaccines, is also responsible for many of the systemic manifestations caused by alterations in signaling pathways.[1]

Local damage to respiratory tract tissue is mediated by several virulence factors, the most important of which is tracheal cytotoxin, which specifically damages and kills ciliated respiratory epithelial cells via local nitric oxide production, causing epithelial sloughing. This damage is believed to contribute to the characteristic paroxysmal cough, although additional unidentified toxins may also be responsible.[1]

Systemic manifestations of pertussis infection, though uncommon, are mediated primarily through PT, which is responsible for a lymphocyte-predominant leukocytosis and pancreatic islet cell sensitization and hyperinsulinemia, which can lead to hypoglycemia, particularly among young infants.[1,14]

EPIDEMIOLOGY

Despite routine vaccination strategies, pertussis remains an important global public health problem, with an estimated 30 to 50 million cases annually; it is responsible for an estimated 300,000 attributable deaths per year. More than 90% of cases occur in developing countries where infant and childhood vaccination rates remain low.[3,15]

Pertussis outbreaks occur in a cyclical pattern, with peaks occurring every 2 to 5 years.[2] Unlike influenza and other respiratory infections, pertussis has no clear seasonal pattern.[2] Before the widespread introduction of the whole-cell pertussis vaccine in the late 1940s, pertussis was a leading cause of death among children worldwide. In the prevaccination period, the average incidence of pertussis in the United States was 157 cases per 100,000 persons, with more than 90% of reported cases occurring in children younger than 10 years. In contrast to current trends, infants younger than 1 year accounted for fewer than 10% of cases.[2] After implementation of vaccination strategies, rates of pertussis infection decreased substantially for several decades, reaching a nadir in the late 1970s. In 1976, only 1010 cases of pertussis were reported in the United States.[2,16]

Since the early 1980s, there has been an increase in the overall annual incidence of pertussis worldwide, particularly among adolescents and adults.[17] Although this increase may reflect a true increase in the number of cases as a result of waning immunity, it also likely reflects increased awareness of pertussis as a cause of prolonged cough in these populations, newer diagnostic testing methods, and improved reporting via national surveillance systems.[18]

Although the incidence of pertussis has increased among adolescents and adults, it has also increased among infants younger than 1 year, in whom rates of hospitalization, serious complications, and mortality are the highest. Recent estimates indicate that up to 90% of pertussis-related hospitalizations[19] and 79% to 90% of pertussis-related deaths occur in infants younger than 1 year **(Fig. 1)**.[20,21]

Recent US Trends

In 2010, more than 27,550 cases of pertussis were reported to the Centers for Disease Control (CDC). This number decreased to 18,719 cases in 2011, but increased dramatically in 2012, with greater than 40,000 provisional cases reported and incidence estimates of 11.6 cases per 100,000 persons.[5] Consistent with recent trends, nearly 50% of these cases occurred in adolescents and adults. US pertussis outbreaks affecting children as well as adolescents and adults have been described in many states and small residential communities, including college campuses.[22,23] Case-fatality rates remain highest among infants younger than 3 months.[5]

CLINICAL MANIFESTATIONS

The clinical presentation of *B pertussis* infection varies by host age, immune status, and coexistent conditions. Children and those not previously immunized are more likely to present with classic symptoms than are adults and children with previous immunity.

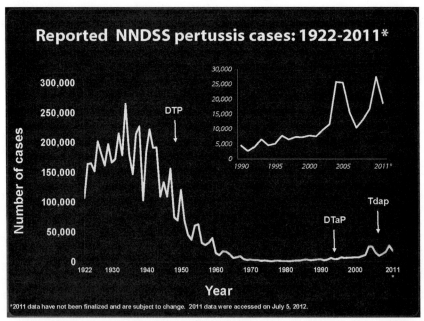

Fig. 1. Reported cases of pertussis in the United States 1922–2011. (*Data from* CDC, National Notifiable Diseases Surveillance System and Supplemental Pertussis Surveillance System and 1922–1949, passive reports to the Public Health Service. Available at: http://www.cdc.gov/media/Pertussis Cases_1922_2011_accessed July 5 2012[1].pdf). Accessed on December 2, 2012.

Classic Presentation

The classic presentation is characterized by 3 well-differentiated phases[1]: the catarrhal (or prodromal) phase, the paroxysmal phase, and the convalescent phase. The catarrhal phase typically begins 7 to 14 days after contact with an infected individual and is marked by signs and symptoms of URI, including rhinorrhea and lacrimation. A low-grade fever may be present and cough, when present, is generally mild. During this stage, affected individuals are highly contagious. The catarrhal stage lasts 1 to 2 weeks; toward the end of these 2 weeks, the cough begins to worsen in both frequency and intensity, and the patient enters the paroxysmal phase, a period marked by coughing fits or paroxysms (average of 15 per 24 hours). These spells of 5 to 10 forceful coughs during a single expiration are frequently followed by a vigorous inspiratory effort with associated whoop, caused by inspiration against a partially closed glottis. Posttussive emesis is common and the cough tends to be worse at night. This prolonged period of cough is a distinguishing feature of pertussis (known as 100-day cough in China), but duration can be highly variable (typically lasting 1–6 weeks). The convalescent phase follows the paroxysmal phase and can last up to 8 weeks; it is characterized by decreased frequency and severity of coughing paroxysms. However, episodic paroxysmal coughing may return, with recurrent upper respiratory infections for up to 1 year (**Table 1**).[24]

Physical Examination, Laboratory, and Radiology Findings

The physical examination is usually normal, without specific findings to differentiate pertussis from other common viral respiratory tract infections.[1] The white blood cell count is often normal. Lymphocytosis can be present, most often between stages 1 and 2, with total lymphocyte count greater than 10,000/mL[25] and is associated with poorer outcomes.[4,19,26] Chest imaging is usually normal. The lack of specific examination, laboratory, and imaging findings emphasizes why it is important for clinicians to have a high clinical suspicion for pertussis based on symptoms alone.

Presentation in Infants, Adolescents, and Adults

Infants represent the most vulnerable population to severe pertussis infection, because of lack of previous or complete immunity through vaccination. Clinical features are often atypical in infants, who are more likely to present with apnea, cyanosis, and poor feeding, as well as shorter duration of cough.[4]

Table 1
Classic phases of pertussis infection

	Catarrhal	Paroxysmal	Convalescent
Onset[a]	7–14 d	2–4 wk	3–10 wk
Clinical features	Rhinorrhea Mild cough Lacrimation Fever absent or low grade Cough later worsens in frequency and intensity	Coughing fits, 5–10 forceful coughs during single expiration Often followed by vigorous inspiratory effort (whoop) Posttussive emesis Cough worse at night	Paroxysms less frequent/severe Paroxysmal cough or inspiratory whoop may recur with repeat upper respiratory infections
Duration	1–2 wk	1–6 wk	Variable

[a] After exposure.

Because most adolescents and adults are immunized against pertussis during childhood, clinical presentation can be atypical, often marked by a prolonged cough in isolation of other symptoms. Most infected adults report a cough of greater than 3 weeks' duration (mean 36–48 days).[18] They may also have episodes of diaphoresis and syncope.[18] Characteristic whoop and posttussive emesis are less common; however, the presence of these symptoms is highly predictive of pertussis in this subset of patients.[27] Because of the atypical features of infection in these patients, many cases of pertussis remain unrecognized. It is estimated that 12% to 32% of cases of cough lasting greater than 1 week in adults are caused by pertussis.[18] Furthermore, adult patients tend to present later, at times when standard diagnostic methods such as culture and PCR are less likely to be positive.[28] The implications of unrecognized infection in this population as a source of ongoing exposure to susceptible individuals have been identified and have influenced immunization schedules in many countries.[29]

Complications

Pneumonia (either primary or secondary) is the most common and most severe complication of pertussis infection, disproportionately affecting infants younger than 6 months of age.[19,20] Respiratory syncytial virus is a common copathogen, with coinfection rates as high as 33% of hospitalized infants.[4] Other complications include neurologic sequelae (seizures and encephalopathy), weight loss, and complications of severe cough, including incontinence, rib fractures, hernias, conjunctival hemorrhage, cerebral artery dissection, and syncope.[19] Pertussis is associated with higher rates of other concurrent infections, such as sinusitis and otitis media.[18] Case-fatality rates approach 1% of infected infants.[19]

DIFFERENTIAL DIAGNOSIS

Because of a lack of specific symptoms, particularly among hosts who present with atypical features, the differential diagnosis of pertussis infection can be refined by duration of cough, as presented in **Table 2**.[30] In the early phase, pertussis is generally indistinguishable from common viral URIs and atypical bacterial pneumonias caused by *Mycoplasma pneumoniae* and *Chlamydia pneumoniae*, all of which

Table 2
Differential diagnosis of pertussis by duration of cough

Acute (<3 wk)	Subacute (3–8 wk)	Chronic (>8 wk)
Viral URI	Postinfectious cough	Postnasal drip
Atypical pneumonia	Bacterial sinusitis	Asthma
Chronic obstructive pulmonary disease exacerbation	Asthma	Chronic obstructive pulmonary disease
Congestive heart failure exacerbation		Angiotensin-converting enzyme inhibitors
Bacterial sinusitis		Gastroesophageal reflux disease
Allergic rhinitis		
Bacterial pneumonia		
Asthma exacerbation		

Data from Mattoo S, Cherry JD. Molecular pathogenesis, epidemiology, and clinical manifestations of respiratory infections due to Bordetella pertussis and other Bordetella subspecies. Clin Microbiol Rev 2005;18(2):326–82; and Irwin RS, Madison JM. The diagnosis and treatment of cough. N Engl J Med 2000;343(23):1715–21.

manifest primarily by rhinorrhea, mild cough, and absent or low-grade fever. Infectious considerations decrease dramatically as the duration of cough increases. Host factors, detailed history taking, and empirical trial of agents such as proton-pump inhibitors for gastroesophageal reflux disease and bronchodilators for asthma can help distinguish pertussis from other common causes of chronic cough (see **Table 2**).

DIAGNOSIS
Clinical Case Definitions

Both the CDC and World Health Organization (WHO) have developed similar case definitions for pertussis for surveillance purposes. WHO defines a clinical case as an individual with cough lasting at least 2 weeks, in addition to at least 1 of the following symptoms: coughing paroxysms, inspiratory whooping, or posttussive vomiting without other apparent cause.[31]

WHO defines a confirmed case as an individual satisfying the above clinical case definition in combination with at least 1 of the following laboratory findings: isolation of B pertussis in culture, detection of genomic sequences by PCR, or positive paired serology (see section on laboratory diagnosis).[31]

The CDC definition for a confirmed case is similar, but does not include paired serology and does include epidemiologic link with a culture-confirmed case of pertussis.[32] The WHO clinical definition is estimated to be 95.2% sensitive and 15.0% specific when compared with laboratory-confirmed cases.[33] With increased number of positive symptoms, the clinical case definition increases in specificity at the expense of decreased sensitivity.

The clinical diagnosis of pertussis is limited by variable disease presentation across age groups, modification of presenting symptoms influenced by previous immunization, and low clinical suspicion by physicians.[1,33] The clinical case definitions described earlier have been criticized as outdated and not universally applicable to all age groups. To more accurately capture the variable clinical presentation, age-specific clinical case definitions for pertussis have been proposed.[34] Based on consensus recommendations developed at the 2011 Global Pertussis Initiative Conference, pertussis should be clinically suspected in patients presenting with cough without fever, and 1 or more age group-specific symptoms (**Fig. 2**).

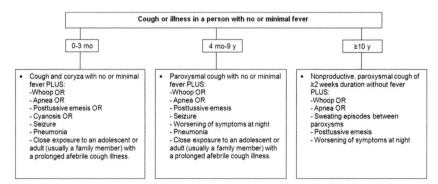

Fig. 2. Clinical case definition of pertussis for surveillance purposes. (*From* Cherry JD, Tan T, Wirsing von Konig CH, et al. Clinical definitions of pertussis: summary of a global pertussis initiative roundtable meeting, February 2011. Clin Infect Dis 2012;54:1762; with permission.)

Laboratory Diagnosis

Once pertussis is clinically suspected based on the criteria described earlier, confirmation may be made via multiple laboratory techniques. There is no universally agreed gold standard for the laboratory diagnosis of pertussis, although traditionally culture has been used because of its high specificity. Several methods exist, each with its own benefits and limitations.

Specimen Collection

Among suspected cases, samples tested for *B pertussis* require proper technique and timing as well as special handling to optimize diagnostic yield. Specimens can be obtained via nasal swab or aspiration. Swabs should be obtained from the posterior nasopharynx, rather than the anterior nasopharynx or throat, to optimize yield of live bacteria or DNA from ciliated respiratory epithelial cells for diagnosis.[24,35] Nasopharyngeal aspiration with saline yields better results than swabs, but aspiration is not always practical in clinical settings.[36] Swabs with Dacron or rayon tips should be used for collection; calcium-alginate and cotton-tipped swabs can inhibit PCR analysis and kill pertussis organisms, respectively.[37] Specimens obtained for culture should be transported in Regan-Lowe agar, a charcoal medium that contains cephalexin to inhibit the growth of other oropharyngeal organisms,[38,39] then plated on either Borget-Genou or Regan-Lowe agar.[38]

Culture

B pertussis can grow on culture media in as little as 2 to 4 days, but growth often takes up to 5 to 7 days,[39] limiting the timeliness for acute management. The specificity of culture for detection of *B pertussis* approaches 100%, but sensitivity ranges from 30% to 70%.[7,39] Sensitivity is limited by improper collection and culturing technique, time delay between specimen collection and culture, previous administration of antibiotics, and previous vaccination status. Cultures tend to be most sensitive in younger patients and if collected early in the disease course, ideally within 2 weeks of symptom onset.[7,38] Advantages include confirmation and strain identification in outbreak settings as well as the ability to perform antimicrobial susceptibility testing.

Molecular Testing

Molecular-based tests offer several advantages over traditional culture techniques, including more rapid diagnosis and improved sensitivity, and are widely used in the diagnosis of pertussis. Many PCR assays are available to detect DNA from various chromosomal regions specific to *B pertussis*. PCR has become an increasingly popular diagnostic technique because of its rapid turnaround time (1–2 days), ability to diagnose pertussis up to 4 weeks after symptom onset (when yield of culture-based techniques is limited), and ability to detect pertussis in patients who have been previously immunized or have already received treatment with up to 5 days of antibiotics. Sensitivity of PCR-based testing ranges from 70% to 99%, with a specificity of 88% to 94%.[7,38] Limitations of PCR testing include availability of laboratory space and properly trained technicians, limited availability of commercial kits, lack of standardized methods, absence of universal thresholds for positivity, and expense of testing.[34] The CDC recommends that PCR be used in conjunction with culture for diagnosis of pertussis, particularly in outbreak situations.[24,40]

Serology

Serologic methods can also be used for the diagnosis of pertussis. Exposure to *B pertussis* results in rapid production of IgA, IgG, and IgM antibodies to various pertussis antigens that can be detected with enzyme-linked immunosorbent assay techniques. These antibodies are typically apparent by the time clinical symptoms manifest. Immune response to pertussis persists for weeks after initial exposure, therefore serology can be useful in diagnosing pertussis in patients with greater than 2 to 4 weeks of symptoms, an advantage over traditional culture-based techniques. Antibodies to the pertussis toxin antigen (anti-PT antibodies) are the most widely used, because the PT antigen is highly immunogenic and specific to *B pertussis*.[41] Immunization results in the production of both IgG and IgM antibodies; therefore, use of serologic testing is more difficult to interpret in patients who have been immunized, particularly in children who have completed the full series or in adolescents and adults who have received a booster in the past year.

Dual-sample serology, based on increase in antibody titer from acute to convalescent samples, is not used clinically because of the high number of previously immunized patients and the usual timing of presentation late in the course of illness. In practice, single-sample serology of anti-PT IgG is used, with a cutoff value based on healthy age-matched controls, to determine a positive test result. There is no universally agreed cutoff value for a positive result, but the European Union reference laboratories suggest a value between 65 and 125 IU/mL. This cutoff range results in a sensitivity of 70% to 80% and a specificity of 95% to 99%.[41]

Serologic diagnosis suffers from a lack of standardized commercially available testing kits and lack of universally agreed cutoff values for interpreting positive results.[7] Further, serologic evaluation is limited in infants, whose ability to generate an antibody response may be limited,[24] and among adolescents and adults, whose booster immunizations may be less remote because of newer vaccination schedules.

Direct Fluorescent Antibody Testing

Direct fluorescent antibody (DFA) testing, which uses fluorochrome-conjugated antibodies to antigens of *B pertussis,* was once widely used for rapid diagnosis of pertussis. This modality has largely been replaced by other diagnostic tests because of limited sensitivity and specificity, with high rates of false-positive results attributable to cross-reactivity with other oropharyngeal flora such as *Haemophilus influenza*.[1,38] The use of DFA is not recommended for the laboratory diagnosis of pertussis.[34]

Guidance regarding optimal testing strategies based on host and timing of presentation is available in **Box 1** and **Fig. 3**.

Box 1
Summary of diagnosis recommendations

- PCR and culture should be performed in all patients with high clinical suspicion of pertussis and cough of less than 2 weeks' duration

- PCR and serology should be performed for adolescent and adult patients with cough of greater than 2 weeks' duration

- Single-sample serology alone should be considered in patients with symptoms for greater than 4 weeks

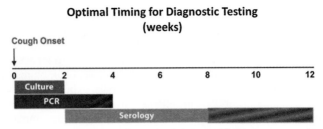

Optimal Timing for Diagnostic Testing (weeks)

Fig. 3. Optimal timing for culture, PCR and serologic diagnosis of pertussis. (*From* Pertussis (whooping cough) diagnosis confirmation. Atlanta (GA): Centers for Disease Control and Prevention, 2012. Available at: http://www.cdc.gov/pertussis/clinical/diagnostic-testing/diagnosis-confirmation.html. Accessed Feb 27, 2013.)

TREATMENT
Antimicrobial Therapy

Efficacy of antimicrobial therapy during the various stages of pertussis infection has been the subject of much debate. Antibiotics are believed to be most effective in limiting symptom severity and duration when administered early in the course of illness.

Macrolides are the treatment of choice for *B pertussis*.[42] Erythromycin, clarithromycin, and azithromycin have all been found to be effective at treating pertussis, with choice of agent primarily based on side effect profile and ease of dosing:

- Azithromycin 500 mg × 1 day, then 250 mg × 4 days
- Clarithromycin 500 mg 2 times/d × 7 days
- Erythromycin 500 mg 4 times/d × 14 days

Newer macrolides including azithromycin and clarithromycin are as effective as erythromycin at eradicating *B pertussis* from nasopharyngeal secretions[43] and are generally preferred because of less frequent dosing and fewer gastrointestinal side effects, which can be particularly severe with erythromycin and can decrease adherence rates.[44–46] Azithromycin is the preferred agent in infants younger than 1 month because of associations between erythromycin use and development of hypertrophic pyloric stenosis.[47] Azithromycin is preferable to clarithromycin and erythromycin in patients on multiple medications, because it has far fewer drug interactions. Resistance to macrolides, although it has been described, is rare, and routine antimicrobial susceptibility testing is not generally performed.

Trimethoprim-sulfamethoxazole can be used as an alternative agent in patients with contraindications or allergies to macrolides.[48] The recommended regimen is:

- Trimethoprim-sulfamethoxazole 1 double-strength tablet 2 times/d x 14 days.

Timing of Treatment

Treatment is most effective at reducing the severity or duration of cough if administered within the first 7 days of symptoms, often before the onset of coughing paroxysms. Treatment initiated after this period has limited impact on symptom duration, but does lead to faster eradication of the organism from the nasopharynx, thus reducing rates of transmission. The CDC recommends treating patients older than 1 year within 21 days of symptom onset. Treatment within 6 weeks of symptom onset is recommended for pregnant women in the third trimester, infants younger than 1 year, and those in close contact with infants. If clinical suspicion for pertussis is high, antibiotic therapy should be initiated at the same time that diagnostic testing is performed.[42]

Symptomatic Treatment of Cough

A Cochrane database systematic review examined the impact of various adjunctive therapies for symptomatic treatment of cough related to pertussis, including corticosteroids, β_2 agonists, leukotriene receptor antagonists, and antihistamines. None of these agents was found to have a significant impact on reducing the frequency or severity of coughing episodes or length of hospital stay.[49]

Postexposure Prophylaxis

The CDC recommends postexposure prophylaxis for all household contacts of an infected patient within 3 weeks of symptom onset in the index patient.[42] The dose and duration of prophylactic antibiotics are the same as those used for treatment. However, a Cochrane review found that postexposure prophylaxis was only marginally effective in preventing development of pertussis in household contacts, and that prophylactic treatment was associated with significant side effects. This study concluded that prophylactic treatment should be instituted only in households with infants younger than 6 months.[43] Clinicians should evaluate on a case-by-case basis the risks and benefits of postexposure prophylaxis. Postexposure prophylaxis should be administered to exposed individuals who have (or are in contact with others with) high-risk characteristics for developing complications from pertussis, including infants younger than 1 year, immunocompromised patients, or patients with chronic pulmonary conditions such as cystic fibrosis or chronic obstructive pulmonary disease.

PREVENTION
Immunization

Routine immunization is recommended to prevent pertussis infection. Historical vaccines using killed whole *B pertussis* organisms in various preparations, in combination with diphtheria and tetanus toxoids, were developed shortly after the cause was identified[1] and were released in the United States in the mid-1940s for routine vaccination of children.[24] Whole-cell vaccines were widely used for many years and resulted in a dramatic decrease in pertussis incidence.[1] Three of the 4 available whole-cell vaccines, evaluated 5 decades after their widespread implementation, were found to be 89% to 96% effective in preventing pertussis infection.[1,24] However, concerns regarding the reactogenicity of whole-cell vaccines, including greater propensity toward both local and systemic reactions as well as controversy surrounding serious neurologic sequelae (now largely refuted), led to the introduction of acellular vaccines in the 1990s.[1] Clinical efficacy of acellular vaccines ranges from 59% to 93%.[1,24]

Vaccination Formulations and Schedules

Current vaccine formulations include DTaP (diphtheria, tetanus, and acellular pertussis), used for the initial childhood vaccine series, and Tdap (which contains reduced doses of diphtheria and pertussis antigens), used for adolescent and adult booster immunizations. Two formulations of Tdap booster are available: Adacel (manufactured by Sanofi Pasteur) and Boostrix (manufactured by GlaxoSmithKline).[50]

Before 2006, infants and children were the only populations routinely immunized against pertussis. As data accumulated supporting the notion of waning immunity after pertussis vaccination[6,51] and the importance of older patients as sources of pertussis transmission to unimmunized infants and children,[10,11] expanded immunization strategies to include adolescents and adults have been investigated. Based on results of the Adult Pertussis Trial, in which the acellular pertussis vaccine was found to be 92%

effective among adolescents and adults,[52] revised vaccination guidelines now include recommendations for pertussis boosters for both adolescents and adults.

The CDC's Advisory Committee of Immunization Practices (ACIP) recommended vaccine schedule for pertussis is summarized in **Box 2**.[8,53] Tdap boosters can be administered at any time, irrespective of timing of the most recent tetanus-containing or diphtheria-containing vaccine.[8] A recent study reported that a Tdap booster in adulthood, 10 years after a previous booster, was safe and elicited a robust immune response.[54] Further refinement of ACIP guidelines may include recommendations for routine decennial Tdap boosters for all adults.[55]

Vaccine Side Effects

The DTap and Tdap vaccines are generally well tolerated and associated with fewer local and systemic reactions than historical whole-cell vaccines. The most common side effects (and their relative frequency) include[56]: injection site pain (67%–75%) or redness (20%); headache (30%–40%) and fatigue (25%–33%); and mild fever less than 100.4°F (1%–4%). Moderate to severe reactions are rare but include: moderate to severe arm pain/swelling (4%–6%); fever greater than 102°F (0.4–1%); seizure (less than 1/14,000); and severe allergic reaction, prolonged seizure, coma, brain damage (less than 1/1,000,000).

Special Populations: Pregnant Women

Pregnant women and those in close contact with infants warrant special consideration. A strategy of vaccinating pregnant women and other household contacts of a neonate to provide partial protection from infection is known as a cocooning strategy.[55] The ACIP, in conjunction with the American College of Obstetrics and Gynecology, recommends that pregnant women who have not previously received a Tdap booster should receive 1 dose of Tdap during the third trimester or late second trimester, or in the immediate postpartum period if it is not administered during pregnancy.[57,58] As noted earlier, all adults, including those aged 65 and older, who anticipate close contact with an infant and who have not received a Tdap booster, are advised to receive 1 dose of Tdap at least 2 weeks before contact with the infant.[8]

Studies have reported detectable levels of antibodies to *B pertussis* antigens in neonates of women immunized during pregnancy, with detectable antibody levels

---

Box 2
Summary recommendations for use of tetanus, diphtheria, and acellular pertussis vaccines

Infants and Children

- Five-dose primary immunization series with DTaP recommended at ages 2, 4, 6, and 18 months, with booster at age 4 to 6 years

Adolescents

- Adolescents 11 to 18 years of age who have completed the recommended childhood DTaP series should receive a single Tdap booster, preferably at their 11-year-old to 12-year-old preventive health visit

Adults

- Adults aged 19 to 64 years should receive a single Tdap booster in lieu of 1 Td booster
- Adults aged 65 and older who have not previously received a Tdap booster should receive 1 booster dose, particularly if contact with infants is anticipated

persisting for up to 6 weeks post partum[59,60] and likely providing partial protection against pertussis initiation of the primary immunization series at age 2 months.

Special Populations: Health Care Workers

Health care workers are at increased risk of exposure to pertussis and have been implicated in nosocomial outbreaks of pertussis.[61] The ACIP recommends that all adult health care workers with direct patient contact receive a Tdap booster.[29]

SUMMARY

- Incidence of pertussis has increased in recent years, particularly among adolescents and adults, as a result of waning immunity and increased recognition/reporting of the disease.
- Infected adults and adolescents serve as a reservoir to transmit pertussis to infants and children, who are at greater risk for morbidity and mortality.
- Previously immunized adolescents and adults are more likely to present with a prolonged cough illness than the classic symptoms of inspiratory whooping and posttussive emesis; they often have no specific examination, laboratory, or radiographic evidence that can distinguish pertussis from other respiratory infections.
- Physicians must have a high level of clinical suspicion to avoid missing the diagnosis of pertussis.
- If pertussis is suspected clinically, attempts should be made to confirm diagnosis. The diagnostic method of choice (culture, PCR, or serology) depends largely on time from symptom onset.
- Prompt initiation of treatment with a macrolide antibiotic may decrease the severity and duration of symptoms, and may also reduce rates of transmission. Treatment should be initiated at the same time that diagnostic testing is performed.
- Routine completion of infant and childhood vaccination series is still critical to prevent pertussis; because of waning immunity over time, booster immunizations are now also necessary for adolescents, adults, pregnant women, and health care workers.

REFERENCES

1. Mattoo S, Cherry JD. Molecular pathogenesis, epidemiology, and clinical manifestations of respiratory infections due to *Bordetella pertussis* and other *Bordetella* subspecies. Clin Microbiol Rev 2005;18(2):326–82.
2. Cherry JD. The epidemiology of pertussis and pertussis immunization in the United Kingdom and the United States: a comparative study. Curr Probl Pediatr 1984;14(2):1–78.
3. Centers for Disease Control and Prevention. Pertussis (whooping cough). Pertussis in other countries. Available at: http://www.cdc.gov/pertussis/countries.html. Accessed November 27, 2012.
4. Crowcroft NS, Booy R, Harrison T, et al. Severe and unrecognised: pertussis in UK infants. Arch Dis Child 2003;88:802–6.
5. Centers for Disease Control and Prevention. Pertussis (whooping cough). Outbreaks. Available at: http://www.cdc.gov/pertussis/outbreaks.html. Accessed December 29, 2012.
6. Jenkinson D. Duration of effectiveness of pertussis vaccine: evidence from a 10 year community study. Br Med J (Clin Res Ed) 1988;296(6622):612–4.

7. Zouari A, Smaoui H, Kechrid A. The diagnosis of pertussis: which method to choose? Crit Rev Microbiol 2012;38(2):111–21.

8. Centers for Disease Control and Prevention. Updated recommendations for use of tetanus toxoid, reduced diphtheria toxoid and acellular pertussis (Tdap) vaccine from the Advisory Committee on Immunization Practices, 2010. MMWR Morb Mortal Wkly Rep 2011;60(1):13–5.

9. Finger H, Wirsing von Konig CH. Bordetella. In: Baron S, editor. Medical microbiology. 4th edition. Galveston (TX): University of Texas Medical Branch at Galveston; 1996. Available at: http://www.ncbi.nlm.nih.gov/books/NBK7813/. Accessed on October 15, 2012.

10. Deen JL, Mink CM, Cherry JD, et al. Household contact study of *Bordetella pertussis* infection. Clin Infect Dis 1995;21(5):1211–9.

11. Mertsola J, Ruuskanen OL, Eerola E, et al. Intrafamiliar spread of pertussis. J Pediatr 1983;103:359–63.

12. Wirsing von Konig CH, Postels-Multani S, Bogaerts H, et al. Factors influencing the spread of pertussis in households. Eur J Pediatr 1998;157:391–4.

13. Pittman M. The concept of pertussis as a toxin-mediated disease. Pediatr Infect Dis 1984;3:467–86.

14. Christie CD, Baltimore RS. Pertussis in neonates. Am J Dis Child 1989;143: 1199–202.

15. Tan T, Trindade E, Skowronski D. Epidemiology of pertussis. Pediatr Infect Dis J 2005;24:S10–8.

16. Centers for Disease Control and Prevention. Pertussis–United States, 2001-2003. MMWR Morb Mortal Wkly Rep 2005;54(50):1283–6.

17. Guris D, Strevel PM, Bardenheier B, et al. Changing epidemiology of pertussis in the United States: increasing reported incidence among adolescents and adults, 1990-1996. Clin Infect Dis 1999;28(6):1230–7.

18. Wirsing von Konig CH, Halperin S, Riffelmann M, et al. Pertussis of adults and infants. Lancet Infect Dis 2002;2(12):744–50.

19. Halperin SA, Wang EE, Law B, et al. Epidemiological features of pertussis in hospitalized patients in Canada, 1991-1997: report of the Immunization Monitoring Program–Active (IMPACT). Clin Infect Dis 1999;28:1238–43.

20. Tanaka M, Vitek CR, Pascual FB, et al. Trends in pertussis among infants in the United States, 1980-1999. JAMA 2003;290(22):2268–75.

21. Vitek CR, Pascual FB, Baughman AL, et al. Increase in deaths from pertussis among young infants in the United States in the 1990s. Pediatr Infect Dis J 2003;22(7):628–34.

22. Centers for Disease Control and Prevention. Pertussis outbreak in an Amish community–Kent County, Delaware, September 2004-February 2005. MMWR Morb Mortal Wkly Rep 2006;55:817–21.

23. Craig AS, Wright SW, Edwards KM, et al. Outbreak of pertussis on a college campus. Am J Med 2007;120:364–8.

24. Waters V, Halperin S. Bordetella pertussis. In: Mandell GL, Bennett JE, Dolin R, editors. Mandell, Douglas, and Bennett's: principles and practice of infectious diseases, vol. 2, 7th edition. Philadelphia: Elsevier; 2010. p. 2955–64.

25. Levene I, Wacogne I. Is measurement of the lymphocyte count useful in the investigation of suspected pertussis in infants? Arch Dis Child 2001;96: 1203–5.

26. Pierce C, Klein N, Peters M. Is leukocytosis a predictor of mortality in severe pertussis infection? Intensive Care Med 2000;26:1512–4.

27. Cornia PB, Hersch AL, Lipsky BA, et al. Does this coughing adolescent or adult patient have pertussis? JAMA 2010;304(8):890–6.

28. Strebel P, Nordin J, Edwards K, et al. Population-based incidence of pertussis among adolescents and adults, Minnesota, 1995-1996. J Invest Dermatol 2001; 183:1353–9.

29. Kretsinger K, Broder R, Cortese M, et al. Preventing tetanus, diphtheria, and pertussis among adults: use of tetanus toxoid, reduced diphtheria toxoid and acellular pertussis vaccine. MMWR Morb Mortal Wkly Rep 2006; 55(RR17):1–33.

30. Irwin RS, Madison JM. The diagnosis and treatment of cough. N Engl J Med 2000;343(23):1715–21.

31. World Health Organization–recommended surveillance standard of pertussis. Available at: http://www.who.int/immunization_monitoring/diseases/pertussis_surveillance/en/index.html. Accessed October 10, 2012.

32. Centers for Disease Control and Prevention. Appendix B. CDC and Council of State and Territorial Epidemiologists (CTSE) pertussis case definition. MMWR Morb Mortal Wkly Rep 2006;55(RR17):35. Available at: http://www.cdc.gov/mmwr/preview/mmwrhtml/rr5517a3.htm. Accessed October 31, 2012.

33. Ghanie RM, Karimi A, Sadeghi H, et al. Sensitivity and specificity of the World Health Organization pertussis clinical case definition. Int J Infect Dis 2010;14: e1072–5.

34. Cherry JD, Tan T, Wirsing von Konig CH, et al. Clinical definitions of pertussis: summary of a global pertussis initiative roundtable meeting, February 2011. Clin Infect Dis 2012;54:1756–65.

35. Marcon MJ, Hamoudi AC, Cannon HJ, et al. Comparison of throat and nasopharyngeal swab specimens for culture diagnosis of Bordetella pertussis infection. J Clin Microbiol 1987;25(6):1109–10.

36. Hallander HO, Reizenstein E, Renemar B, et al. Comparison of nasopharyngeal aspirates with swabs for culture of Bordetella pertussis. J Clin Microbiol 1993; 31(1):50–2.

37. Cloud JL, Hymas W, Caroll KC. Impact of nasopharyngeal swab types of detection of Bordetella pertussis by PCR and culture. J Clin Microbiol 2002;40(10): 3838–40.

38. Muller FM, Hoppe JE, Wirsing von Konig CH. Laboratory diagnosis of pertussis: state of the art in 1997. J Clin Microbiol 1997;35(10):2435–43.

39. Young SA, Anderson GL, Mitchell PD. Laboratory observations during an outbreak of pertussis. Clin Microbiol Newsl 1987;9:176–9.

40. Centers for Disease Control and Prevention. Outbreaks of respiratory illness mistakenly attributed to pertussis–New Hampshire, Massachusetts, and Tennessee, 2004-2006. MMWR Morb Mortal Wkly Rep 2007;56(33):837–42.

41. Guiso N, Berbers G, Fry NK, et al. What to do and what not to do in serological diagnosis of pertussis: recommendations from EU reference laboratories. Eur J Clin Microbiol Infect Dis 2011;30:307–12.

42. Tiwari T, Murphy TV, Moran J. Recommended antimicrobial agents for the treatment and post-exposure prophylaxis of pertussis; 2005 CDC Guidelines. MMWR Morb Mortal Wkly Rep 2005;54(RR-14):1–16.

43. Altunaiji S, Kukuruzovic R, Curtis N, et al. Antibiotics for whooping cough (pertussis). Cochrane Database Syst Rev 2007;(3):CD004404.

44. Aoyama T, Sunakawa K, Iwata S, et al. Efficacy of short-term treatment of pertussis with clarithromycin and azithromycin. J Pediatr 1996;129(5):761–4.

45. Langley JM, Halperin SA, Boucher FD, et al. Azithromycin is as effective as and better tolerated than erythromycin for the treatment of pertussis. Pediatrics 2004;114(1):e96–101.

46. Lebel MH, Mehra S. Efficacy and safety of clarithromycin versus erythromycin for the treatment of pertussis: a prospective, randomized, single blind trial. Pediatr Infect Dis 2001;20(12):1149–54.

47. Maheshwai N. Are young infants treated with erythromycin at risk for developing hypertrophic pyloric stenosis? Arch Dis Child 2007;92:271–3.

48. Hoppe JE, Halm U, Hagedorn HJ. Comparison of erythromycin ethylsuccinate and co-trimoxazole for treatment of pertussis. Infection 1989;4:227–31.

49. Bettiol S, Wang K, Thompson MJ, et al. Symptomatic treatment of the cough in whooping cough. Cochrane Database Syst Rev 2012;(5):CD003257.

50. Centers for Disease Control and Prevention. FDA approval of expanded age indication for a tetanus toxoid, reduced diphtheria toxoid and acellular Pertussis Vaccine. MMWR Morb Mortal Wkly Rep 2011;60(37):1279–80.

51. Le T, Cherry JD, Chang SJ, et al. Immune responses and antibody decay after immunization of adolescents and adults with an acellular pertussis vaccine: the APERT study. J Infect Dis 2004;190:535–44.

52. Ward JL, Cherry JD, Chang SJ, et al. Efficacy of an acellular pertussis vaccine among adolescents and adults. N Engl J Med 2005;353(15):1555–63.

53. Centers for Disease Control and Prevention. Use of diphtheria toxoid-tetanus toxoid-acellular pertussis vaccine as a five-dose series: supplemental recommendations of the Advisory Committee on Immunization Practices (ACIP). MMWR Morb Mortal Wkly Rep 2000;49(RR-13):1–8.

54. Mertsola J, Van Der Meeren O, He Q, et al. Decennial administration of a reduced antigen content diphtheria and tetanus toxoids and acellular pertussis vaccine in young adults. Clin Infect Dis 2010;51(6):656–62.

55. Cherry JD. The present and future control of pertussis. Clin Infect Dis 2010; 51(6):663–7.

56. Centers for Disease Control and Prevention. Possible side effects from vaccines. Available at: http://www.cdc.gov/vaccines/vac-gen/side-effects.htm#td. Accessed November 14, 2012.

57. Centers for Disease Control and Prevention. Updated recommendations for use of tetanus toxoid, reduced diphtheria toxoid and acellular pertussis vaccine (Tdap) in pregnant women and persons who have or anticipate having close contact with an infant aged <12 months–Advisory Committee on Immunization Practices (ACIP), 2011. MMWR Morb Mortal Wkly Rep 2011;60(41):1424–6.

58. Committee on Obstetric Practice. Committee Opinion: update on immunization and pregnancy: tetanus, diphtheria, and pertussis vaccination. Obstet Gynecol 2012;119(3):690–1.

59. Gall SA, Myers J, Pichichero M. Maternal immunization with tetanus-diphtheria-pertussis vaccine: effect on maternal and neonatal serum antibody levels. Am J Obstet Gynecol 2011;204(4):334.e1.

60. Shakib JH, Ralson S, Raissy HH, et al. Pertussis antibodies in postpartum women and their newborns. J Perinatol 2010;30:93–7.

61. Calugar A, Ortega-Sánchez IR, Tiwari T, et al. Nosocomial pertussis: costs of an outbreak and benefits of vaccinating health care workers. Clin Infect Dis 2006; 42(7):981–8.

Multidrug-resistant Tuberculosis

John B. Lynch, MD, MPH

KEYWORDS

- Tuberculosis • Drug resistance • Drug-susceptibility testing • HIV/AIDS

KEY POINTS

- Multidrug-resistant tuberculosis (MDR-TB) is replacing drug-susceptible tuberculosis in many areas of the world.
- This development is the result of the mismanagement of drugs with activity against *Mycobacterium tuberculosis* at the individual and programmatic level.
- MDR-TB disproportionately affects poor and marginalized populations, including individuals with human immunodeficiency virus/acquired immunodeficiency syndrome.
- MDR-TB is not usually diagnosed because of availability of testing in the most affected areas.
- Current testing modalities for detection of MDR-TB are insufficient to address the epidemic.
- Treatment of MDR-TB is more toxic and longer than treatment of drug-susceptible tuberculosis and outcomes are worse.
- Although several new drugs have recently become available, these are the first new antituberculosis drugs in decades. New drugs and drug combinations need to be developed.
- Prevention of new infections, both in the community and in the health care setting, is critical to controlling the epidemic.
- The spread of MDR-TB is inevitable unless action on every level is taken.

...results show that the alarming levels of drug-resistant TB recently detected in Minsk are not confined to the capital city but are widespread throughout the country.

—*Alena Skrahina, and colleagues, Bull World Health Organ 2013[1]*

BACKGROUND

The quote from Skrahina and colleagues[1] comes from a recent study that found nearly 1 in 2 patients with tuberculosis (TB) in Belarus in 2009 to 2010 were infected with multidrug-resistant strains.[1] Belarus, as one of the former Soviet states, has among

Disclosures: The author has no funding sources, and no conflicts of interest.
Division of Allergy and Infectious Diseases, Department of Medicine, Harborview Medical Center, University of Washington, 325 9th Avenue, Box 359930, Seattle, WA, USA
E-mail address: jblynch@uw.edu

Med Clin N Am 97 (2013) 553–579
http://dx.doi.org/10.1016/j.mcna.2013.03.012
0025-7125/13/$ – see front matter © 2013 Elsevier Inc. All rights reserved.

the highest levels of multidrug-resistant TB (MDR-TB) in the world, a significant burden to an already challenged public health system. However, Belarus is not alone in facing this widespread problem. At the same time that the global response to TB is having a positive impact, drug-resistant TB is increasing in incidence, threatening to reduce these gains (World Health Organization [WHO] report). With an estimated 2 billion individuals infected with TB in the world and nearly 2 million dying every year, any step backward will have profound effects on those populations disproportionately affected by this pathogen: the poor and marginalized.[2–4]

The development of antibiotic drug resistance is the result of social, political, and clinical decision making since the introduction of the first drug with activity against *Mycobacterium tuberculosis*.[5–8] As with all bacteria, the genetic mechanisms that facilitate drug resistance existed before the advent of chemotherapy, but it has been the application of these lifesaving drugs that has created the current problem.[9–11] This coevolution is, as Dr Joshua Lederberg[12] wrote, between "our wits and their genes," and humanity has not always been using its wits in how antibiotics are used to shape the pathogenic microbiome.

In the last 20 years, many organizations and countries have recognized the ongoing problem of TB, leading to efforts to diagnose, treat, and cure cases, most often with community and countrywide public health–driven programs. However, aside from costs and resource allocation, there are significant barriers at each of these steps to cure, including, but not limited to:

- Identification of affected individuals
- Diagnosis often relies on the century-old technique of stained sputum smears (sensitivity ~60%, specificity ~98%) and mycobacterial culture (the gold standard)
- Treatment requires 4 drugs for at least 2 months and 2 drugs for an additional 4 months, continuously
- Failure to cure can go undetected for months or years

With a disease as widespread as TB disproportionately affecting largely poor populations, programs have focused on efficiently detecting and treating as many people as possible, with the goals of both curing cases and preventing further transmission.[13,14] These efforts are complex, but can be done effectively, even in the poorest populations in the world.[15,16] At the same time, large countrywide programs can have problems with access to medications and equipment and technological expertise in diagnosis, leading to treatment interruptions, continuing cycles of transmission, and failures to cure. On a global level these large-scale programs seem to have turned the tide, with fewer TB cases each year since 2004.[17] Although much work remains to be done, the current approach to drug-sensitive TB is considered to be on the right track and headed for success. The only problem is that the mistakes of the last 20 years have led to a new epidemic of progressively more drug-resistant TB.

HOW DID WE GET HERE? A HISTORICAL PERSPECTIVE

In March of 1882, H.H. Robert Koch presented 2 groundbreaking ideas to the Berlin Physiologic Society. One was the set of postulates that defined an infectious agent and the second was the causal (*die aetiologie*) agent of TB.[18] Although *M tuberculosis* was accepted as the cause of TB as a result, no drug treatment was possible until 1944 when Schatz and Waksman[19] described the effects of streptomycin on the organism in vitro. This discovery was followed by one of the first randomized controlled trials: a study of the effect of streptomycin on humans with pulmonary

TB.[20] It was in this group of trial participants, among the first people with TB ever treated, that resistance to streptomycin was discovered and treatment success was linked to the development of resistance.[5]

Nearly all of the drugs currently considered first or second line and used in combination therapy were discovered in the subsequent 15 years, including p-aminosalicylic acid (1949), isoniazid (1952), pyrazinamide (1954), cycloserine (1955), ethionamide (1956), rifampin (1957), and ethambutol (1962). Recognition of the rapid development of resistance[21,22] led to combination treatment, initially using the newer drugs para-aminosalicylic acid and thiacetazone,[23] and later isoniazid (isonicotinic acid hydrazide).[24] However, resistance to each of these classes of antibiotics was quickly seen, most importantly to isoniazid and rifampin, considered the most potent of the anti-TB drugs.[25] At the same time, many clinicians continued to use isoniazid monotherapy and other drug combinations depending on drug availability, leading to the emergence of drug-resistant TB, just as effective combination therapy was being implemented.[8]

By the 1960s, concern arose on the public health front as reports of drug resistance in various populations were published. A 1961 United States Public Health Service survey of patients with no history of treatment of TB found that 1.6% of cases were resistant to isoniazid and 2.8% were resistant to streptomycin.[26] At the same time, patients presenting at Veteran's Administration hospitals for the first time with TB were found to be infected with drug-resistant isolates (5% resistance to streptomycin, 6% resistance to isoniazid, and 8% resistance to p-aminosalicylic acid).[27] In 1966, Steiner and Cosio[28] reported the recovery of drug-resistant TB from gastric lavage samples from children who had never been treated, indicating transmission of already-resistant strains. This same group later found that 15.2% of infected children followed at Kings County Medical Center in New York City had isoniazid resistance, 9.2% had streptomycin resistance, and 3.4% had resistance to p-aminosalicylic acid.[29,30] A harbinger of things to come, a 1961 study of patients in New York City who had previously been treated for TB found that 38.9% were infected with TB resistant to all 3 major drugs tested.[31]

Although not as many data from outside the United States for this time period is accessible, a 1975 survey of TB drug susceptibility was performed in Canada and compared with one from 1963 to 1964. During that 10-year period, primary drug resistance increased from 4.9% to 6.3%. That report attributed much of the increase to immigrants arriving with already-resistant infections, implying that drug resistance was already a significant problem in countries of origin for these individuals.[32] Asian-born immigrants to Melbourne, Australia, also disproportionately had higher rates of isoniazid-resistant TB compared with nonimmigrants.[33] In Poland, approximately 5.3% of patients were resistant to 1 or 2 drugs (isoniazid, streptomycin, ethambutol, rifampicin).[34] Conflicting data were reported in Japan,[35] but in Hong Kong 20% of previously untreated patients had resistance to at least 1 drug.[36] A Medical Research Council report found a similar level of resistance in East Africa during the same time period.[37]

Even with drug-resistant TB being widespread, the US Federal Government ended the practice of providing public health funds specifically for TB treatment in 1972.[8] With decreased attention to funding research and attention directed away from infectious diseases, the drug supply also shut down, leading to 40 years without a new drug approved for the treatment of TB. In 1985, Iseman[7] wrote about his concern for the development of drug-resistant TB on an epidemic scale as a result of ineffective TB control programs, which he called "tailoring a time bomb." In the 1980s, as the incidence of TB started to increase relative to decreasing public health efforts, limited access to care, poverty, and the increasing human immunodeficiency virus (HIV)/acquired immunodeficiency syndrome (AIDS) epidemic.[38–41] Although outbreaks of drug-resistant TB had been reported in the United States, it was not until multiple outbreaks of TB and MDR-TB were reported in the early 1990s[42,43] that the attention of policy makers was captured.[44] In 1993, the US Centers for Disease Control and Prevention (CDC) and the New York City Department of Health reported an increase in MDR-TB from 3% to 9% compared with the prior decade.[42]

The CDC expanded TB surveillance to include drug-susceptibility results in 1993. Although total MDR-TB cases peaked in the United States in 1993 with 407 (2.5%) of all cases of TB compared with 120 (1%) in 1998, cases of primary infection slowly increased over the next 2 decades.[45] Most patients diagnosed with MDR-TB and extremely-drug-resistant TB (XDR-TB) have been exposed to first-line and second-line drugs for treatment.[46] Other patient characteristics that predict MDR-TB include being in a hospital, cavitary lung disease, unemployment, history of imprisonment, alcohol abuse, and tobacco use.[46] However, these factors do not explain the larger problem and origin of the epidemic.

Although the United States was able to respond, the associated costs were large, estimated to have been about $1 billion. In low-income and middle-income countries with fewer resources in the 1970s and 1980s, the focus was on primary care, to the exclusion of diseases like TB requiring lengthy treatment courses. This de-emphasis was apparent at places like the WHO, which, by the end of the 1980s, had only 2 individuals in the TB program.[8]

This approach was reversed in the early 1990s concurrent with the outbreaks in the United States and Europe, often associated with HIV infection, and globally.[47–49] In response, TB was declared a global health emergency in 1993 by the WHO.[50] The response was the introduction of a new program, Directly Observed Therapy-Short Course (DOTS) for the treatment of TB in 1994, focused on identification of cases by sputum smear microscopy, an insensitive test for pulmonary TB, and completion of standard 4-drug therapy in the absence of drug-susceptibility testing. This response was successful and led to a turn in the tide of global TB over the ensuing decade.[51] As the higher-income countries realized that additional funding was necessary to meet the goals of the global TB program, the Global Fund was established in 2002, soon after the first Global Plan to Stop TB 2001 to 2005 was released by the WHO and the Stop TB Partnership, all focused on keeping the momentum going. Aside from MDR-TB, the global response to TB was headed in the right direction (**Box 1**).

CURRENT EPIDEMIOLOGY

The most recent estimates of TB report nearly 9 million new cases per year and 1.4 million deaths per year).[17] Twenty-two low-income and middle-income countries account for more than 80% of all cases globally. The number of TB deaths and cases decreased at a rate of 2.2% between 2010 and 2011. Since 1990, mortality caused by TB has decreased by 41% and is approaching the Millennium Development Goal of a

---

Box 1
Definitions

MDR-TB = drug resistance to at least rifampin and isoniazid

XDR-TB = MDR-TB plus resistance to the injectables (kanamycin, capreomycin, amikacin) and fluoroquinolones (gatifloxacin, levofloxacin, oflaxacin, moxifloxacin).

50% reduction by 2015 (except in Africa and Europe). Since 1995, 51 million individuals with TB have been cured and 20 million lives saved in the last 15 years as a result of the standardized approach to TB. The HIV pandemic continues to have an impact on TB cases and deaths, with coinfection in 13% of cases but in nearly one-third of deaths. HIV plays a larger role in some areas, such as Africa, where 80% of coinfected individuals live. As a result, TB continues to be the most common cause of death in people with HIV infection in sub-Saharan Africa.[52]

In settings in which there are barriers to detection, including costs associated with diagnosis and treatment, and under-resourced health systems, distance, conflict and violence, social stigma, or lack of resources, obtaining a reliable incidence rate is difficult.[53–55] In some instances, cases may be based only on clinical diagnoses, leading to potential overestimation, or at least estimates of disease prevalence that are difficult to replicate. Beyond the diagnosis of TB, testing of drug resistance traditionally requires culturing of the organism in the presence of the drug. This technique has been replaced for some drugs in some areas with molecular testing, but these techniques are not yet widespread, nor do they address testing all first-line and second-line drugs. With the introduction of rapid molecular diagnostics, there may be the ability to both diagnose TB and detect resistance within the space of hours.

As a result, it is unclear how large the MDR-TB problem is given the challenges inherent in the systems of detection and diagnosis and the barriers to identifying drug resistance in the individual cases. According to the 2012 WHO report, 74 countries with at least 2 years of data could not report whether MDR-TB rates were changing. Several countries with likely high burdens have no data or no data in the last 10 years (2011 most recent reviewed). The best estimate is that less than 3% of patients diagnosed with TB have had drug-susceptibility testing.

When evaluating the prevalence and incidence of MDR-TB and XDR-TB in populations, definitions are commonly presented as total population, MDR-TB in new cases of TB (never or <1 month of treatment), MDR-TB in previously treated cases (or >1 month of treatment), and XDR-TB as a proportion of all MDR-TB cases. These data are often stratified by HIV infection given the importance of coinfection. The WHO, representing 182 member states, 204 countries and territories, and 99% of the global disease burden, provides reports on TB rates, including MDR-TB and XDR-TB cases. Countries with more robust surveillance and research programs provide firmer estimates of disease prevalence and incidence. This consideration is important when reviewing available data; as of 2010, 58 countries had at least 1 case of XDR-TB, but this reporting cannot assume that each of those 58 reporting systems have the same capabilities for case detection.[56]

Given the limitations discussed earlier, there are an estimated 500,000 incident cases of MDR-TB and 50,000 incident cases of XDR-TB per year, cumulatively accounting for 3.6% of all TB cases.[17] Of the MDR-TB cases, 300,000 are new cases (primary drug resistance) and 200,000 are previously treated (acquired drug resistance). The 10 countries with the largest populations of MDR-TB included the former Soviet republics, India, China, South Africa, and Bangladesh. China and India accounted for approximately 50% of all MDR cases. In the former Soviet states in Eastern Europe, the rates of XDR-TB among MDR-TB cases ranged from 6.6% to 23.7%.[46] The prevalence of MDR-TB does not seem to be limited to cities where treatment programs are often concentrated. Following a report measuring the prevalence of MDR-TB in Minsk, Belarus, a countrywide survey found a similar level of drug resistance in nonurban areas of the country.[1,57] The prevalence of MDR-TB was highest among previously treated cases (76.5%), but more than one-third of new cases also had MDR-TB (35.3%) compared with a prevalence of 47.8% in Minsk.

Surveys of MDR-TB in China report that 34.2% of all TB cases had some drug resistance (not meeting the definition of MDR-TB), 5.7% to 8.32% had MDR-TB, and 0.5% to 0.68% had XDR-TB.[58,59] Among previously treated TB cases, 25.6% were MDR-TB and 2.1% were XDR-TB.[58] Another study limited to hospitalized patients found MDR-TB in 20.2% and XDR-TB in 1.4%. Many of these patients had experienced years of infection (52.6% had ≥4 years of infection).[60] In contacts of patients with MDR-TB or XDR-TB in Peru, 242 of 4503 contacts developed active TB. XDR-TB contacts TB 2X MDR. Of 142 individuals with tested isolates, 129 had MDR-TB.[61]

As with any transmissible disease, MDR-TB does not respect borders or income. High-income countries also have cases of MDR-TB and XDR-TB.[62] Most of these occur in individuals emigrating from TB-endemic countries and so resistance patterns reflect the patterns seen in the country of origin.

DIAGNOSIS OF MDR-TB

Patients with pulmonary MDR-TB present with the same symptoms and signs as other patients with TB. Classic symptoms of infection include fever, prolonged cough (>2–3 weeks), unexplained weight loss (typically >10% of body weight), night sweats, loss of appetite, and fatigue, but can also be minimal to absent.[63,64] Patients with more advanced pulmonary disease may have hemoptysis and chest pain. Extrapulmonary TB can occur at any site, and symptoms and signs depend on where the infection occurs (tender lymphadenopathy with lymphadenitis, change in mental status with TB meningitis, abdominal pain and distention with peritoneal TB, and so forth). Although patients with HIV may present with more advanced disease when infected with MDR-TB, there are no clinical clues that increase or decrease the suspicion for MDR-TB.

All of the barriers associated with initial testing for drug-sensitive TB also apply for MDR-TB. Sputum smears, long advocated as the diagnostic test of choice, miss between 50% and 70% of active pulmonary infection. In addition, standard sputum smears may be negative more often in patients with HIV infection compared with smears from patients without HIV.[65] Because this is the test most commonly available in high-burden settings, many cases of pulmonary TB go undiagnosed.[66] More importantly, neither sputum microscopy nor isolation of M tuberculosis in culture detects drug resistance.

Although WHO guidelines recommend rapid drug-sensitivity testing (DST) for isoniazid and rifampin within 2 days, it is estimated that only 1 in 20 people with MDR-TB are diagnosed using currently available tools and systems.[67] In low-income and middle-income countries (LMIC), where the burden of MDR-TB is the highest, definitive diagnosis relies on sputum culture and DST using the indirect 1% proportion method[68,69] on solid media. Although long considered the standard for testing of drug resistance, this method takes 3 to 6 weeks and there are some data that indicate that MDR-TB clinical isolates grow poorly on solid media,[70] which may inhibit the ability to complete the assay. Time in culture can be decreased to 10 to 14 days using liquid medium, if available.[71] Regardless of the medium, these tests require technological skills and laboratory facilities that are not available evenly around the world. Even in the ideal situation, diagnosis can take 8 to 16 weeks (or longer) from the time the sputum is obtained until the drug sensitivities are reported. As a result, patients may be started on standard 4-drug therapy (isoniazid, rifampin, pyrazinamide, and ethambutol) for presumptive infection only to learn later that 1 or more of these drugs are not effective. Of equal concern is the potential of this approach to generate more drug-resistant TB that can then be transmitted.

Drug resistance can considered as acquired and primary resistance. Acquired resistance occurs when drug resistance develops on therapy, typically when a person is treated with too few active drugs, allowing the mycobacteria to mutate. Compared with acquired resistance, primary resistance occurs when a person is infected with an already drug-resistant strain. Unlike many other bacteria with quiescent drug-resistance genes, *M tuberculosis* develops resistance by spontaneous mutations. The rate of resistance mutations to many of the drugs used against TB has been measured and is predictable.[72] In a manner analogous to infection with HIV, a person infected with *M tuberculosis* develops drug-resistant strains in the absence of drug pressure.[73,74] However, these drug-resistant strains only become clinically meaningful with the application of anti-TB drugs. Although initial studies seemed to find a fitness cost to drug resistance for *M tuberculosis*, most recent studies are not supportive.[75,76] Acquisition of drug-resistance mechanisms does not seem to affect virulence or transmission, although there may be exceptions.[77,78]

Tests for drug susceptibility can be broadly separated into 2 categories: phenotypic/culture-based assays and genotypic/molecular assays. Within each category are several assays that address barriers to more rapid detection of drug resistance and have the potential for use in LMIC.

Phenotypic/Culture-based Diagnostic Tests of Drug Susceptibility

Phenotypic assays using inexpensive, culture-based, noncommercial assays have long been the method of choice for detecting drug resistance. Although the major issue has been availability of resources, when the assays are available and performed correctly, the time to results is many weeks to months. As a result, new methods to simplify and speed up culture-based methods have been developed, including the nitrate reductase assay (NRA),[79] microscopic-observation drug susceptibility (MODS)[80] using liquid media, and thin-layer agar (TLA) assays.[81] NRA detects reduction of nitrate to nitrite by the bacteria using a colorimetric assay. MODS and TLA are both culture based, allow the direct inoculation of the medium with patient specimens, and rely on microscopic evaluation for bacterial growth. As with conventional DST, growth in the presence of drugs at a standard concentration indicates resistance. In a meta-analysis, Minion and colleagues[81] found MODS to be accurate for rifampicin resistance, slightly less accurate for isoniazid, and to have low sensitivity for ethambutol and streptomycin. In the few studies available, TLA was 100% concordant with standard DST and had a rapid turnaround time. Compared side by side with MODS using reference strains, NRA was slightly more sensitive for the detection of isoniazid, rifampin, streptomycin, and ethambutol.[82] Time to availability of results for MODS and NRA ranged from 5 to 18 days (in addition to culture), with slightly longer times in the MODS arm, in part because of contamination of specimens, a known concern for directly inoculated specimens.[81] All three methods offer drug-susceptibility results faster than conventional proportion DST and do not require expensive proprietary equipment, although training and certain equipment is needed (such as an inverted microscope).

There are also several commercial assays for the detection of TB and drug-resistance testing, including epsilometer tests (E-tests), the BACTEC460 radiometric system (Becton Dickinson Diagnostic Instruments, Sparks, MD), and Mycobacteria Growth Indicator Tube (MGIT) 960 (Becton Dickinson Diagnostic Instruments, Sparks, MD), a fluorometric assay (Lemus 2004). Both the BACTEC460 and MGIT960 systems automatically compare growth in liquid media with drugs with a control tube without drugs. These assays are quick (<14 days) but are expensive and are concentrated in high-income counties. In a review of testing using automated methods in laboratories in the United States, agreement between laboratories using the same methods varied between 82.6% (MGIT) and 93% (BACTEC460). Compared with standard DST, the BACTEC system provided data on pyrazinamide (not available on conventional DST), similar sensitivity for isoniazid and rifampin, and was significantly better for the detection of ethambutol.[83] The MGIT system was less sensitive for the detection of resistance to rifampin and ethambutol compared with either conventional DST or BACTEC460 results, but was also able to provide results on pyrazinamide resistance. Turnaround time for both the BACTEC460 ands MGIT systems is on average 7 to 8 days.[84] In a rollout of the MGIT960 system in the Korean Institute for Tuberculosis, total time for mycobacterial culture and DST using the MGIT 960 system was 27 days compared with 70 days for culture and DST on solid medium.[85] Given the burden of MDR-TB in LMIC, there is an urgent need for rapid DST in settings that are not able to afford these commercial systems.

Genotypic/Molecular Tests

Genotypic testing relies on the detection of specific gene sequences associated with *M tuberculosis* for the diagnosis and the detection of genetic sequences associated with specific drug resistance.[86] Although there are several technologies available, ranging from locally derived polymerase chain reaction (PCR) assays to complex 1-step commercial assays, the key benefit is the rapid turnaround time (2–48 hours) to diagnosis and detection of drug resistance. The 2 main classes are line probe assays (LPAs) and nucleic acid amplification tests.

LPA

In 2008, the WHO approved the use of the LPA for rapid diagnosis of MDR-TB on direct smear-positive clinical or cultured specimens. The GenoType MTBDR*plus* (Hain Lifescience), a commercial LPA, uses multiplex PCR to amplify pathogen DNA followed by reverse hybridization to identify *M tuberculosis* and isoniazid and rifampin resistance (mutations in *rpoB*, *katG*, and *inhA*). Turnaround time is approximately 5 hours from start to finish. A 2008 review found the MTBDR*plus* assay to be both sensitive and specific (≥97% and ≥99% for rifampin and ≥90% and ≥99% for isoniazid using either cultured isolates or smear-positive sputum). Concordance with standard DST was 99%.[87] The GenoType MTBDR*plus* assay was also compared with conventional DST in a cohort of 604 patients with TB in Stockholm, Sweden, using samples prepared using standard PCR extraction techniques.[88] Compared with DST, this test was 95.2% sensitive and 100% specific for the detection of MDR-TB, similar to prior findings.[89,90] More promising was the decrease in turnaround time, from 21 days with conventional DST to 7 days with the MTBDR*plus* assay for smear-negative cases in culture. Consistent with prior studies, the cases of drug resistance missed were primarily isoniazid resistance that mapped to mutations less commonly seen and are not detected by this assay.

Performing an LPA requires extraction of DNA in an appropriate laboratory followed by PCR and hybridization in a setting that minimizes contamination. Training of technologists to perform successful assays can take as few as 4 days, although one study found invalid results likely caused by operator error and recommended slightly longer periods of supervision.[91] The same group recommended 3 separate rooms to minimize contamination risk as well as access to molecular-grade water. In a comparison of genotypic tests, the MTBDR*plus* assay was 58% sensitive for the detection of disease in smear-negative cases. This finding is important given the greater proportion of smear-negative cases and ongoing risk of transmission, particularly in high HIV prevalence areas.[92] Following implementation of the MTBDR*plus* in 25 public health clinics in South Africa, the number of cases diagnosed with MDR-TB increased dramatically, particularly new cases.[93] Culture conversion at 8 months was also significantly improved in patients with MDR-TB. As with all new technologies, innovative approaches to financing such as that developed by Foundation for Innovative Diagnostics (www.finddiagnostics.org) and others, will likely need to be continued.

Automatic nucleic acid amplification
Nucleic acid amplification assays are also available in standardized commercial products. The best studied is the GeneXpert MTB/RIF assay, a self-contained, cartridge-based technological platform integrating sputum processing, DNA extraction, and amplification that detects the presence of TB and resistance to rifampin based on mutations in the *rpoB* gene. Testing takes less than 2 hours, high-level biosafety facilities are not needed, the risk of cross-contamination is minimal and training to perform the assay takes only 1 to 2 days. In a study conducted from July 2008 to March 2009 on 1462 symptomatic patients in 5 trial sites (Lima, Peru; Baku, Azerbaijan; Cape Town and Durban, South Africa; and Mumbai, India).[94] Of these cases, 720 (41.6%) were suspected to have MDR-TB. Technologists without previous molecular assay experience underwent 2 to 3 days of training. Three sputum samples from each patient were obtained, 2 of which underwent standard preparation with Ziehl-Neelson staining, cultivation on solid and liquid media, and the MTB/RIF test. The third specimen underwent staining and direct microscopy and the MTB/RIF test without standard decontamination (NALC-NaOH [N-acetyl-L-cysteine-sodium hydroxide]). Positive cultures were confirmed by antigen detection and indirect drug-susceptibility testing on Lowenstein-Jensen medium or MGIT. Sites also performed other tests (LPA) depending on local protocols and availability. The MTB/RIF test was 97.6% sensitive for culture-positive patients, 99.8% for smear-positive and culture-positive cases, and 90.2% for smear-negative and culture-positive cases (when multiple samples were evaluated). Sensitivity was slightly lower in HIV-positive patients (93.9%). Specificity was 99.2% for a single test and slightly lower for more than 1 sample. The sensitivity of detection of rifampin resistance was 97.6% and the specificity was 98.1% compared with phenotypic drug-susceptibility testing. Among the 15 patients with discrepant results (resistance by the MTB/RIF test, sensitive by phenotypic testing), resistance was detected by sequencing in 9 cases, increasing the susceptibility to 99.1% and 100% specificity. Among 115 cases with culture-negative TB with suspected MDR-TB, on treatment the TB-RIF test detected 52 positive cases and 8 with rifampin resistance (newly detected). Using a more frontline approach, another group used the TB-RIF assay in a high-MDR, high-prevalence setting using single spot sputum samples in South Africa and reported a sensitivity of 95% and specificity 94% for smear-positive cases and 50% in smear-negative cases, leading to earlier diagnosis and potentially reduced transmission of drug-sensitive and drug-resistant TB.[95]

Detection of resistance to other first-line drugs is not as straightforward. Testing conditions for the detection of resistance to pyrazinamide, a critical drug for shortening the course of therapy and active against nonreplicating MTB, is challenging because the activity of the drug depends on an acidic pH that inhibits the growth of MTB. Pyrazinamide susceptibility testing is lacking in many areas because there are no reliable, accessible testing methods available and no external quality assurance, unlike for other first-line drugs.[96] The BACTEC460 and MGIT960 are currently the only WHO-approved methods for detection of resistance, although there are also genotypic and colorimetric tests available.[97] Detection of *pncA* gene mutations associated with resistance has been shown to be 93% specificity and 87% sensitive, but is not currently part of automated testing.[98]

Detection of Resistance to Second-line Drugs (Diagnosing XDR-TB)

Resistance to second-line drugs, including the injectables (amikacin, kanamycin, capreomycin) and the fluoroquinolones, is a significant challenge for most areas with the highest burdens of MDR-TB and XDR-TB. A second-generation LPA, the genotype MTBDRsl, detects fluoroquinolone resistance (based on mutations in QRDR in the gyrase A region), resistance to the injectable drugs (based on mutations in the rrs gene), and ethambutol resistance (based on mutations in the emb gene). This kit was compared with standard DST using the MGIT960 method using smear-positive specimens with varying bacillary burdens.[99] Like the MRTBDRplus assay, the MTBDRsl assay required DNA extraction followed by PCR and reverse hybridization and a test strip provides a visual indicator of both wild-type and drug-resistance mutations. This genotypic test was 91% sensitive and 98.4% specific for fluoroquinolone resistance (positive predictive value [PPV] 99%, negative predictive value [NPV] 88%), 100% concordant for the injectables, and 56.2% sensitive and 81% specific for ethambutol (PPV 88.1%, NPV 43.2%). The low sensitivity of the test to detect ethambutol resistance is similar to that found in other studies using this assay.[100–103] Twenty out of 21 (95.2%) XDR-TB cases were detected. In another, larger study in 4 countries, the line probe diagnostic assay was useful in screening resistance to individual second-line drugs.[104]

Implementation of standardized, inexpensive testing close to the patient is sorely needed in affected areas. Given the difficulty associated with performing DST on patients with TB and the WHO goal of performing DST on more patients, new tools are needed. Large-scale implementation and cost-effectiveness studies are underway to best deploy DST methods and technologies. Given what has already been experienced with resurgent TB in the 1980s and 1990s, the costs associated with not addressing drug-resistance testing have the potential to be enormous.

TREATMENT

Treatment of MDR-TB requires more complex therapy compared with standard TB therapy using 4 drugs, with longer time to culture conversion, lower overall cure rates, more adverse drug reactions, and more deaths.[105–108] The second-line drugs needed to treat MDR-TB are more expensive, toxic (common side effects include ototoxicity, neuropathy, renal injury, and psychiatric side effects), and the treatment course is longer (typically 24 months).[109] Given these additional burdens in highly affected settings, the strain on health systems is significant.[93,110–114] The prevalence of MDR-TB is linked to the improper use of standard drugs for the treatment of TB and lower quality TB control programs. These geographic areas are the same places that most need to address MDR-TB. However, as has been proved multiple times in the last 20 years, complexity should not deter action. In the case of TB, this was most famously shown by the nongovernmental organization Partners in Health in the late 1990s, when they moved ahead with a program to treat patients with MDR-TB in the slums in Lima, Peru[115] that was effective.

Health care providers have few resources for definitive guidance for the treatment of MDR-TB. As part of the Integrated Management of Adolescent and Adult Illness project, WHO and Partners in Health published a field guide for treatment in low-resource settings built on directly observed therapy (DOT) standards.[116] In this guideline, treatment is the last of the 5 As: assess, advise, agree, assist, and arrange for treatment. It is only with the patient's education, understanding, cooperation, and support of the community that treatment can optimally be started. The history of prior anti-TB therapy is critical because the use of any drug for more than 1 month is associated with drug resistance.[117] Before starting antimicrobials, basic laboratory tests should be checked to establish baselines, including aspartate aminotransferase, alanine aminotransferase (ALT), total bilirubin, serum creatinine, potassium, thyroid-stimulating hormone level, and a pregnancy test. Once treatment is started, smear-positive patients should have repeat smears every month and all patients should have TB culture repeated every 3 months with DST every 6 months. Monitoring of smear-negative patients is indicated as well because up to 18% of previously negative smears convert to positive status during treatment.[118]

Treatment of MDR-TB can be given as standardized or individualized regimens, the former when no DST data are available and the latter based on DST results. As per WHO recommendations, patients who are not cured by combination first-line treatment receive the same four drugs plus streptomycin. For patients with undiagnosed MDR-TB, this approach is not as effective.[119] In patients at risk for drug-resistant infection, treatment can be initiated before DST results are known using a standardized regimen that includes 4 second-line drugs likely to be effective plus pyrazinamide.[109] A typical empiric regimen would include pyrazinamide, kanamycin, levofloxacin, ethionamide, cycloserine (or p-amino salicylic acid), and pyridoxine. All drugs are continued for 6 to 8 months, depending on when sputum cultures are negative on more than 1 sample, and clinical improvement. Following culture conversion, the injectable can be stopped and the patient continues on oral medications for 12 to 18 months. More generally, the regimen should incorporate any first-line drugs that are available, a later generation quinolone (levofloxacin or moxifloxacin), and 1 injectable (capreomycin, kanamycin, or amikacin). Adding additional drugs is not recommended unless clinical improvement does not occur and the effectiveness of the drugs being used is not known. If DST results find additional susceptibilities or no drug resistance, patients can be transitioned to standard 4-drug therapy. In the setting of known DST results or transmission from another person with MDR-TB and known DST results, treatment can be initiated based on those results.

Patients on treatment should know the symptoms to look for and which to report immediately. Nausea, vomiting, diarrhea, and neuropathylike sensations are usually not urgent and can be addressed as needed. Patients with more concerning symptoms, such as jaundice, rash, dyspnea, or hallucinations, need to be evaluated urgently. Ethionamide and PAS (para-aminosalicylic acid) are commonly associated with nausea and vomiting, the former more acutely and the latter later. PAS is also associated with diarrhea. Cycloserine can have psychiatric side effects including depression, anxiety, and psychosis.

These recommendations are based on low-quality evidence and few studies are available to help guide therapy for MDR-TB. Three reviews of treatment of MDR-TB are available at the time of this writing, but only observational data are included because no randomized trials have been published.[106,120] A fourth review[121] used the same collection of studies to conduct an individual patient data meta-analysis instead of pooled data. Patients with XDR-TB were excluded from analysis. Using a variety of treatment approaches, the success rate for treatment was approximately 75%, but there was wide variance. In their analysis, older age, HIV infection, extensive disease, and prior therapy were associated with death. The use of 4 active drugs was also associated with successful treatment and the addition of more drugs did not improve outcomes. This latter finding was also seen in a retrospective study of hospitalized patients in China.[60] Treatment completion/cure has been higher in some settings with more resources, such as Canada (71% vs the global average of 60%). A Canadian study also found a higher than expected rate (10.3%) of fluoroquinolone resistance and unpredictable variation of resistance to other drugs, including pyrazinamide (43.4%) and ethionamide (38.6%), all parts of the recommended treatment regimen for MDR-TB.[62] A retrospective cohort study of patients with MDR-TB in Bangladesh found a successful outcome in 87.9% of patients treated with a gatifloxacin and clofazimine–based regimen for only 9 months.[122] There are potentially effective anti-TB drug combinations that are yet to be discovered.

Treatment of drug-resistant TB is more costly than treating drug-sensitive TB. In South Africa, the per-patient cost of treatment of XDR-TB was $26,392; for MDR-TB, $6772; and for drug-sensitive TB, $257.[123] MDR-TB treatment was one-third of the national TB budget even though ~2% of cases were MDR-TB. In the same country, a study of hospitalized patients with MDR-TB found a mean hospital length of stay of 105 days and an average cost per patient of $17,164. Eighty-six percent of these patients had a conversion of cultures to no growth and were discharged to home.[124] Considering the larger context, analyses using models of MDR-TB treatment in Peru found that treatment with second-line drugs was cost-effective.[125,126]

In Botswana, treatment of HIV-infected patients with individualized MDR-TB and HIV therapy seems to have similar outcomes compared with non–HIV-infected patients being treated for MDR-TB.[127] MDR-TB treatment in this same population in the absence of antiretroviral therapy is associated with worse outcomes compared with non–HIV-infected populations.[128–130] The high early mortality seen in this cohort argues strongly for early initiation of second-line TB drugs in patients with MDR-TB.[131–133] One common theme in prior studies of HIV-positive patients with MDR-TB is the rapidity of death in the absence of effective treatment. Several studies in the 1980s and 1990s of MDR-TB in HIV-coinfected patients from Europe and the United States reported mortalities exceeding 70%, often within 4 to 8 weeks of diagnosis, and before laboratory confirmation of MDR-TB. In a 2006 report from the KwaZulu-Natal province of South Africa, 52 of 53 (98%) patients with XDR-TB died a median of 16 days from the time of diagnosis.[134] It is critical that patients with HIV and MDR-TB start treatment of both diseases as soon as is safe (**Box 2**).[135]

New Drugs for MDR-TB

Linezolid, a member of the recently introduced class of oxazolidinone antibiotics, has been shown to have bacteriostatic activity against MTB in vitro.[136] Although results in the murine model were not promising,[137] a series of studies indicated some activity in humans infected with TB.[138–140] In 2012, Lee and colleagues[141] published the results of a randomized study of HIV-negative patients in South Korea with sputum culture–positive XDR-TB (including patients with genotypic/phenotypic resistance and treatment nonresponders with drug susceptibility). Linezolid was added to failing regimens at 600 mg orally per day (standard bacterial dosing is 600 mg by mouth twice daily), added immediately or following a 2-month delay. Patients continued on linezolid until sputum culture conversion for 2 weeks or they completed 4 months of linezolid treatment. A total of 41 patients underwent randomization (50% to immediate start and 50% to delayed start). At the end of the study, 34 of 38 patients had culture conversion on solid media by 6 months. At the time of publication, 13 patients had completed treatment and 3 had no relapses at the 12-month follow-up. Testing of the 4 patients who did not respond to treatment found a 3-fold increase in the minimum inhibitory concentration to linezolid. Perhaps unsurprisingly for clinicians who have some experience with linezolid, 87% of patients experienced an adverse event, although only 3 patients had to discontinue the drug as a result. Drug resistance to linezolid was seen in 11% of patients who received the drug for 6 months or more.[141]

A second drug, delamanid, a member of the nitro-dihydro-imidazooxazole class of drugs, also shows promise for the treatment of drug-resistant TB. Early studies found

Box 2 Anti-TB drugs	
First-line drugs	
Rifampicins	
Isoniazid	
Ethambutol	
Pyrazinamide	
Streptomycin	
Second-line drugs	
Injectables (kanamycin, amikacin, capreomycin)	
Fluoroquinolones	
p-Aminosalicylic acid	
Cycloserine	
Ethionamide	
Group 5 drugs	
Clofazimine	
Macrolides	
Linezolid	
Thiacetazone	
Amoxicillin/clavulanate	
Clarithromycin	

a decrease in sputum bacterial burden, which led to a randomized clinical trial of the drug in adults with pulmonary MDR-TB in the Philippines, Peru, Latvia, Estonia, China, Japan, Korea, Egypt, and the United States.[142] Patients with HIV infection and a CD4 count greater than 349 were included. Delamanid was added to the optimized background regimen for 8 weeks and patients were monitored for sputum culture conversion. At the end of the study period, sputum culture conversion in the delamanid group was 45.4% and 29.6% in the placebo group, a 53% increase (95% confidence interval, 11–112). Culture conversion at 2 months, a known surrogate associated with treatment success,[143,144] was also statistically greater in the treatment arm. This time point is associated with improved long-term outcomes, providing additional support for the effect of the drug.[118,143,144] Reported toxicity included more QT-prolongation but no clinical events in the treatment group.

Early in 2013, the US Food and Drug Administration approved bedaquiline (previously known as TMC027/R207910) for the treatment of drug-resistant TB, the first drug to be approved for TB since 1971. This drug belongs to the diarylquinoline class of drugs and inhibits the mycobacterial ATP synthase. A randomized study of the drug was conducted in South Africa among hospitalized adult patients with MDR-TB. Patients with XDR-TB were excluded, as were patients with HIV with CD4+ counts of fewer than 300 cells per microliter or who were on antiretrovirals.[145] Bedaquiline was added to a standard background regimen, initially at a higher daily dose that was then decreased to a thrice-weekly lower dose for a total of 8 weeks. Nausea was significantly more common in the treatment group (26% vs 4%, $P = .04$). Culture conversion in a liquid culture system was greater in the treatment group (10 of 21 patients, 48%) compared with the placebo group (2%).

In an effort to develop new first-line regimens that could be effective against MDR-TB, the Global Alliance for TB Drug Development (TB Alliance) performed a randomized trial in South Africa of various combinations of drug therapy: bedaquiline alone, bedaquiline plus PA-824 (a novel nitroimidazo-oxazine, the same class that includes delamanid), bedaquiline plus pyrazinamide, PA-824 plus pyrazinamide, and PA-824 plus moxifloxacin plus pyrazinamide. The end point was early bactericidal activity at day 14 and all patients had drug-sensitive TB and were treatment-naive. The 3-drug combination of PA-824/pyrazinamide/moxifloxacin was comparable with standard 4-drug therapy based on early bactericidal activity. Although promising, whether this combination of drugs is effective for long-term treatment and cure of MDR-TB depends on future studies.[146]

For the first time in decades, there is a great deal of activity in the development of new drugs and the application of existing antimicrobials for the treatment of TB. The reasons for this development are beyond the scope of this article, but it seems that public-private partnerships like the TB Alliance (www.tballiance.org) have been instrumental in moving candidate drugs forward in studies.

Surgery for MDR-TB

Although surgery was once commonly used for the treatment of TB, the advent of effective drug treatment virtually eliminated the need for such drastic interventions. At present, surgery for TB occurs in an estimated 5% of cases.[121] Most commonly, surgical intervention is for the treatment of complications of disease, such as pneumothorax, empyema, fistula, and massive hemoptysis. In the setting of MDR-TB, surgery may play a larger role in decreasing the bacillary burden, removing tissue that has poor drug penetration, treating complications, and possibly shortening the course of treatment. Pulmonary cavities caused by TB have been shown to have between 10^7 to 10^9 organisms, making direct removal of affected tissue a potentially effective option. Which patients should go on to surgery remains unclear and is usually determined by local practice and expertise. Criteria for surgery published in 1990 by Iseman and colleagues[147] listed 3 indications for surgery in the setting of MDR-TB infection: (1) drug resistance is extensive and there is a high failure of treatment failure with medications alone; (2) disease is localized, allowing resection and sufficient lung function subsequently; and (3) effective drug therapy is available to treat residual disease. With careful selection of patients, modern techniques, and continued effective drug therapy, postoperative mortality has decreased to <3%.[147,148]

In a series of 45 patients with MDT-TB undergoing treatment in Romania, most were men (72%) and tobacco users (70%), the mean time of chemotherapy for TB was 4 months, and all were sputum smear positive at the time of surgery.[149] Procedures included lobectomy in 30 patients, segmentectomy in 4 patients, and cavernoplasty (speleoplasty) in 11 patients. By 1 month after surgery, 83% were sputum smear negative. In an earlier study from Seoul of 27 surgical patients with MDR-TB, cavitary lesions were seen in 92.6% of patients and more than half (59.3%) of patients underwent lobectomy.[150] Complications occurred in 26% of patients, including reoperation in 2 patients. During the early postoperative period, 81.5% of patients had a sputum conversion and, by completion of all treatment, 96.3% were sputum culture negative. Similar results have been reported from Japan[151] and China.[152] Although surgery may play a role in MDR-TB treatment, especially as new resistance arises, patient access to trained surgeons in high MDR-TB burden areas is limited.

Beyond XDR-TB: Totally Drug-resistant TB

Several reports have been published documenting patients with TB who have failed treatment with all available drugs or are infected with strains that are resistant in vitro to all available drugs.[153–156] In these articles, some investigators have used the term totally-drug resistant to describe the isolates, the latest in a rapidly growing lexicon used to describe increasingly drug-resistant TB isolates. The introduction of new terms to describe classes of drug resistance is complex, especially given the challenges inherent in drug-susceptibility testing and prognosis for patients.[83,157,158] It is rare to have isolates tested against every drug with possible activity against TB (including WHO group 5 drugs), even in one of the 14 Supranational Reference Laboratories[159] and there are no standardized methods for all old or new drugs (eg, bedaquiline and delaminid). Depending on the location of the patient, the range of drug-susceptibility testing available, and access to drugs, the isolate may be functionally totally drug resistant[160] but not resistant to all drugs. This is the case for many patients with MDR-TB who are not being treated currently. Given these limitations, the WHO working group on drug-resistant TB recommends not yet adding this term to the lexicon.[161]

The isolates from 4 patients described in the study from India were resistant to all first-line and second-line drugs (isoniazid, rifampicin, ethambutol, streptomycin, pyrazinamide, ofloxacin, moxifloxacin, amikacin, capreomycin, kanamycin, para-aminosalicylic acid, and ethionamide) tested by MGIT DST and genotypic DST (MTBDR*plus* and MTBDRsl LiPA) in a major referral laboratory.[153] Review of each case revealed mismanaged treatment of MDR-TB in the private sector. As pointed out by the investigators, patients with MDR-TB are not included in the national TB program, leaving them to seek care by inexpert providers.

Shah and colleagues[156] performed a cross-sectional study of patients with suspected TB (inpatient and outpatient) in Tugela Ferry district hospital in 2008 to 2009. This site is the origin of a previous report of XDR-TB in patients with HIV infection leading to nearly 100% mortality. Testing for susceptibility to isoniazid, rifampin, ethambutol, streptomycin, ofloxacin, kanamycin, capreomycin, and ethionamide were performed by phenotypic DST using the 1% proportional method on solid media. Of the 209 patients with culture-confirmed TB, 30 (14%) had MDR-TB and 19 (9%) had XDR-TB. Thirteen were also resistant to capreomycin and ethionamide. Four of the XDR-TB isolates were resistant to both capreomycin and kanamycin. None of the patients with XDR-TB had a history of treatment with second-line drugs and most (92%) were coinfected with HIV. At the time of the report, 4 were known to be alive and on treatment of XDR-TB.

In the early report from Italy, 2 patients were infected with very drug-resistant strains following extensive exposure to multiple anti-TB drugs.[154] One patient was exposed to an infected family member with MDR-TB and received suboptimal treatment, leading to the development of additional resistance, progression of disease, and death. The infection was also transmitted to her daughter, requiring 3 years of combined medical and surgical treatment. The second patient also died of TB after being hospitalized for nearly 2 years for continuous treatment. Extensive drug-susceptibility testing was performed at the Supranational Reference Laboratory and the isolates met criteria for XDR-TB plus resistance to all first-line and second-line drugs that could be tested.

INFECTION PREVENTION AND CONTROL

TB is most commonly transmitted from one to person to another when the infection is either not treated or inadequately treated, as often occurs with MDR-TB.[162–164] In environments with more MDR-TB, the likelihood of primary infection with MDR-TB (primary resistance) is greater than that associated with development of resistance on therapy (acquired resistance).[156,165,166] This realization is critical because it has historically been simpler to lay the blame on patients when they are found to have MDR-TB and focus on adherence.[6,167,168] The epidemic of MDR-TB may now be at sufficient density to be spreading predominantly as primary infections.

Prevention of transmission relies on infection control practices, including identification of cases, administrative practices, environmental practices, and personal protective equipment (PPE) use. Health care facilities, both inpatient and outpatient, need to be designed and built to minimize the risk of transmission, particularly in areas with large populations of immunocompromised patients (eg, HIV infection). Given the history of MDR-TB, it is not surprising that outbreaks of MDR-TB in congregate settings date back decades.[169–173] Although there were responses to these outbreaks, including recommendation for improved infection control practices,[174–176] they were not commonly put into place, especially in areas with the greatest burden of MDR-TB. In many parts of the world, treatment of TB, and especially MDR-TB, historically has taken place in hospitals, putting other patients and health care workers (HCWs) at risk of infection (WHO policy on TB infection control in health care facilities, 2009). Given this understanding, moving patients back into the outpatient setting is becoming accepted and experience in treating patients with complex MDR-TB in the community setting is accumulating.[16,177–180] However, the decision to treat a patient in a specific setting is often determined by policy decisions and concerns for transmission in the community. Regardless, there are not enough beds to accommodate all the patients with MDR-TB, so alternatives need to be developed.[181]

Social network analysis was used to show a transmission network associated with a serial outbreak of XDR-TB in patients in the 355-bed Tugela Ferry district hospital,[182] an area with an incidence of 119 MDR-TB cases and 53 XDR-TB cases per 100,000 individuals.[170] Patients were infected while hospitalized and in turn became sources for ongoing transmission. Consistent with prior findings, only 59% had smear-positive disease. The study showed that there was at least 1 patient with unrecognized XDR-TB on the ward on 91% of days over the 2 years studied, creating a dangerous environment for both patients and HCWs. This hospital-associated outbreak of life-threatening XDR-TB revealed deficiencies in diagnosis and infection control practices, even though the hospital followed a policy for diagnosis and DST that was more aggressive than the national policy.

There are simple, low-cost interventions that decrease the risk of MDR-TB transmission. The most common first-line level of protection is the use of surgical-type masks on patients to prevent aerosolization of droplet nuclei.[183,184] These masks are used to prevent transmission of potential pathogens by the respiratory route of the wearer, in contrast with respirators worn to protect the wearer. Using a classic experimental method involving guinea pigs exposed to air exhaust from rooms housing patients with TB, transmission of MDR-TB was reduced by 56% when the source patients remained masked from 7 AM to 7 PM for the 12-week study period.[183,185]

Adoption of infection control recommendations in health care settings is challenging. HCWs are at significant risk of infection given the lack of infection control practices and availability of PPE.[186,187] Systems that put HCWs at risk for MDR-TB are at risk of decreased morale and loss of these highly trained, hard-to-replace individuals.[188,189] What works in one setting may not work in another, particularly moving from high-income to low-income hospitals and clinics. The South African government implemented a national infection control plan for drug-resistant TB, but a cross-sectional study by anonymous questionnaire and structured interviews found highly variant adherence to infection control recommendations.[190] One in 5 of the 24 facilities had no infection control officer, and most (89%) of the infection control officers thought that they had no authority to make changes to prevent nosocomial transmission. Similar lack of adherence to recommended guidelines has been described in the United States as well,[191,192] despite data supporting using a bundled infection control approach including isolation, negative pressure rooms, and PPE use by HCWs leading to fewer MDR-TB cases and fewer tuberculin skin-test conversions in HCWs.[175,176,193]

THE FUTURE

Global action to control the devastation of TB infection is on target to achieve gains. The successes of the DOTS program illustrate that complex care can be developed, delivered, and scaled up in a meaningful way. At the same time, it is also an example of how well-intentioned efforts can lead to unexpected outcomes. Drug-resistant TB has the potential to become the predominant type of TB in some parts of the world and to do so under the watch of the global health community and many disease experts. This same community has come to realize the magnitude of the problem and, in doing so, has started the difficult task of responding. In 2009, the 62nd World Health Assembly endorsed actions to control MDR-TB and XDR-TB focused on access to DR-TB diagnostics and drugs. Public-private partnerships like the TB Alliance and the Foundation for Innovative New Diagnostics (FIND, www. finddiagnostics.org), together with strengthening local, regional, national, and international public health agencies, have the potential to respond to the needs of these patients. Just as importantly, recognition of the social determinants of TB acquisition remains, as ever, critical to any response. As a result, attention to human rights, justice, and equity is as important as the biologic response. Although palliative care has been proposed as a potential option for patients with drug-resistant TB, TB is primarily an infectious disease that can be prevented and cured if only the effort is made.[194]

REFERENCES

1. Skrahina A, Hurevich H, Zalutskaya A. Multidrug-resistant tuberculosis in Belarus: the size of the problem and associated risk factors. Bull World Health Organ 2013;91(1):36–45.
2. Centers for Disease Control and Prevention (CDC). Interruptions in supplies of second-line antituberculosis drugs - United States, 2005-2012. MMWR Morb Mortal Wkly Rep 2013;62:23–6.
3. Hirsch-Moverman Y, Daftary A, Franks J, et al. Adherence to treatment for latent tuberculosis infection: systematic review of studies in the US and Canada. Int J Tuberc Lung Dis 2008;12:1235–54.
4. Lalloo UG, Pillay S. Managing tuberculosis and HIV in sub-Sahara Africa. Curr HIV/AIDS Rep 2008;5:132–9.
5. Crofton J, Mitchison DA. Streptomycin resistance in pulmonary tuberculosis. Br Med J 1948;2:1009–15.
6. Keshavjee S, Farmer PE. Tuberculosis, drug resistance, and the history of modern medicine. N Engl J Med 2012;367:931–6.
7. Iseman MD. Tailoring a time-bomb. Inadvertent genetic engineering. Am Rev Respir Dis 1985;132:735–6.
8. Cegielski JP. Extensively drug-resistant tuberculosis: "there must be some kind of way out of here". Clin Infect Dis 2010;50(Suppl 3):S195–200.

9. Bhullar K, Waglechner N, Pawlowski A, et al. Antibiotic resistance is prevalent in an isolated cave microbiome. PLoS One 2012;7:e34953.

10. Wright GD, Poinar H. Antibiotic resistance is ancient: implications for drug discovery. Trends Microbiol 2012;20:157–9.

11. D'Costa VM, et al. Antibiotic resistance is ancient. Nature 2011;477:457–61.

12. Lederberg J. Infectious history. Science 2000;288:287–93.

13. Dye C, Lönnroth K, Jaramillo E. Trends in tuberculosis incidence and their determinants in 134 countries. Bull World Health Organ 2009;87(9):683–91.

14. Raviglione M, et al. Scaling up interventions to achieve global tuberculosis control: progress and new developments. Lancet 2012;379:1902–13.

15. Keshavjee S, et al. Treating multidrug-resistant tuberculosis in Tomsk, Russia: developing programs that address the linkage between poverty and disease. Ann N Y Acad Sci 2008;1136:1–11.

16. Mitnick C, et al. Community-based therapy for multidrug-resistant tuberculosis in Lima, Peru. N Engl J Med 2003;348:119–28.

17. WHO. Global tuberculosis report 2012. Geneva (Switzerland): World Health Organization; 2012.

18. Daniel TM. The history of tuberculosis. Respir Med 2006;100:1862–70.

19. Smith DG, Waksman SA. Tuberculostatic and tuberculocidal action of streptomycin. J Bacteriolo 1947;54(1):67.

20. McDougall JB. Streptomycin and tuberculous meningitis. Br Med J 1948; 1(4540):74.

21. Velu S, et al. A controlled comparison of streptomycin plus pyrazinamide and streptomycin plus PAS in the retreatment of patients excreting isoniazid-resistant organisms. Tubercle 1964;45:144–59.

22. Kristenson A. Treatment of cavernous pulmonary tuberculosis with a combination of chemotherapy and antibiotics. Acta Tuberc Scand Suppl 1950;26:15–25.

23. Fox W, Ellard GA, Mitchison DA. Studies on the treatment of tuberculosis undertaken by the British Medical Research Council tuberculosis units, 1946-1986, with relevant subsequent publications. Int J Tuberc Lung Dis 1999;3:S231–79.

24. Selikoff IJ, Robitzek EH, Ornstein GG. Treatment of pulmonary tuberculosis with hydrazide derivatives of isonicotinic acid. J Am Med Assoc 1952;150:973–80.

25. Manten A, Van Wijngaarden LJ. Development of drug resistance to rifampicin. Chemotherapy 1969;14:93–100.

26. Conway H. Prevalence of drug resistance in previously untreated patients United States Public Health Service Cooperative Investigation. Am Rev Respir Dis 1964;89:327–36.

27. Hobby GL. Primary drug resistance in tuberculosis. A review. I. Am Rev Respir Dis 1962;86:839–46.

28. Steiner M, Cosio A. Primary tuberculosis in children. 1. Incidence of primary drug-resistant disease in 332 children observed between the years 1961 and 1964 at the Kings County Medical Center of Brooklyn. N Engl J Med 1966; 274:755–9.

29. Sen A. Fertility and coercion. Univ Chic Law Rev 2007;63:1035–61.

30. Steiner P, Rao M, Victoria MS, et al. A continuing study of primary drug-resistant tuberculosis among children observed at the Kings County Hospital Medical Center between the years 1961 and 1980. Am Rev Respir Dis 1983; 128:425–8.

31. Chaves AD, Dangler G, Abeles H, et al. The prevalence of drug resistance among strains of M. tuberculosis isolated from ambulatory patients in New York City. Am Rev Respir Dis 1961;84:744–5.

32. Hershfield ES, Eidus L, Helbecque DM. Canadian survey to determine the rate of drug resistance to isoniazid, PAS and streptomycin in newly detected untreated tuberculosis patients and retreatment cases. Int J Clin Pharmacol Biopharm 1979;17:387–93.

33. Hurley JC, Uren EM, Andrew JH, et al. Culture-positive tuberculosis at St Vincent's Hospital, Melbourne, 1962-1989. Aust N Z J Med 1993;23:7–11.

34. Janowiec M, Zwolska-Kwiek Z, Bek E. Drug resistance in newly discovered untreated tuberculosis patients in Poland, 1974-1977. Tubercle 1979;60: 233–7.

35. Tsukamura M. Annual change of drug resistance cases viewed through a Japanese National Sanatorium. Acta Tuberc Pneumol Scand 1964;45:149–53.

36. Pines A, Richardson RJ. Drug-resistance in patients with pulmonary tuberculosis presenting at chest clinics in Hong Kong. Tubercle 1964;45:77–95.

37. Pepys J, Mitchison DA, Kinsley BJ. The prevalence of bacterial resistance to isoniazid and to PAS in patients with acute pulmonary tuberculosis presenting for treatment in East Africa. Tubercle 1960;41:32–6.

38. Cantwell MF, Snider DE, Cauthen GM, et al. Epidemiology of tuberculosis in the United States, 1985 through 1992. JAMA 1994;272:535–9.

39. Brudney K, Dobkin J. Resurgent tuberculosis in New York City. Human immunodeficiency virus, homelessness, and the decline of tuberculosis control programs. Am Rev Respir Dis 1991;144:745–9.

40. Barnes PF, Bloch AB, Davidson PT, et al. Tuberculosis in patients with human immunodeficiency virus infection. N Engl J Med 1991;324:1644–50.

41. Cantwell MF, McKenna MT, McCray E, et al. Tuberculosis and race/ethnicity in the United States: impact of socioeconomic status. Am J Respir Crit Care Med 1998;157:1016–20.

42. Frieden TR, Sterling T, Pablos-Mendez A. The emergence of drug-resistant tuberculosis in New York City. N Engl J Med 1993;328(8):521–6.

43. Pearson ML, et al. Nosocomial transmission of multidrug-resistant *Mycobacterium tuberculosis*. A risk to patients and health care workers. Ann Intern Med 1992;117:191–6.

44. McKenna MT, McCray E, Jones JL, et al. The fall after the rise: tuberculosis in the United States, 1991 through 1994. Am J Public Health 1998;88:1059–63.

45. CDC. Reported tuberculosis in the United States, 2011. Atlanta (GA): Center for Disease Control and Prevention; 2011.

46. Dalton T, et al. Prevalence of and risk factors for resistance to second-line drugs in people with multidrug-resistant tuberculosis in eight countries: a prospective cohort study. Lancet 2012;380:1406–17.

47. Centers for Disease Control (CDC). Nosocomial transmission of multidrug-resistant tuberculosis among HIV-infected persons–Florida and New York, 1988-1991. MMWR Morb Mortal Wkly Rep 1991;40:585–91.

48. Centers for Disease Control (CDC). Tuberculosis outbreak among persons in a residential facility for HIV-infected persons–San Francisco. MMWR Morb Mortal Wkly Rep 1991;40:649–52.

49. From the Centers for Disease Control. Nosocomial transmission of multidrug-resistant tuberculosis among HIV-infected persons–Florida and New York, 1988-1991. JAMA 1991;266:1483–5.

50. WHO. TB. A global emergency. Geneva (Switzerland): World Health Organization; 1994.

51. Watts G. WHO annual report finds world at a crossroad on tuberculosis. BMJ 2012;345:e7051.

52. Mukadi YD, Maher D, Harries A. Tuberculosis case fatality rates in high HIV prevalence populations in sub-Saharan Africa. AIDS 2001;15:143–52.
53. Huffman SA, Veen J, Hennink MM, et al. Exploitation, vulnerability to tuberculosis and access to treatment among Uzbek labor migrants in Kazakhstan. Soc Sci Med 2012;74:864–72.
54. Long Q, et al. Barriers to accessing TB diagnosis for rural-to-urban migrants with chronic cough in Chongqing, China: a mixed methods study. BMC Health Serv Res 2008;8:202.
55. Storla DG, Yimer S, Bjune GA. A systematic review of delay in the diagnosis and treatment of tuberculosis. BMC Public Health 2008;8:15.
56. WHO. Toward universal access to diagnosis and treatment of multidrug-resistant and extensively drug-resistant tuberculosis by 2015. Geneva (Switzerland): World Health Organization; 2011.
57. Skrahina A, et al. Alarming levels of drug-resistant tuberculosis in Belarus: results of a survey in Minsk. Eur Respir J 2012;39:1425–31.
58. Zhao Y, et al. National survey of drug-resistant tuberculosis in China. N Engl J Med 2012;366:2161–70.
59. He GX, et al. Multidrug-resistant tuberculosis, People's Republic of China, 2007-2009. Emerg Infect Dis 2011;17:1831–8.
60. Liu CH, et al. Characteristics and treatment outcomes of patients with MDR and XDR tuberculosis in a TB referral hospital in Beijing: a 13-year experience. PLoS One 2011;6(4):e19399.
61. Becerra MC, et al. Tuberculosis burden in households of patients with multidrug-resistant and extensively drug-resistant tuberculosis: a retrospective cohort study. Lancet 2011;377:147–52.
62. Minion J, Gallant V, Wolfe J, et al. Multidrug and extensively drug-resistant tuberculosis in Canada 1997-2008: demographic and disease characteristics. PLoS One 2013;8:e53466.
63. Hoa NB, et al. National survey of tuberculosis prevalence in Viet Nam. Bull World Health Organ 2010;88:273–80.
64. Lawn SD, Zumla AI. Tuberculosis. Lancet 2011;378:57–72.
65. Magee MJ, et al. Prevalence of drug resistant tuberculosis among patients at high-risk for HIV attending outpatient clinics in Delhi, India. Southeast Asian J Trop Med Public Health 2012;43:354–63.
66. Zhang Y, Yew WW. Mechanisms of drug resistance in *Mycobacterium tuberculosis*. Int J Tuberc Lung Dis 2009;13:1320–30.
67. Caws M, Ha DT. Scale-up of diagnostics for multidrug resistant tuberculosis. Lancet Infect Dis 2010;10:656–8.
68. Martin A, et al. The nitrate reductase assay for the rapid detection of isoniazid and rifampicin resistance in *Mycobacterium tuberculosis*: a systematic review and meta-analysis. J Antimicrob Chemother 2008;62:56–64.
69. Canetti G, Rist N, Grosset J. Measurement of sensitivity of the tuberculous bacillus to antibacillary drugs by the method of proportions. Methodology, resistance criteria, results and interpretation. Rev Tuberc Pneumol (Paris) 1963;27:217–72.
70. Katiyar SK, Bihari S, Prakash S, et al. A randomised controlled trial of high-dose isoniazid adjuvant therapy for multidrug-resistant tuberculosis. Int J Tuberc Lung Dis 2008;12:139–45.
71. Parsons LM, Somoskövi Á, Gutierrez C. Laboratory diagnosis of tuberculosis in resource-poor countries: challenges and opportunities. Clin Microbiol Rev 2011;24(2):314–50.

72. Mlambo CK, et al. Genotypic diversity of extensively drug-resistant tuberculosis (XDR-TB) in South Africa. Int J Tuberc Lung Dis 2008;12:99–104.
73. David HL. Probability distribution of drug-resistant mutants in unselected populations of *Mycobacterium tuberculosis*. Appl Microbiol 1970;20:810–4.
74. Gillespie SH. Evolution of drug resistance in *Mycobacterium tuberculosis*: clinical and molecular perspective. Antimicrob Agents Chemother 2002;46: 267–74.
75. Andersson DI, Levin BR. The biological cost of antibiotic resistance. Curr Opin Microbiol 1999;2:489–93.
76. Pym AS, Saint-Joanis B, Cole ST. Effect of katG mutations on the virulence of *Mycobacterium tuberculosis* and the implication for transmission in humans. Infect Immun 2002;70:4955–60.
77. Gandhi NR, et al. Multidrug-resistant and extensively drug-resistant tuberculosis: a threat to global control of tuberculosis. Lancet 2010;375:1830–43.
78. Zignol M, Gemert W, Falzon D. Surveillance of anti-tuberculosis drug resistance in the world: an updated analysis, 2007-2010. Bull World Health Organ 2012; 90(2):111–119D.
79. Angeby KA, Klintz L, Hoffner SE. Rapid and inexpensive drug susceptibility testing of *Mycobacterium tuberculosis* with a nitrate reductase assay. J Clin Microbiol 2002;40:553–5.
80. Moore DA, et al. Microscopic-observation drug-susceptibility assay for the diagnosis of TB. N Engl J Med 2006;355:1539–50.
81. Minion J, Leung E, Menzies D, et al. Microscopic-observation drug susceptibility and thin layer agar assays for the detection of drug resistant tuberculosis: a systematic review and meta-analysis. Lancet Infect Dis 2010;10:688–98.
82. Dixit P, Singh U, Sharma P, et al. Evaluation of nitrate reduction assay, resazurin microtiter assay and microscopic observation drug susceptibility assay for first line antitubercular drug susceptibility testing of clinical isolates of *M. tuberculosis*. J Microbiol Methods 2012;88:122–6.
83. Angra PK, et al. Performance of tuberculosis drug susceptibility testing in U.S. laboratories from 1994 to 2008. J Clin Microbiol 2012;50:1233–9.
84. Ardito F, Posteraro B, Sanguinetti M, et al. Evaluation of BACTEC Mycobacteria Growth Indicator Tube (MGIT 960) automated system for drug susceptibility testing of *Mycobacterium tuberculosis*. J Clin Microbiol 2001;39:4440–4.
85. Koh WJ, Ko Y, Kim CK, et al. Rapid diagnosis of tuberculosis and multidrug resistance using a MGIT 960 system. Ann Lab Med 2012;32:264–9.
86. Müller B, Borrell S, Rose G, et al. The heterogeneous evolution of multidrug-resistant *Mycobacterium tuberculosis*. Trends Genet 2012. http://dx.doi.org/ 10.1016/j.tig.2012.11.005.
87. Ling DI, Zwerling AA, Pai M. GenoType MTBDR assays for the diagnosis of multidrug-resistant tuberculosis: a meta-analysis. Eur Respir J 2008;32:1165–74.
88. Chryssanthou E, Angeby K. The GenoType® MTBDR*plus* assay for detection of drug resistance in *Mycobacterium tuberculosis* in Sweden. APMIS 2012;120: 405–9.
89. Anek-Vorapong R, et al. Validation of the GenoType MTBDR*plus* assay for detection of MDR-TB in a public health laboratory in Thailand. BMC Infect Dis 2010;10:123.
90. Hillemann D, Rüsch-Gerdes S, Richter E. Evaluation of the GenoType MTBDR*plus* assay for rifampin and isoniazid susceptibility testing of *Mycobacterium tuberculosis* strains and clinical specimens. J Clin Microbiol 2007;45: 2635–40.

91. Albert H, et al. Rapid screening of MDR-TB using molecular Line Probe Assay is feasible in Uganda. BMC Infect Dis 2010;10:41.

92. Getahun H, Harrington M, O'Brien R, et al. Diagnosis of smear-negative pulmonary tuberculosis in people with HIV infection or AIDS in resource-constrained settings: informing urgent policy changes. Lancet 2007;369:2042–9.

93. Hanrahan CF, et al. The impact of expanded testing for multidrug resistant tuberculosis using genotype MTBDR*plus* in South Africa: an observational cohort study. PLoS One 2012;7:e49898.

94. Boehme CC, et al. Rapid molecular detection of tuberculosis and rifampin resistance. N Engl J Med 2010;363:1005–15.

95. Theron G, et al. Evaluation of the Xpert MTB/RIF assay for the diagnosis of pulmonary tuberculosis in a high HIV prevalence setting. Am J Respir Crit Care Med 2011;184:132–40.

96. Van Deun A, Wright A, Zignol M, et al. Drug susceptibility testing proficiency in the network of supranational tuberculosis reference laboratories. Int J Tuberc Lung Dis 2011;15:116–24.

97. Zhou M, et al. Rapid colorimetric testing for pyrazinamide susceptibility of *M. tuberculosis* by a PCR-based in-vitro synthesized pyrazinamidase method. PLoS One 2011;6(11):e27654.

98. Chang KC, Yew WW, Zhang Y. Pyrazinamide susceptibility testing in *Mycobacterium tuberculosis*: a systematic review with meta-analyses. Antimicrob Agents Chemother 2011;55:4499–505.

99. Ajbani K, et al. Evaluation of genotype MTBDRsl assay to detect drug resistance associated with fluoroquinolones, aminoglycosides and ethambutol on clinical sediments. PLoS One 2012;7(11):e49433.

100. Hillemann D, Rüsch-Gerdes S, Richter E. Feasibility of the GenoType MTBDRsl assay for fluoroquinolone, amikacin-capreomycin, and ethambutol resistance testing of *Mycobacterium tuberculosis* strains and clinical specimens. J Clin Microbiol 2009;47:1767–72.

101. Miotto P, Bigoni S, Migliori GB. Early tuberculosis treatment monitoring by Xpert® MTB/RIF. Eur Respir J 2012;39(5):1269–71.

102. Lacoma A, et al. GenoType MTBDRsl for molecular detection of second-line-drug and ethambutol resistance in *Mycobacterium tuberculosis* strains and clinical samples. J Clin Microbiol 2012;50:30–6.

103. Brossier F, Veziris N, Aubry A, et al. Detection by GenoType MTBDRsl test of complex mechanisms of resistance to second-line drugs and ethambutol in multidrug-resistant *Mycobacterium tuberculosis* complex isolates. J Clin Microbiol 2010;48:1683–9.

104. Ignatyeva O, et al. Detection of resistance to second-line antituberculosis drugs by use of the genotype MTBDRsl assay: a multicenter evaluation and feasibility study. J Clin Microbiol 2012;50:1593–7.

105. Mukherjee JS, Rich ML, Socci AR, et al. Programmes and principles in treatment of multidrug-resistant tuberculosis. Lancet 2004;363(9407):474–81.

106. Orenstein EW, et al. Treatment outcomes among patients with multidrug-resistant tuberculosis: systematic review and meta-analysis. Lancet Infect Dis 2009;9:153–61.

107. Rajbhandary SS, Marks SM, Bock NN. Costs of patients hospitalized for multidrug-resistant tuberculosis. Int J Tuberc Lung Dis 2004;8:1012–6.

108. Bloss E, et al. Adverse events related to multidrug-resistant tuberculosis treatment, Latvia, 2000-2004. Int J Tuberc Lung Dis 2010;14:275–81.

109. WHO. Guidelines for the programmatic management of drug-resistant tuberculosis-2011 update. Geneva: WHO; 2011.

110. Eang MT, et al. The multi-step process of building TB/HIV collaboration in Cambodia. Health Res Policy Syst 2012;10:34.

111. Brostrom R, et al. Islands of hope: building local capacity to manage an outbreak of multidrug-resistant tuberculosis in the Pacific. Am J Public Health 2011;101:14–8.

112. Perumal R, Padayatchi N, Stiefvater E. The whole is greater than the sum of the parts: recognising missed opportunities for an optimal response to the rapidly maturing TB-HIV co-epidemic in South Africa. BMC Public Health 2009;9:243.

113. van der Werf MJ, Langendam MW. Multidrug resistance after inappropriate tuberculosis treatment: a meta-analysis. Eur Respir J 2012;39(6):1511–9.

114. Menzies NA, Cohen T, Lin HH, et al. Population health impact and cost-effectiveness of tuberculosis diagnosis with Xpert MTB/RIF: a dynamic simulation and economic evaluation. PLoS Med 2012;9:e1001347.

115. Mitnick CD, Shin SS, Seung KJ, et al. Comprehensive treatment of extensively drug-resistant tuberculosis. N Engl J Med 2008;359(6):563–74.

116. Seung KJ, Satti H. Management of MDR-TB: a field guide.

117. Caminero JA, World Health Organization, American Thoracic Society, British Thoracic Society. Treatment of multidrug-resistant tuberculosis: evidence and controversies. Int J Tuberc Lung Dis 2006;10:829–37.

118. Gammino VM, et al. Bacteriologic monitoring of multidrug-resistant tuberculosis patients in five DOTS-Plus pilot projects. Int J Tuberc Lung Dis 2011;15: 1315–22.

119. Mak A, et al. Influence of multidrug resistance on tuberculosis treatment outcomes with standardized regimens. Am J Respir Crit Care Med 2008;178: 306–12.

120. Johnston JC, Shahidi NC, Sadatsafavi M, et al. Treatment outcomes of multidrug-resistant tuberculosis: a systematic review and meta-analysis. PLoS One 2009;4(9):e6914.

121. Ahuja SD, et al. Multidrug resistant pulmonary tuberculosis treatment regimens and patient outcomes: an individual patient data meta-analysis of 9,153 patients. PLoS Med 2012;9:e1001300.

122. Van Deun A, et al. Short, highly effective, and inexpensive standardized treatment of multidrug-resistant tuberculosis. Am J Respir Crit Care Med 2010; 182:684–92.

123. Pooran A, Pieterson E, Davids M, et al. What is the cost of diagnosis and management of drug resistant tuberculosis in South Africa? PLoS One 2013;8: e54587.

124. Schnippel K, Rosen S, Shearer K. Costs of inpatient treatment for multi-drug-resistant tuberculosis in South Africa. Trop Med Int Health 2013;18(1):109–16.

125. Resch SC, Salomon JA, Murray M, et al. Cost-effectiveness of treating multidrug-resistant tuberculosis. PLoS Med 2006;3:e241.

126. Suarez PG, et al. Feasibility and cost-effectiveness of standardised second-line drug treatment for chronic tuberculosis patients: a national cohort study in Peru. Lancet 2002;359:1980–9.

127. Hafkin J, et al. Impact of the human immunodeficiency virus on early multidrug-resistant tuberculosis treatment outcomes in Botswana. Int J Tuberc Lung Dis 2013. http://dx.doi.org/10.5588/ijtld.12.0100.

128. Farley JE, et al. Outcomes of multi-drug resistant tuberculosis (MDR-TB) among a cohort of South African patients with high HIV prevalence. PLoS One 2011;6: e20436.
129. Seung KJ, et al. Early outcomes of MDR-TB treatment in a high HIV-prevalence setting in Southern Africa. PLoS One 2009;4:e7186.
130. Wells CD, et al. HIV infection and multidrug-resistant tuberculosis: the perfect storm. J Infect Dis 2007;196(Suppl 1):S86–107.
131. Akksilp S, et al. Antiretroviral therapy during tuberculosis treatment and marked reduction in death rate of HIV-infected patients, Thailand. Emerg Infect Dis 2007;13:1001–7.
132. Manosuthi W, Chottanapand S, Thongyen S, et al. Survival rate and risk factors of mortality among HIV/tuberculosis-coinfected patients with and without antiretroviral therapy. J Acquir Immune Defic Syndr 2006;43:42–6.
133. dos Santos AP, et al. Safety and effectiveness of HAART in tuberculosis-HIV co-infected patients in Brazil. Int J Tuberc Lung Dis 2013;17:192–7.
134. Gandhi NR, et al. Extensively drug-resistant tuberculosis as a cause of death in patients co-infected with tuberculosis and HIV in a rural area of South Africa. Lancet 2006;368:1575–80.
135. Palacios E, et al. HIV-positive patients treated for multidrug-resistant tuberculosis: clinical outcomes in the HAART era. Int J Tuberc Lung Dis 2012;16:348–54.
136. Tato M, et al. In vitro activity of linezolid against *Mycobacterium tuberculosis* complex, including multidrug-resistant *Mycobacterium bovis* isolates. Int J Antimicrob Agents 2006;28:75–8.
137. Cynamon MH, Klemens SP, Sharpe CA. Activities of several novel oxazolidinones against *Mycobacterium tuberculosis* in a murine model. Antimicrob Agents Chemother 1999;43(5):1189–91.
138. Anger HA, et al. Linezolid use for treatment of multidrug-resistant and extensively drug-resistant tuberculosis, New York City, 2000-06. J Antimicrob Chemother 2010;65:775–83.
139. Condos R, Hadgiangelis N, Leibert E. Case series report of a linezolid-containing regimen for extensively drug-resistant tuberculosis. Chest 2008; 134(1):187–92.
140. Fortún J, et al. Linezolid for the treatment of multidrug-resistant tuberculosis. J Antimicrob Chemother 2005;56:180–5.
141. Lee M, Lee J, Carroll MW, et al. Linezolid for treatment of chronic extensively drug-resistant tuberculosis. N Engl J Med 2012;367(16):1508–18.
142. Gler MT, Skripconoka V. Delamanid for multidrug-resistant pulmonary tuberculosis. N Engl J Med 2012;366(23):2151–60.
143. Wallis RS, et al. Biomarkers and diagnostics for tuberculosis: progress, needs, and translation into practice. Lancet 2010;375:1920–37.
144. Holtz TH, et al. Time to sputum culture conversion in multidrug-resistant tuberculosis: predictors and relationship to treatment outcome. Ann Intern Med 2006;144:650–9.
145. Diacon AH, Pym A, Grobusch M. The diarylquinoline TMC207 for multidrug-resistant tuberculosis. N Engl J Med 2009;360(23):2397–405.
146. Diacon AH, et al. 14-day bactericidal activity of PA-824, bedaquiline, pyrazinamide, and moxifloxacin combinations: a randomised trial. Lancet 2012;380: 986–93.
147. Iseman MD, Madsen L, Goble M, et al. Surgical intervention in the treatment of pulmonary disease caused by drug-resistant *Mycobacterium tuberculosis*. Am Rev Respir Dis 1990;141:623–5.

148. Rizzi A, et al. Results of surgical management of tuberculosis: experience in 206 patients undergoing operation. Ann Thorac Surg 1995;59:896–900.

149. Man MA, Nicolau D. Surgical treatment to increase the success rate of multidrug-resistant tuberculosis. Eur J Cardiothorac Surg 2012;42:e9–12.

150. Sung SW, et al. Surgery increased the chance of cure in multi-drug resistant pulmonary tuberculosis. Eur J Cardiothorac Surg 1999;16:187–93.

151. Shiraishi Y, Katsuragi N, Kita H, et al. Different morbidity after pneumonectomy: multidrug-resistant tuberculosis versus non-tuberculous mycobacterial infection. Interact Cardiovasc Thorac Surg 2010;11:429–32.

152. Yew WW, Leung CC. Management of multidrug-resistant tuberculosis: update 2007. Respirology 2008;13:21–46.

153. Udwadia ZF. MDR, XDR, TDR tuberculosis: ominous progression. Thorax 2012; 67(4):286–8.

154. Migliori GB, De Iaco G, Besozzi G, et al. First tuberculosis cases in Italy resistant to all tested drugs. Euro Surveill 2007;12:E070517.1.

155. Velayati AA, et al. Emergence of new forms of totally drug-resistant tuberculosis bacilli: super extensively drug-resistant tuberculosis or totally drug-resistant strains in Iran. Chest 2009;136:420–5.

156. Shah NS, et al. Increasing drug resistance in extensively drug-resistant tuberculosis, South Africa. Emerg Infect Dis 2011;17:510–3.

157. Kim SJ. Drug-susceptibility testing in tuberculosis: methods and reliability of results. Eur Respir J 2005;25:564–9.

158. Jacobson KR, Tierney DB, Jeon CY, et al. Treatment outcomes among patients with extensively drug-resistant tuberculosis: systematic review and meta-analysis. Clin Infect Dis 2010;51:6–14.

159. Shah NS, et al. Worldwide emergence of extensively drug-resistant tuberculosis. Emerg Infect Dis 2007;13:380–7.

160. Cegielski P, et al. Challenges and controversies in defining totally drug-resistant tuberculosis. Emerg Infect Dis 2012;18:e2.

161. Drug-resistant tuberculosis. (World Health Organization). Available at: http://www.who.int/tb/challenges/mdr/tdrfaqs/en/index.html. Accessed on February 1, 2013.

162. Brooks SM, Lassiter NL, Young EC. A pilot study concerning the infection risk of sputum positive tuberculosis patients on chemotherapy. Am Rev Respir Dis 1973;108:799–804.

163. Gunnels JJ, Bates JH, Swindoll H. Infectivity of sputum-positive tuberculous patients on chemotherapy. Am Rev Respir Dis 1974;109:323–30.

164. Jensen PA, Lambert LA, Iademarco MF, et al, CDC. Guidelines for preventing the transmission of Mycobacterium tuberculosis in health-care settings, 2005. MMWR Recomm Rep 2005;54:1–141.

165. Cox HS, Sibilia C, Feuerriegel S, et al. Emergence of extensive drug resistance during treatment for multidrug-resistant tuberculosis. N Engl J Med 2008; 359(22):2398–400.

166. Shin SS, et al. Development of extensively drug-resistant tuberculosis during multidrug-resistant tuberculosis treatment. Am J Respir Crit Care Med 2010; 182:426–32.

167. Gelmanova IY, et al. Barriers to successful tuberculosis treatment in Tomsk, Russian Federation: non-adherence, default and the acquisition of multidrug resistance. Bull World Health Organ 2007;85:703–11.

168. Nodieva A, et al. Recent nosocomial transmission and genotypes of multidrug-resistant Mycobacterium tuberculosis. Int J Tuberc Lung Dis 2010; 14:427–33.

169. Moro ML, et al. An outbreak of multidrug-resistant tuberculosis involving HIV-infected patients of two hospitals in Milan, Italy. Italian Multidrug-Resistant Tuberculosis Outbreak Study Group. AIDS 1998;12:1095–102.

170. Gandhi NR, et al. HIV coinfection in multidrug- and extensively drug-resistant tuberculosis results in high early mortality. Am J Respir Crit Care Med 2010; 181:80–6.

171. Edlin BR, et al. An outbreak of multidrug-resistant tuberculosis among hospitalized patients with the acquired immunodeficiency syndrome. N Engl J Med 1992;326:1514–21.

172. Frieden TR, et al. A multi-institutional outbreak of highly drug-resistant tuberculosis: epidemiology and clinical outcomes. JAMA 1996;276:1229–35.

173. Rullán JV, et al. Nosocomial transmission of multidrug-resistant *Mycobacterium tuberculosis* in Spain. Emerg Infect Dis 1996;2:125–9.

174. Frieden TR, Fujiwara PI, Washko RM, et al. Tuberculosis in New York City–turning the tide. N Engl J Med 1995;333:229–33.

175. Wenger PN, et al. Control of nosocomial transmission of multidrug-resistant *Mycobacterium tuberculosis* among healthcare workers and HIV-infected patients. Lancet 1995;345:235–40.

176. Maloney SA, et al. Efficacy of control measures in preventing nosocomial transmission of multidrug-resistant tuberculosis to patients and health care workers. Ann Intern Med 1995;122:90–5.

177. Kangovi S, Mukherjee J, Bohmer R, et al. A classification and meta-analysis of community-based directly observed therapy programs for tuberculosis treatment in developing countries. J Community Health 2009;34:506–13.

178. Shin S, et al. Community-based treatment of multidrug-resistant tuberculosis in Lima, Peru: 7 years of experience. Soc Sci Med 2004;59:1529–39.

179. Farmer P, Kim JY. Community based approaches to the control of multidrug resistant tuberculosis: introducing "DOTS-plus". BMJ 1998;317:671–4.

180. Wandwalo E, Kapalata N, Egwaga S, et al. Effectiveness of community-based directly observed treatment for tuberculosis in an urban setting in Tanzania: a randomised controlled trial. Int J Tuberc Lung Dis 2004;8:1248–54.

181. Nardell E, Dharmadhikari A. Turning off the spigot: reducing drug-resistant tuberculosis transmission in resource-limited settings. Int J Tuberc Lung Dis 2010;14:1233–43.

182. Gandhi NR, et al. Nosocomial transmission of extensively drug-resistant tuberculosis in a rural hospital in South Africa. J Infect Dis 2013;207:9–17.

183. Riley RL. Airborne infection. Am J Med 1974;57:466–75.

184. Wells WF, Ratcliffe HL, Grumb C. On the mechanics of droplet nuclei infection; quantitative experimental air-borne tuberculosis in rabbits. Am J Hyg 1948;47: 11–28.

185. Dharmadhikari AS, et al. Surgical face masks worn by patients with multidrug-resistant tuberculosis: impact on infectivity of air on a hospital ward. Am J Respir Crit Care Med 2012;185:1104–9.

186. Escombe AR, et al. Tuberculosis transmission risk and infection control in a hospital emergency department in Lima, Peru. Int J Tuberc Lung Dis 2010;14:1120–6.

187. O'Donnell MR, et al. High incidence of hospital admissions with multidrug-resistant and extensively drug-resistant tuberculosis among South African health care workers. Ann Intern Med 2010;153:516–22.

188. Padayatchi N, Daftary A, Moodley T, et al. Case series of the long-term psychosocial impact of drug-resistant tuberculosis in HIV-negative medical doctors. Int J Tuberc Lung Dis 2010;14:960–6.

189. Harrington M. Health systems failing health workers: time for a change. Int J Tuberc Lung Dis 2010;14:935–6.
190. Kanjee Z, Catterick K, Moll AP, et al. Tuberculosis infection control in rural South Africa: survey of knowledge, attitude and practice in hospital staff. J Hosp Infect 2011;79:333–8.
191. Sutton PM, Nicas M, Harrison RJ. Tuberculosis isolation: comparison of written procedures and actual practices in three California hospitals. Infect Control Hosp Epidemiol 2000;21:28–32.
192. Bratcher DF, Stover BH, Lane NE, et al. Compliance with national recommendations for tuberculosis screening and immunization of healthcare workers in a children's hospital. Infect Control Hosp Epidemiol 2000;21:338–40.
193. Stroud LA, et al. Evaluation of infection control measures in preventing the nosocomial transmission of multidrug-resistant Mycobacterium tuberculosis in a New York City hospital. Infect Control Hosp Epidemiol 1995;16:141–7.
194. Upshur R. Apocalypse or redemption: responding to extensively drug-resistant tuberculosis. Bull World Health Organ 2009;87:481–3.

Infections in Transplant Patients

Genevieve L. Pagalilauan, MD[a],*, Ajit P. Limaye, MD[b]

KEYWORDS

- Solid organ transplant • Common infections • Primary care
- Opportunistic infections

KEY POINTS

- Primary care providers must prepare themselves to care for an increasing population of solid organ transplant (SOT) patients.
- SOT recipients require lifelong immunosuppression, and therefore are chronically at increased risk for infections.
- Typical signs of infection may be subtle or absent in the setting of immunosuppressive medications.
- Expedited, comprehensive diagnostic testing for infectious symptoms is important, and sometimes invasive procedures may be warranted.

Generalists must learn to care for infectious complications in solid organ transplant patients.

Primary care providers (PCPs) in North America must prepare themselves to see a growing number of solid organ transplant (SOT) patients. More SOTs are being performed, and SOT patients are living longer.[1] Based on transplant data analyzed from 2008 for 104 countries, around 100,800 SOTs are performed every year worldwide: 69,400 kidney transplants (46% from living donors), 20,200 liver transplants (14.6% from living donors), 5400 heart transplants, 3400 lung transplants, and 2400 pancreas transplants.[2]

Data from the Health Resources and Services Administration showed that more than 27,000 solid organs were transplanted in the United States in 2008.[3] Over the past decade, graft survival and patient survival has improved for nearly every organ. The most gains occurred in living liver donor recipients and heart-lung transplants, with 11% to 34% increased survival. More manifestations of chronic diseases

The authors have no disclosures relevant to this work.
[a] Division of General Internal Medicine, University of Washington School of Medicine, 4245 Roosevelt Way Northeast, Seattle, WA 98115, USA; [b] Division of Allergy and Infectious Disease, University of Washington School of Medicine, University of Washington, Box 356174, 1959 Northeast Pacific Street, Seattle, WA 98195, USA
* Corresponding author.
E-mail address: jadepag@uw.edu

http://dx.doi.org/10.1016/j.mcna.2013.03.002
0025-7125/13/$ – see front matter © 2013 Elsevier Inc. All rights reserved.
medical.theclinics.com

commonly seen by generalists now qualify patients for SOT, including symptomatic chronic conditions such as congestive heart failure (CHF), chronic obstructive lung disease (COPD), chronic hepatitis, and chronic kidney disease (CKD). Given the prevalence of these chronic conditions, more than 100,000 people are on waiting lists in the United States for SOTs. While wait-list length is influenced by changes in demand, listing practices, death rates, donation rates, and allocation policies, it is important to be aware that the demand for SOT is increasing (**Fig. 1**).[3]

SOT recipients are at risk for infections in the short and long term, resulting in higher morbidity and mortality.[4]

Unlike the vast majority of hematopoietic cell transplant recipients who eventually have immunosuppressive medications discontinued, SOT patients require lifelong immunosuppression and therefore remain at lifelong increased risk of infection.[5] To avoid transplant rejection the commonly used immunosuppression regimens are broadly acting, decreasing both cellular and humoral immunity. Reduced cellular immunity leaves hosts susceptible to viral, fungal, and intracellular pathogens while decreased humoral immunity increases the risk for encapsulated bacteria. In most SOT recipients the degree of immunosuppression, and hence the infectious risk, tends to decrease over time, but never returns to a normal baseline. For those who develop recurrent or chronic organ rejection and require intensification of their immunosuppressive regimen, the risk for infection remains high. Usual immunosuppressive regimens include a corticosteroid, a calcineurin inhibitor, and an antimetabolite.[5]

More care is decentralized from major transplant centers.

Even patients who live in rural and geographically isolated areas are receiving SOTs. Because the risk of many transplant-related complications tends to decrease after 3 to

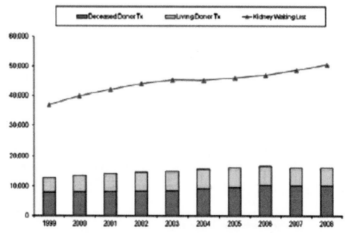

Fig. 1. Number of transplants and size of active waiting list. There was a very large gap between the number of patients waiting for a transplant and the number receiving a transplant. This gap widened over the decade, meaning that the waiting times from listing to transplant continued to increase. The number of living-donor transplants grew until 2004 while the number of decreased donor transplants continued to rise gradually until 2006. (*Data from* Harper SA, Bradley JS, Englund JA, et al. Seasonal influenza in adults and children—diagnosis, treatment, chemoprophylaxis, and institutional outbreak management: Clinical practice guidelines of the Infectious Diseases Society of America. Clin Infect Dis 2009;48(8):1003–32.)

6 months posttransplant, patients generally are referred back to their PCPs/specialists by around 3 months after the transplant. Hence, subacute and long-term management is now being done by generalists with the transplant center providing a consultative role if needed. Most transplant centers will provide the patient and primary physician a packet with transplant-specific care guidelines, recommended monitoring, and follow-up requirements. PCPs of new SOT patients should request this information from the transplant center (**Box 1**).

PRACTICAL ISSUES IN THE MANAGEMENT OF SOT INFECTION

Typical signs and symptoms of infection are muted by immunosuppressive agents.

In immunocompetent hosts, the signs and symptoms of inflammation (rubor, dolor, calor) can be important clues to infection. However, the immunosuppressive agents that SOT recipients receive can blunt this inflammatory response (the mechanism by which they prevent rejection), thereby making the signs and symptoms of inflammation much more subtle.[5] Thus, it is important for PCPs and patients to remain vigilant of even subtle manifestations of infections. Common urgent-visit concerns such as low-grade fevers, new cough, or diarrhea can portend serious infections. This article reviews common presenting symptoms that should be approached differently in SOT patients than in immunocompetent persons.

In this time of heightened awareness of medical costs and growing resistance to antimicrobial therapy, the usual approach to average-risk ambulatory patients is to be judicious and pragmatic in our use of diagnostic and therapeutic interventions.[6] Several features of infection in SOT patients mandate a different approach than is used in immunocompetent patients (the clinical presentation can be more subtle,

---

Box 1
What the PCP should expect from the transplant center

Checkout Materials, Including the Following Information:

- Standard monitoring
  - Labs, immunosuppressive level targets, imaging
  - Frequency of routine clinic appointments
  - Frequency of transplant clinic appointments
  - Assessment for common complications/side effects
    - Hypertension, hyperlipidemia, osteoporosis, diabetes, dental disease
    - Secondary cancer surveillance
- Troubleshooting recommendations for common presentation of infection
  - Fever, cytomegalovirus, typical infections
- Preventive care issues
  - Vaccinations
  - Nutrition, activity, travel
  - Pregnancy
  - Cancer screening

Adapted from UWMC SOT patient/provider materials.

multiple pathogens may be present concomitantly, and the progression of infection may be more rapid). As a result, in general more comprehensive diagnostic testing and earlier escalation to advanced imaging and invasive diagnostic procedures are warranted for SOT patients.[5] Although empiric therapeutic interventions have their place in SOT patients, thorough efforts to identify and characterize the etiologic agent(s) of infection are imperative.

Some tests used to diagnose infections in immunocompetent patients are much less sensitive in SOT patients. For example, tests that rely on the host's immune system (eg, serology) may be less sensitive than direct detection of the pathogen. Although serologic tests can help identify latent infections, antibody development to acute infections may be delayed or never develop in immunosuppressed patients. Instead, direct detection of pathogens using culture, polymerase chain reaction (PCR), and so forth, from optimal specimens is preferred.[5,7]

To add to the complexity, SOT patients are more likely than immunocompetent patients to have rapid progression of infection because of the lack of an appropriate immune response. An example is pneumonia, which can be safely treated in the ambulatory setting in most immunocompetent patients but can often result in hospitalization in SOT patients.[8] SOT patients are more likely to have multiple pathogens and resistance patterns that complicate the choice of antimicrobial therapy.[7] Early involvement of infectious disease specialists may be warranted.

PCPs should familiarize themselves with the timeline of susceptibility to infections.

In general, the intensity of immunosuppression decreases with the time from transplant and, as a result, the risk for serious opportunistic infections tends to decrease with time. However, if episodes of rejection occur, immunosuppressive medications are intensified and patients again become more vulnerable to opportunistic infections that might more typically be seen in the earlier period posttransplant.[5,7]

The first month after transplant is a vulnerable time for nosocomial infections with multidrug-resistant organisms, including those related to complicated surgery.

Nosocomial infections may be related to the transplant surgery itself or exposures to the hospital environment.[5,7] Many such infections are the results of venous and urinary catheterization as well as intubation. Most SOT patients are aggressively treated for known infections before transplantation, given the risks of immunosuppression. protocols exist to screen donors for infections, but the short time frame necessitates limited diagnostic testing. Although serologic testing for viral hepatitis, human immunodeficiency virus (HIV), herpesviruses, and microbiological testing with blood and urine cultures can identify active bacterial and fungal infections, donor-related infections are well described.[9] During the first posttransplant month, bacterial and fungal infections are more common than viral infections, and often these nosocomial pathogens are drug-resistant strains. SOT patients in this time frame will typically still be under the direct care of the transplant center.

The effects of immunosuppressive medications typically manifest in months 1 to 6, so this is when opportunistic infections tend to be most common.

Donor-acquired conditions, or reactivation of recipient infections such as hepatitis B and C, are apt to infect the patient after the first month.[7,9] By 3 months posttransplant, if all is going well, immunosuppression will typically be tapered and most patients will leave the direct care of the transplant program. Patients will be receiving prophylaxis for *Pneumocystis jiroveci* pneumonia (PJP) (trimethoprim/sulfamethoxazole or dapsone, or monthly inhaled pentamidine) and cytomegalovirus (CMV) (commonly valganciclovir).[5] Reactivation of latent infections can occur during this time period, including *Mycobacterium tuberculosis* and *Strongyloides stercoralis*. SOT patients are susceptible during this period to endemic mycoses including *Coccidioides*, *Histoplasma*, *Blastomyces*, and *Cryptococcus*.[7] Prophylactic medications are typically discontinued by 6 to 12 months after transplant. The need for prophylaxis diminishes over time, but SOT patients will always be susceptible to typical community-acquired viral and bacterial infections.

Further concerns are raised 6 months or more posttransplant.

Most stable SOT patient are on reduced doses of immunosuppression, and therefore have decreased risk for opportunistic infections. CMV, Epstein-Barr virus, herpes simplex virus, and hepatitis viruses remain a concern, but more commonly SOT patients are infected with seasonal respiratory and gastrointestinal viruses, community-acquired pneumonias, and urinary tract infections during this period.[7,10] In patients who experience allograft rejection, doses of immunosuppressive medication are increased. In those who require higher levels of immunosuppression, the risk for opportunistic infections may be as high as during the 1- to 6-month posttransplant period; this would include an increased risk for PJP, *Nocardia*, *Varicella*, and *Aspergillus* (**Fig. 2**).[7]

CASES OF INFECTIOUS DISEASE IN SOT PATIENTS

Case 1

A 45-year-old man, 2 years post orthotopic liver transplant, presents to your clinic in January with 5 days of rhinorrhea, mild sore throat, dry cough, mild headache, and chills. ROS is negative for pleurisy or dyspnea, but positive for fatigue. Vital signs (VS): temperature (T) 37.7°C, heart rate (HR) 100 beats/min, blood pressure (BP) 110/70 mm Hg, respiratory rate (RR) 22 breaths/min, oxygen saturation (O_2 sat) 98%. His examination shows clear nasal secretions, mild pharyngeal erythema, and no adenopathy, and his lungs are clear to auscultation bilaterally. His transplanted liver is nontender on palpation, and he is hydrating orally and urinating without difficulty. He had an influenza vaccination 2 months prior.

You recommend:

A. Chest radiograph (CXR), rapid influenza test, empiric therapy with levofloxacin

B. Reassurance, conservative measures, acetaminophen 500 mg every 6 hours for headache push fluids, strict return precautions

C. CXR, rapid influenza test, empiric oseltamivir

D. Sinus computed tomography (CT) scan, levofloxacin

E. Lumbar puncture, admission with ceftriaxone, ampicillin, acyclovir, fluconazole

Correct answer: C.

The Infectious Disease Society of America (IDSA) guidelines recommend that clinicians consider influenza for all patients with acute onset of fever and respiratory symptoms during the influenza season.[11] The IDSA does not have a unique diagnostic algorithm for immunosuppressed patients during or outside of the influenza season, but does warn that chronically ill/immunosuppressed patients could present atypically and have more severe consequences of infection with influenza.[11] Otherwise healthy patients can forgo diagnostic testing and be treated empirically if they present for care

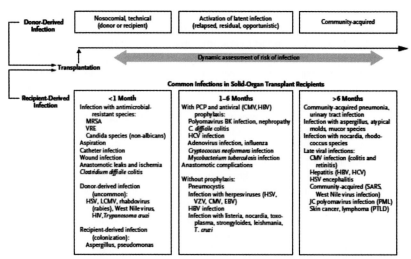

Fig. 2. Changing timeline of infection after organ transplantation. Infections occur in a generally predictable pattern after solid organ transplantation. The development of infection is delayed by prophylaxis and accelerated by intensified immunosuppression, drug toxic effects that may cause leukopenia, or immunomodulatory viral infections such as infection with cytomegalovirus (CMV), hepatitis C virus (HCV), or Epstein-Barr virus (EBV). At the time of transplantation, a patient's short-term and long-term risk of infection can be stratified according to donor and recipient screening, the technical outcome of surgery, and the intensity of immunosuppression required to prevent graft rejection. Subsequently, an ongoing assessment of the risk of infection is used to adjust both prophylaxis and immunosuppressive therapy. HBV, hepatitis B virus; HIV, human immunodeficiency virus; HSV, herpes simplex virus; LCMV, lymphocytic choriomeningitis virus; MRSA, methicillin-resistant *Staphylococcus aureus*; PCP, *Pneumocystis carinii* pneumonia; PML, progressive multifocal leukoencephalopathy; PTLD, posttransplantation lymphoproliferative disorder; SARS, severe acute respiratory syndrome; VZV, varicella zoster virus; VRE, vancomycin-resistant *Enterococcus faecalis*. (*From* Fishman JA. Infection in solid-organ transplant recipients. N Engl J Med 2007;357(25):2601–1; with permission. Copyright © 2007 Massachusetts Medical Society.)

within 48 to 72 hours of the onset of symptoms, but SOT patients should be approached differently.

Although the rate of influenza infection in SOT patients appears to be similar to the general population (2%–4% in SOT vs 3%–5% in the general population), the severity of infections is higher.[12] The type of organ transplant may influence the risk of complications. Lung transplant recipients are most vulnerable, followed by liver, then kidney transplant patients.[13] Whereas healthy patients typically shed the virus 1 day prior and up to 1 week following the onset of symptoms, SOT patients can be infectious for weeks to months because of their inability to clear the virus,[14] and are more likely to present with atypical symptoms including no or only a low-grade fever (50%–80% of SOT patients with influenza present with fever). Hence, symptoms of rhinorrhea, dry cough, sore throat, or gastrointestinal symptoms of stomach upset and diarrhea commonly seen in noninfluenza respiratory or gastrointestinal viral infections may be the only presenting symptoms of influenza. When fever is present in the setting of symptoms of upper respiratory tract infection, it is a very predictive sign for influenza in SOT patients.[12]

SOT patients are more prone to develop lower respiratory tract infections, including influenza pneumonia (47% of hospitalized SOT patients), secondary bacterial pneumonia (*Streptococcus* and *Staphylococcus*, 17% of hospitalized SOT patients), other bacterial superinfections, and extrarespiratory manifestations such as central nervous system or myocardial involvement.[12] As a result, SOT patients may require hospitalization and aggressive management of influenza infection more commonly than immunocompetent patients.

Whereas empiric therapy or supportive therapy alone is acceptable in many otherwise healthy ambulatory patients, SOT patients benefit from specific identification of the pathogen(s). Immunocompetent patients should be tested as soon as symptoms begin, ideally within less than 5 days. However, regardless of the timing of symptom onset, it is appropriate to test SOT patients for influenza when the suspicion arises. Whereas nasopharyngeal washes and aspirates are superior in immunocompetent patients, upper and lower respiratory tract specimens can be helpful in SOT patients.[11]

What is the appropriate workup of transplant patients suspected of influenza?

Rapid antigen tests have limited sensitivity for the diagnosis of influenza, and a negative test does not exclude the diagnosis. More sensitive tests such as respiratory virus PCR panels are becoming the gold standard at many laboratories. These tests are appropriate for use in symptomatic patients but can cause confusion by identifying multiple viruses in asymptomatic patients, making it difficult to determine if the identified viruses are pathogens. If patients have lower respiratory tract symptoms or clinical or radiographic evidence of lower tract infection, they should undergo bronchoscopy with testing.[12] For more information on testing, the reader is advised to visit the seasonal flu Web site of the Centers for Disease Control and Prevention: (http://www.cdc.gov/flu/professionals/diagnosis/labprocedures.htm).

Because of increasing resistance patterns to M2 inhibitors such as amantadine in influenza A and H1N1, neuraminidase inhibitors such as oral oseltamivir and inhaled zanamivir are considered the first-line therapy. The optimal duration of therapy is not well defined. In immunocompetent individuals the typical course is 5 days. However, SOT patients can continue to shed the virus for a longer duration. Active treatment for 10 to 14 days with weekly PCR monitoring should be considered.[12] Given the higher rate of bacterial superinfection or coinfection, antibiotics should be considered, especially in SOT patients with lower respiratory infection symptoms, while awaiting results of diagnostic studies.

What is the best way to handle influenza vaccination in transplant patients?

SOT patients should be vaccinated with an inactivated influenza vaccine before and after transplantation. There is some controversy about the optimal timing of vaccination posttransplant, but the prudent approach is to vaccinate SOT patients as soon as the seasonal vaccine is available before influenza season. The efficacy of vaccination may be lower in SOT patients than in immunocompetent patients, but does appear to be safe. One study found that of the population of SOT patients diagnosed with influenza, 50% had received the vaccination and none of these patients had protective levels of antibodies against influenza at the time of admission. The same study showed that influenza vaccination decreased the risk of associated pneumonia (relative risk 0.3) in comparison with SOT patients who were not immunized.[15] There is no evidence that additional benefit is gained from high-dose vaccines or intradermal inoculation. The live attenuated nasal vaccine is contraindicated in immunocompromised persons, including those who have received a SOT. Evidence does not show an increased risk for graft rejection or failure with influenza vaccination.[16]

Case 2

A 52-year-old woman 3.5 months status post living-related kidney transplant presents to your clinic to reestablish care after her transplant. She reports 7 days of subjective fevers and a nonproductive cough. She has no rhinorrhea, sore throat, nausea, vomiting, diarrhea, or body ache, but she has had anorexia and some mild night sweats. She has had many well-wishers at her home since returning and suspects she could have had an infectious exposure. VS: T 38.1°C, HR 96, BP 132/90, RR 24, O_2 sat 94% on room air. On examination she is speaking in full sentences but looks tired. She has scattered shoddy cervical adenopathy, no nuchal rigidity, and some scattered inspiratory crackles bilaterally. There are wheezes, and her lungs are equally resonant on percussion. Her heart is regular without a murmur, she has a reassuring soft abdominal examination, and her transplant kidney is nontender on palpation.

Allergies: sulfamethoxazole

CXR: bilateral nodular infiltrates

Which management strategy would you choose?

A. Empiric treatment with azithromycin, calculate CURB-65 and if less than 2, treat as an outpatient with 1 week follow-up

B. Admit for workup including CT scan and likely bronchoscopy

C. Empiric treatment with levofloxacin, calculate CURB-65 and if less than 2, treat was an outpatient with 1 week follow-up

D. Empiric treatment with azithromycin and oseltamivir, calculate CURB-65 and if less than 2, treat as an outpatient

Correct answer: B.

The differential diagnosis for nodular infiltrates in SOT patients includes:

- Fungal infections (*Aspergillus, Cryptococcus*)
- Mycobacterial infections (*Mycobacterium tuberculosis, Mycobacterium avium intracellulare complex*)
- Bacterial infections (*Nocardia, Legionella, Rhodococcus equi*)
- Malignancy (lymphoma)

Features of this case that mandate an aggressive diagnostic evaluation include immunosuppression, onset within the posttransplant period at highest risk for opportunistic infection, and the nodular nature of the pulmonary infiltrates.

Community-acquired pneumonia (CAP) in SOT patients is common (3 times higher incidence than in immunocompetent individuals) and dangerous (11%–43% mortality rate).[17,18] A Canadian case-control study found that immunosuppressive medications increased the risk for CAP, with an odds ratio of 15.[17] Despite the uniquely higher risk facing SOT patients, the IDSA and the American Thoracic Society (ATS) do not specifically consider immunosuppressed patients in their consensus guidelines for CAP. Rather, the guidelines address CAP and separate guidelines address nosocomial pneumonia (recent hospitalization or institutional settings).[19] For this patient, the presentation in the 3- to 6-month posttransplant period increases her risk for opportunistic infections, given the effects of longer duration and higher dose of immunosuppressive medications. Viral infections such as CMV and respiratory viruses can cause primary lung infections during this time, and can also complicate matters by further decreasing immunity and increasing the risk for opportunistic infections such as *Aspergillus fumigatus* and PJP.[10]

Causes of CAP in immunocompromised patients, in order of frequency, are[17]:

- *Streptococcus pneumoniae*
- *Legionella pneumophila*
- *Haemophilus influenzae*
- Gram-negative rods (GNRs): *Pseudomonas aeruginosa*
- *Nocardia* spp
- *Staphylococcus aureus*
- Viral (influenza, respiratory syncytial virus)

ATS and IDSA recommend the use of assessment tools of pneumonia severity to determine the appropriate care setting: ambulatory, inpatient, or ICU. CURB-65 is a recommended tool that gives 1 point for Confusion, Uremia, Respiratory rate greater than 30/min, Blood pressure less than 90 mm Hg, and age 65 or older. A score greater than or equal to 2 on CURB-65 should spur providers to consider hospitalizing patients. The pneumonia severity index (PSI) is the other recommended tool, and has 11 initial elements to the assessment. If patients have any of the 11 elements they are risk stratified into 4 higher-risk classes that correlate to 30-day mortality risk, as does CURB-65.[19] PSI has a higher discriminatory power and is more accurate in lower-risk patients. Neither tool specifically considers immunosuppression or SOT as a risk factor for severe disease. Hence, it is important for PCPs to use such tools with caution in SOT patients. Current guidelines recommend these tools be used for supplemental data, and that the physician's determination of the patient's global risk be the primary determinant of the treatment plan.[19]

In SOT patients with lower respiratory symptoms of cough, dyspnea, increased respiratory rate, or fever, testing should include complete blood count, chemistry panel, blood cultures, sputum culture, and a chest radiograph. Although chest radiographs have lower sensitivity in immunosuppressed people, the pattern of disease on radiography can still be helpful. Focal airspace disease is correlated with bacterial (and mycobacterial) pneumonia. Multifocal airspace disease and nodular infiltrates have a much broader differential (as discussed earlier). Diffuse and interstitial patterns are concerning for pneumocystis or viral infections. In immunocompromised patients with pulmonary infiltrates, chest CT scan and bronchoscopy have clearly shown benefit in distinguishing among infectious and noninfectious causes.[20,21]

Consensus guidelines recommend empiric treatment with institutionally tailored antibiotic choices that should reflect the resistance in the community. PCPs should not delay empiric therapy while waiting for testing. Usual choices of a respiratory fluoroquinolone, macrolides, or broader-spectrum β-lactams + a macrolide are also reasonable empiric therapy for SOT patients.[19] Depending on clinical presentation, severity scores, reliability and level of home support, some patients can be treated as an outpatient with very close follow-up, whereas others need to be managed in the inpatient setting. Hospitalizing immunosuppressed SOT patients and putting them at risk for nosocomial infections is an important consideration. Early consultation with pulmonary and infectious disease specialists, very close follow-up, and rapid escalation of the intensity of both diagnostic and therapeutic efforts depending on response are appropriate.

Regarding follow-up, because this patient is in the highest-risk time frame for opportunistic infections, and has nodular infiltrates on her chest radiograph conferring a broader range and possibly higher-risk situation, an infectious disease consultation should be initiated as well as hospitalization for intensified diagnostic and therapeutic interventions. Typically recommended regimens for CAP requiring hospitalization (ceftriaxone + azithromycin, respiratory fluoroquinolone) would not be active against the cause of this patient's pneumonia.

Nocardia was diagnosed on Gram stain (beaded, branching, filamentous gram-positive rod) and culture of a bronchial alveolar lavage (BAL) sample. Invasive procedures are often necessary to make the diagnosis of pulmonary nocardosis (44% in one study).[22] *Nocardia* is a soil-borne bacterium that more commonly presents as an opportunistic infection in immunosuppressed patients, although it can cause self-limited indolent disease in immunocompetent patients. SOT patients are particularly vulnerable when their T-cell immunity is suppressed, often when corticosteroid doses are higher.[23] Because *Nocardia* has a propensity to disseminate to other sites (brain, bones, skin), the patient should be carefully clinically assessed for these complications, with further imaging clinically appropriate. The primary treatment is typically with sulfamethoxazole-based antibiotics. This patient had no evidence of dissemination outside her lungs and was treated with imipenem initially, given her sulfamethoxazole allergy, then converted to linezolid orally for 6 months.

Case 3

A 48-year-old woman, 2 years post liver transplant for autoimmune hepatitis, presents with watery, profuse diarrhea for 3 days, resulting in 3 lb (1.36 kg) of unintentional weight loss. She reports no nausea, vomiting, blood in the stool, or tenesmus, but has had a low-grade fever. She has no recent travel, change in her medications, or unusual or risky food ingestions or sexual behavior. However, on further questioning she is a girl-scout leader for her 10-year-old daughter's group, and they recently had a day outing to a local water park. On examination she is tired, without jaundice. VS: T 38.1°C, HR 95, BP 110/65. Her abdominal examination is minimally tender without guarding or rigidity, and her liver is nontender on examination.

What testing would you pursue?

A. None indicated. Treat her with supportive therapy as she has no blood, or severe VS abnormality.

B. Ova and parasite stool sample × 3

C. Enteric pathogen stool culture

D. Enteric pathogens, *Clostridia difficile*, *Giardia* and *Cryptosporidium*, *Isospora*, *Cyclospora* × 3

Correct answer: D.

Diarrhea is a common symptom in both the general and SOT populations. Noninfectious and infectious causes are prevalent, but morbidity and mortality in susceptible immunocompromised SOT patients is much higher.[24] SOT patients can present with infectious causes of diarrhea, with acute onset and chronic presentations. The differential diagnosis favors infectious causes, then medication side effects, and in the setting of prolonged immunosuppression, posttransplant lymphoproliferative disease (PTLD) should be considered.[24] Unlike in stem cell transplant recipients, graft-versus-host disease is an uncommon reason for diarrhea following solid organ transplantation. CMV, *C difficile*, and bacterial pathogens are common infectious causes; parasitic infections are less common (**Table 1**).[25]

C difficile–associated diarrhea (CDAD) is the most common nosocomial antibiotic-associated diarrhea in SOT populations.[26] In the general population we worry about risk factors such as hospitalizations, gastrointestinal surgery, advanced age, uremia, and multiple comorbidities. Most cases of CDAD in SOT patients occur during the first 3 months, owing to associated risk factors of prolonged hospitalization, prolonged

Table 1	
Differential diagnosis of diarrhea in SOT patients	
Infectious	
Viral	Cytomegalovirus, rotavirus, norovirus, herpesviruses, adenovirus
Bacterial	*Escherichia coli* (shiga toxin–producing strains), *Salmonella, Shigella, Clostridium difficile, Yersinia, Campylobacter, Vibrio*
Parasite	Cryptosporidia, *Isospora, Cyclospora, Giardia*
Fungal	Microsporidia
Noninfectious	
Medications	Antibiotics, azathioprine, mycophenolate mofetil, sirolimus, tacrolimus
Other	Idiopathic enteritis or colitis, inflammatory bowel disease, posttransplant lymphoproliferative disease, graft-vs-host disease

antibiotic exposure, and the intensity of immunosuppression. Late-onset CDAD in SOT can happen months to years after transplantation, and is associated with intensification of immunosuppression to address rejection or antibiotic exposure.[9,26] The presentation can vary from mild diarrhea to life-threatening sepsis.

A prospective Canadian study of more than 1300 SOT patients found that the incidence of CDAD increased from 4.5% in 1999 to 21% in 2005, and with interventions decreased to 9.5% in 2010. The study showed that CDAD resulting in graft loss, colectomy, or death was more likely in those with a white blood cell count of greater than 25,000, and the finding of pancolitis on CT scan. The presence of both conferred an increased risk for these complicated events by 42%. In such patients, disease progressed despite timely and appropriate antimicrobial therapy.[26] PCPs should be aggressive in their approach to diagnosis and treatment of SOT patients with suspected CDAD and should have a low threshold for hospitalizing SOT patients for expedited care.

Recommendations for diagnostic testing and the initial treatment of acute diarrhea, including *C difficile*, have been previously published. IDSA guidelines specifically consider immunosuppression for diarrhea lasting 7 days or more. However, SOT patients are at higher risk than immunocompetent populations, and for acute diarrhea, regardless of duration, providers should have a high suspicion of bacterial, viral, and parasitic causes.[24] The unique risks in SOT (chronic immunosuppression, medications that commonly cause diarrhea, risk of exposure to antibiotics) can make finding a diagnosis a complex process. Endoscopy with biopsy should be considered in those with a negative noninvasive evaluation. Reported rates of abnormality on colonoscopy and histology range from 20% to 40%, but only 10% of colonoscopy findings lead to a change in medical management.[25]

Regarding follow-up, this patient was diagnosed with cryptosporidiosis via special staining and PCR of a fresh stool sample. Supportive therapy and antimotility agents were initiated alongside a cautious reduction in immunosuppression.

Cryptosporidium is a fecal-orally transmitted, water-borne protozoan found worldwide, including in the United States. It is a highly resistant parasite whose oocysts can survive for 3 to 10 days in water despite appropriate levels of iodine and chlorine treatment.[27] Water-borne outbreaks of cryptosporidiosis have been traced to water parks and public fountains. Food-borne outbreaks have also been linked to infected food handlers and unpasteurized apple cider, and person-to-person contact has been described at daycare centers.[27] Whereas it can cause self-limited mild diarrhea in the general population, in children and immunocompromised people

---

Box 2
Diarrhea pearls

- Routine diagnostic studies for the workup of diarrhea in the general population should be used for SOT patients but, if the etiology remains obscure and symptoms persist, meticulously assess for viral, bacterial, and parasitic infections including abdominal imaging and colonoscopy.

- Consider *C difficile* in patients with risk factors, even for community-acquired diarrhea.

- Consider cryptosporidiosis in SOT patients with a history of travel or exposures to water parks.

- *Cryptosporidium* can shed oocysts intermittently, so serial testing on 3 separate days is appropriate. Providers should ask specifically for *Cryptosporidium* testing, as it may not be included on standard ova and parasite testing.

- Immunosuppressive medications may cause diarrhea. Monitor immunosuppressive levels closely, and proactively adjust doses to avoid related toxicities.

- Hand washing with water and soap is an important preventive strategy. Many causes of infectious diarrhea (rotavirus, norovirus, *Cryptosporidium*) are not effectively killed with alcohol-based hand sanitizers.

---

cryptosporidiosis can cause severe and prolonged diarrhea. A literature review showed *Cryptosporidium* to be an important cause of more severe infectious diarrhea in the SOT population; this is especially true for children with SOT or recipients of intestinal grafts. A retrospective cohort found an increased risk for cryptosporidiosis in men, and in those with a longer duration of diarrheal symptoms and increased tacrolimus (TAC) levels. Cases of cryptosporidiosis that were associated with higher TAC levels also correlated with a self-limited but important increase in creatinine (**Box 2**).[28]

UTIs are very common in adult renal, and kidney-pancreas (K-P) transplant patients (6%–86%),[29,30] being reported in up to 40% of pediatric renal SOT patients.[31] UTIs also affect other SOT recipients but typically occur in the first month posttransplant, owing to the inherent risks of urinary catheterization.[29] In nonrenal SOT patients risk

---

Case 4

A 37-year-old woman with history of renal transplant 5 months ago and history of recurrent urinary tract infections presents with concern for a urinary tract infection (UTI). She endorses 2 days of frequency, urgency, and dysuria. She is mildly nauseated but has no chills, vomiting, or flank pain. She thinks her urine is mildly malodorous and cloudy. Her medications include tacrolimus, prednisone, mycophenolate mofetil, amlodipine, and trimethoprim/sulfamethoxazole SS as pneumocystis prophylaxis. VS: T 38.2°C, HR 88, BP 115/70. She appears well, has no rash or flank tenderness, she has mild tenderness over her surgical site and transplanted kidney, and in the suprapubic area. Her urine dipstick is positive for leukocyte esterase and nitrites.

In addition to sending urinalysis and urine culture, you should treat her empirically with:

A. Nitrofurantoin ER

B. Trimethoprim/sulfamethoxazole DS

C. Ciprofloxacin

D. Fosfomycin

E. Amoxicillin

Correct answer: C.

factors include female gender, increased age, and diabetes. In renal and K-P transplant patients, the risk or UTI is high for the first year after transplantation. Risk factors include a history of posttransplant dialysis, age, and female gender.[29] Factors that may increase the risk for recurrent UTI include ureteric stricture, vesicoureteral reflux, prolonged urinary catheterization, and overimmunosuppression.[29]

UTIs occur at higher frequency with increased morbidity in renal transplant recipients. Studies are mixed, and have not convincingly demonstrated an increased risk for graft rejection or increased mortality due to UTIs.[29,31,32] Whereas some studies have found that specific immunosuppressive regimens and intensity of immunosuppression appear to increase the risk of UTIs, other studies do not support the notion that UTIs are opportunistic infections in SOT patients. Rather, the increased risk is thought to be due to other factors (**Table 2**) and posttransplant anatomic changes that effectively define all UTIs in renal transplant patients as "complicated UTIs."[29,30]

Asymptomatic bacteriuria (ASB) without signs and symptoms of infection is common in renal transplant patients. ASB has been associated with increased risk for UTI in the first year, but significant controversy exists about whether it should be treated within that time frame.[33] Candiduria is common, affecting up to 10% of renal transplant patients, but it is mostly asymptomatic.[33] The approach to asymptomatic candiduria is also controversial, given the paucity of available data on this topic. No convincing data exist to show that graft survival, morbidity, or mortality improves with treatment of asymptomatic candiduria in kidney transplant patients.[33]

The diagnosis of cystitis is the same in SOT patients as it is for the general population. The important caveats are that urine culture should be obtained in all SOT patients given the higher risk of multidrug-resistant bacterial infections, and that upper tract (ie, kidney allograft) infections are very common in kidney transplant recipients. Pyelonephritis should be considered in kidney transplant patients with signs/symptoms of cystitis accompanied by fever, bacteremia, increased creatinine, leukocytosis, chills, or pain/tenderness over the transplanted kidney.[29]

Table 2
Major risk factors for bacterial urinary tract infection and pyelonephritis in renal transplant recipients

Risk Factor[Refs]	OR (95% CI)
Bacterial urinary tract infection[13,24,54,57]	
Female gender	5.8 (3.79–8.89)
Age (per year)	0.02 (1.01–1.04)
Reflux kidney disease before transplantation	3.0 (1.05–8.31)
Deceased donor	3.64 (1.0–12.7)
Duration of bladder catheterization	1.50 (1.1–1.9)
Length of hospitalization before UTI	0.92 (0.88–0.96)
Increase in immunosuppression	17.04 (4.0–71.5)
Acute pyelonephritis[4,25]	
Female gender	5.14 (1.86–14.20)
Acute rejection episodes	3.84 (1.37–10.79)
Number of UTIs	1.17 (1.06–1.30)
Mycophenolate mofetil	1.9 (1.2–2.3)

Abbreviations: CI, confidence interval; OR, odds ratio; UTI, urinary tract infection.
Data from Rice J, Safdar N. Urinary tract infections in solid organ transplant recipients. Am J Transplant 2009;9(Suppl 4):S267–72.

Many transplant centers use trimethoprim/sulfamethoxazole as prophylaxis against *Pneumocystis* in renal transplant patients during the first 6 to 12 months after transplantation, and this appears to also decrease the risk of UTI. However, this has also been associated with breakthrough infections caused by trimethoprim/sulfamethoxazole-resistant organisms. Long-term prophylaxis has been shown to decrease the incidence of UTI, although the growing resistance to trimethoprim/sulfamethoxazole among GNRs, reportedly more than 80% in some settings, limits the utility of long-term antibiotic prophylaxis.[29,33]

A multicenter, prospective cohort study followed 4000 SOT patients over 2 years of follow-up, during which 208 episodes of UTI occurred in renal transplant recipients. The vast majority were due to GNRs (>50% *Escherichia coli*, 10% *Pseudomonas aeruginosa* and *Klebsiella pneumoniae*, 6% other gram negatives) and only 7% due to *Enterococcus* species.[29] Several studies also identify *Staphylococcus* species as common pathogens in renal SOT patients.[30,33] An alarming amount of antibiotic resistance was observed, with more than one-quarter identified as extended-spectrum β-lactamase resistance (ESBL). Carbapenem-resistant *Klebsiella*, *Pseudomonas aeruginosa*, and vancomycin-resistant *Enterococcus* are all increasing in frequency.[34]

Regarding follow-up, this patient has typical symptoms of cystitis; however, she also has tenderness over her transplanted kidney and fever, suggesting associated allograft pyelonephritis. It is inappropriate to use antibiotics that are effective only for lower UTIs (eg, nitrofurantoin and fosfomycin). The infection has occurred while receiving prophylactic trimethoprim/sulfamethoxazole, making this inappropriate empiric therapy. Despite evidence of growing resistance in some strains, fluoroquinolones remain a reasonable option for empiric therapy.[29] However, at centers with high rates of resistance to fluoroquinolones, treatment with broader-spectrum antibiotics might be appropriate. Other common pathogens causing cystitis/graft pyelonephritis in kidney transplant patients include *Enterococcus* and *Pseudomonas*.

Clinically stable SOT patients without signs of sepsis but with evidence of cystitis can be appropriately managed in the ambulatory setting. However, any concern for graft pyelonephritis should trigger hospitalization and further evaluation. The rate of predisposing anatomic abnormalities is relatively high in kidney transplant recipients with graft pyelonephritis, so further diagnostic workup typically includes CT imaging of the kidneys and/or urological evaluation (for structural or functional abnormalities).[30]

Case 5

A 48-year-old woman with history of renal transplant 6 years ago requests a routine preventive care examination. In addition to her usual SOT monitoring, she also requests "booster" shots of any vaccinations you recommend.

Past immunization history: influenza last year, Td 3 years ago, standard childhood vaccinations.

You recommend:

A. Intramuscular influenza vaccination only

B. Td only

C. Flumist (nasal flu vaccine), check titers for tetanus and diphtheria, and revaccinate if low

D. Yearly influenza vaccination, pneumococcal vaccination with pneumococcal vaccine 13 (PCV13) then pneumococcal polysaccharide vaccine 23 (PPSV23), one-time Tdap (tetanus, diphtheria, acellular pertussis)

Correct answer: D.

As more SOT patients are living longer, PCPs should be prepared to address preventive care concerns. This section focuses on vaccine preventive care issues unique to the infectious risks facing SOT patients, and does not cover noninfectious preventive care.

The key pearls for vaccination in SOT patients are that in general, live vaccines are contraindicated posttransplant, and that the immunologic response to routine vaccinations may be diminished, especially in the first 3 to 6 months after transplantation.[35] This situation suggests that PCPs must be proactive; if a patient's chronic disease condition progresses on a path toward possible SOT, then appropriate live vaccinations (this may include measles, mumps, rubella, zoster, and varicella) should be administered pretransplant, before the patient is immunosuppressed. The American Society of Transplantation (AST) 2009 guidelines recommend that any live vaccines be administered at least 4 weeks before transplant.[36] Even inactivated/killed vaccinations should be considered pretransplant when possible, because of the anticipated better response rate. Although end-stage chronic illnesses that necessitate SOT might be associated with reduced immune response to vaccinations, immunologic response to vaccinations is thought to be even further suppressed in the posttransplant period.[35]

Influenza

Three of 4 studies on the response to vaccination to influenza in SOT patients reported significantly reduced protective titers in comparison with normal controls. Lower responses were correlated to SOT patients on combination immunosuppressive therapy. Specifically, mycophenolate mofetil (MMF) and cyclosporine were implicated.[37] Given the substantial morbidity and mortality associated with influenza in immunosuppressed populations, yearly inactivated influenza vaccination is recommended.[35] Live attenuated influenza vaccine is contraindicated in SOT patients.

Pneumococcal

SOT patients are at higher risk than the general population for invasive pneumococcal infections.[8] Although pneumococcal vaccination has been shown to be safe in SOT patients, response rates to vaccination are reduced, ranging from 13% to 50% depending on the serotype measured.[38] Major guidelines (AST, ACIP) recommend pneumococcal vaccination in immunosuppressed patients, including those who have received a solid organ transplant, and recent updated guidelines that incorporate both the polysaccharide and conjugate vaccines have recently been published.[39]

- Vaccine-naïve SOT patients are advised to have PCV13 followed by PCV23 8 weeks later.
- In SOT patients who have previously received PPSV23, a dose of PCV13 should be given at least 1 year after the dose of PCV23.
- SOT patients younger than 65 years should have a repeat PPSV23 at 5 years, and those vaccinated before age 65 should have a repeat PCV23 at 65 or 5 years after the first dose.

Tetanus/Diphtheria/Pertussis

Immunologic response to tetanus is close to normal in SOT patients, and should be repeated every 10 years as per IDSA/ACIP guidelines. Diphtheria immunity wanes significantly even after the first year, but current guidelines do not recommend checking titers for diphtheria.[36] A single booster dose of pertussis vaccine (Tdap) should be given to adults older than 19 years.[35,40]

Human Papilloma Virus

The human papilloma virus (HPV) vaccine has not been well studied in SOT patients. It is not a live vaccine and should therefore theoretically be safe in the posttransplant population. The indications for HPV vaccination are similar to those in non-SOT patients.[36,40]

It is safe to give hepatitis A and B, meningococcal, and *H influenzae* B vaccinations after transplant in patients with indications. The first 6 months after SOT, when immunosuppression is at its peak, is not the ideal time for vaccination administration because the immunologic response is significantly diminished.[35]

Because household/other close contacts are presumed to be a primary source for many important infections, it is important for PCPs to counsel SOT patients' families and close contacts on the importance for them to be appropriately immunized. PCPs should add this to their list of annual preventive care reminders for their SOT patients (**Table 3**).

The risk for cervical cancer is reportedly increased (up to 11-fold) in immunosuppressed patients in comparison with the general population.[41] As such, the recommendation from the United States Preventive Task Force Service (USPSTF) and the American College of Obstetrics and Gynecology is for yearly Papanicolaou smear and pelvic examination for cervical cancer screening in immunosuppressed patients.[42,43] However, this practice is best supported for people immunosuppressed

Table 3
Vaccination recommendations in adults with SOT, and household contacts, before and after solid organ transplantation

Vaccination	SOT Recipients		Household Contacts	
	Pre	Post	Pre	Post
Inactive				
Influenza	Yes	Yes	Yes	Yes
Hepatitis A	Yes	Yes	Yes	Yes
Hepatitis B	Yes	Yes	Yes	Yes
Td	Yes	Yes	Yes	Yes
Tdap	Yes	Yes	Yes	Yes
Streptococcus pneumoniae	Yes	Yes	Yes	Yes
Haemophilus influenzae[a]	Yes	Yes	Yes	Yes
Human papilloma virus[a]	Yes	Yes	Yes	Yes
Polio (inactive)[a]	Yes	Yes	Yes	Yes
Neisseria meningitides[a]	Yes	Yes	Yes	Yes
Live Attenuated				
Influenza (nasal)		No	Yes	No
Varicella (Varivax)[a]	Yes	No	Yes	Yes
Varicella (Zostavax)[a]	Yes	No	Yes	Yes
Measles[a]	Yes	No	Yes	Yes
Mumps[a]	Yes	No	Yes	Yes
Rubella[a]	Yes	No	Yes	Yes

[a] Optional based on risk factors.

Adapted from ATS 2009 immunization guidelines for SOT, ATS 2009 immunization guidelines for household members of SOT.

by HIV infection. The evidence that HPV causes cervical cancer is excellent, and the increased risk of cervical cancer evidenced in HIV immunosuppression has been extrapolated to apply to SOT patients. However, in 2011 Engels and colleagues[44] evaluated data from a United States registry of more than 400,000 SOT patients and found no increased risk of cervical cancer. In addition, a 10-year prospective case-control study of 48 renal and K-P SOT patients showed no increased risk of cervical cancer in the SOT patients.[45]

Despite the emerging data that immunosuppression in SOT recipients might not necessarily increase the risk of cervical cancer, at present PCPs should follow updated USPSTF cervical cancer screening guidelines from 2012, which explicitly exclude immunosuppressed patients from lengthening the screening interval beyond 1 year.[43]

SUMMARY

SOT recipients need PCPs who are familiar with their unique needs. Understanding the lifelong infectious risks faced by SOT patients because of their need for lifelong immunosuppressive medications is fundamental. SOT recipients can present with atypical and muted manifestations of infections. The savvy, prepared PCP will keep a careful eye on the patient and initiate a comprehensive evaluation for infectious etiology. PCPs should work together with their local (infectious disease and other) specialists to generate care plans if the diagnosis or management is in question.

REFERENCES

1. Lodhi SA, Lamb KE, Meier-Kriesche HU. Solid organ allograft survival improvement in the United States: the long-term does not mirror the dramatic short-term success. Am J Transplant 2011;11(6):1226–35. http://dx.doi.org/10.1111/j.1600-6143.2011.03539.x.
2. GKT1 activities and practices. World Health Organization Web site. Available at: http://www.who.int/transplantation/gkt/statistics/en/. Accessed November 14, 2012.
3. Wolfe RA, Roys EC, Merion RM. Trends in organ donation and transplantation in the United States, 1999-2008. Am J Transplant 2010;10(4 Pt 2):961–72. http://dx.doi.org/10.1111/j.1600-6143.2010.03021.x.
4. Cervera C, Fernandez-Ruiz M, Valledor A, et al. Epidemiology and risk factors for late infection in solid organ transplant recipients. Transpl Infect Dis 2011;13(6): 598–607. http://dx.doi.org/10.1111/j.1399-3062.2011.00646.x.
5. Fishman JA. Infection in solid-organ transplant recipients. N Engl J Med 2007; 357(25):2601–14. http://dx.doi.org/10.1056/NEJMra064928.
6. Kale MS, Bishop TF, Federman AD, et al. Trends in the overuse of ambulatory health care services in the United States. Arch Intern Med 2012;1–7. http://dx.doi.org/10.1001/2013.jamainternmed.1022.
7. Fishman JA. Infections in immunocompromised hosts and organ transplant recipients: essentials. Liver Transpl 2011;17(Suppl 3):S34–7. http://dx.doi.org/10.1002/lt.22378.
8. Kumar D, Humar A, Plevneshi A, et al. Invasive pneumococcal disease in solid organ transplant recipients—10-year prospective population surveillance. Am J Transplant 2007;7(5):1209–14. http://dx.doi.org/10.1111/j.1600-6143.2006.01705.x.
9. Fishman JA, Greenwald MA, Grossi PA. Transmission of infection with human allografts: essential considerations in donor screening. Clin Infect Dis 2012;55(5): 720–7. http://dx.doi.org/10.1093/cid/cis519.

10. Hoyo I, Sanclemente G, Cervera C, et al. Opportunistic pulmonary infections in solid organ transplant recipients. Transplant Proc 2012;44(9):2673–5. http://dx.doi.org/10.1016/j.transproceed.2012.09.067.

11. Harper SA, Bradley JS, Englund JA, et al. Seasonal influenza in adults and children—diagnosis, treatment, chemoprophylaxis, and institutional outbreak management: clinical practice guidelines of the Infectious Diseases Society of America. Clin Infect Dis 2009;48(8):1003–32. http://dx.doi.org/10.1086/598513.

12. Weigt SS, Gregson AL, Deng JC, et al. Respiratory viral infections in hematopoietic stem cell and solid organ transplant recipients. Semin Respir Crit Care Med 2011;32(4):471–93. http://dx.doi.org/10.1055/s-0031-1283286.

13. Gainer SM, Patel SJ, Seethamraju H, et al. Increased mortality of solid organ transplant recipients with H1N1 infection: a single center experience. Clin Transplant 2012;26(2):229–37. http://dx.doi.org/10.1111/j.1399-0012.2011.01443.x.

14. Martin ST, Torabi MJ, Gabardi S. Influenza in solid organ transplant recipients. Ann Pharmacother 2012;46(2):255–64. http://dx.doi.org/10.1345/aph.1Q436.

15. Perez-Romero P, Aydillo TA, Perez-Ordonez A, et al. Reduced incidence of pneumonia in influenza-vaccinated solid organ transplant recipients with influenza disease. Clin Microbiol Infect 2012;18(12):E533–40. http://dx.doi.org/10.1111/1469-0691.12044.

16. Avery RK. Influenza vaccines in the setting of solid-organ transplantation: are they safe? Curr Opin Infect Dis 2012;25(4):464–8. http://dx.doi.org/10.1097/QCO.0b013e328355a79b.

17. Sousa D, Justo I, Dominguez A, et al. Community-acquired pneumonia in immunocompromised older patients: incidence, causative organisms and outcome. Clin Microbiol Infect 2012. http://dx.doi.org/10.1111/j.1469-0691.2012.03765.x.

18. Cervera C, Agusti C, Angeles Marcos M, et al. Microbiologic features and outcome of pneumonia in transplanted patients. Diagn Microbiol Infect Dis 2006;55(1):47–54. http://dx.doi.org/10.1016/j.diagmicrobio.2005.10.014.

19. Mandell LA, Wunderink RG, Anzueto A, et al. Infectious Diseases Society of America/American Thoracic Society consensus guidelines on the management of community-acquired pneumonia in adults. Clin Infect Dis 2007;44(Suppl 2): S27–72. http://dx.doi.org/10.1086/511159.

20. Ramirez P, Valencia M, Torres A. Bronchoalveolar lavage to diagnose respiratory infections. Semin Respir Crit Care Med 2007;28(5):525–33. http://dx.doi.org/10.1055/s-2007-991524.

21. Waite S, Jeudy J, White CS. Acute lung infections in normal and immunocompromised hosts. Radiol Clin North Am 2006;44(2):295–315. http://dx.doi.org/10.1016/j.rcl.2005.10.009, ix.

22. Georghiou PR, Blacklock ZM. Infection with Nocardia species in Queensland. A review of 102 clinical isolates. Med J Aust 1992;156(10):692–7.

23. Tan CK, Lai CC, Lin SH, et al. Clinical and microbiological characteristics of nocardiosis including those caused by emerging Nocardia species in Taiwan, 1998-2008. Clin Microbiol Infect 2010;16(7):966–72. http://dx.doi.org/10.1111/j.1469-0691.2009.02950.x.

24. Krones E, Hogenauer C. Diarrhea in the immunocompromised patient. Gastroenterol Clin North Am 2012;41(3):677–701. http://dx.doi.org/10.1016/j.gtc.2012.06.009.

25. Rice JP, Spier BJ, Cornett DD, et al. Utility of colonoscopy in the evaluation of diarrhea in solid organ transplant recipients. Transplantation 2009;88(3):374–9. http://dx.doi.org/10.1097/TP.0b013e3181ae98ab.

26. Boutros M, Al-Shaibi M, Chan G, et al. *Clostridium difficile* colitis: increasing incidence, risk factors, and outcomes in solid organ transplant recipients. Transplantation 2012;93(10):1051–7. http://dx.doi.org/10.1097/TP.0b013e31824d34de.

27. Yoder JS, Wallace RM, Collier SA, et al. Centers for Disease Control and Prevention (CDC). Cryptosporidiosis surveillance—United States, 2009-2010. MMWR Surveill Summ 2012;61(5):1–12.

28. Bonatti H, Barroso Ii LF, Sawyer RG, et al. *Cryptosporidium enteritis* in solid organ transplant recipients: multicenter retrospective evaluation of 10 cases reveals an association with elevated tacrolimus concentrations. Transpl Infect Dis 2012; 14(6):635–48. http://dx.doi.org/10.1111/j.1399-3062.2012.00719.x.

29. Vidal E, Torre-Cisneros J, Blanes M, et al. Bacterial urinary tract infection after solid organ transplantation in the RESITRA cohort. Transpl Infect Dis 2012; 14(6):595–603. http://dx.doi.org/10.1111/j.1399-3062.2012.00744.x.

30. Saemann M, Horl WH. Urinary tract infection in renal transplant recipients. Eur J Clin Invest 2008;38(Suppl 2):58–65. http://dx.doi.org/10.1111/j.1365-2362.2008.02014.x.

31. Silva A, Rodig N, Passerotti CP, et al. Risk factors for urinary tract infection after renal transplantation and its impact on graft function in children and young adults. J Urol 2010;184(4):1462–7. http://dx.doi.org/10.1016/j.juro.2010.06.028.

32. Iqbal T, Naqvi R, Akhter SF. Frequency of urinary tract infection in renal transplant recipients and effect on graft function. J Pak Med Assoc 2010;60(10):826–9.

33. Rice JC, Safdar N, AST Infectious Diseases Community of Practice. Urinary tract infections in solid organ transplant recipients. Am J Transplant 2009;9(Suppl 4): S267–72. http://dx.doi.org/10.1111/j.1600-6143.2009.02919.x.

34. Neuner EA, Sekeres J, Hall GS, et al. Experience with fosfomycin for treatment of urinary tract infections due to multidrug-resistant organisms. Antimicrob Agents Chemother 2012;56(11):5744–8. http://dx.doi.org/10.1128/AAC.00402-12.

35. Masters JM, Thomsen AK, Hayney MS. Vaccinations in solid-organ transplant patients: what a health professional should know. J Am Pharm Assoc (2003) 2009; 49(3):458–9. http://dx.doi.org/10.1331/JAPhA.2009.09508.

36. Danzinger-Isakov L, Kumar D, AST Infectious Diseases Community of Practice. Guidelines for vaccination of solid organ transplant candidates and recipients. Am J Transplant 2009;9(Suppl 4):S258–62. http://dx.doi.org/10.1111/j.1600-6143.2009.02917.x.

37. Agarwal N, Ollington K, Kaneshiro M, et al. Are immunosuppressive medications associated with decreased responses to routine immunizations? A systematic review. Vaccine 2012;30(8):1413–24. http://dx.doi.org/10.1016/j.vaccine.2011.11.109.

38. Kumar D, Rotstein C, Miyata G, et al. Randomized, double-blind, controlled trial of pneumococcal vaccination in renal transplant recipients. J Infect Dis 2003; 187(10):1639–45. http://dx.doi.org/10.1086/374784.

39. Centers for Disease Control and Prevention (CDC). Use of 13-valent pneumococcal conjugate vaccine and 23-valent pneumococcal polysaccharide vaccine for adults with immunocompromising conditions: recommendations of the advisory committee on immunization practices (ACIP). MMWR Morb Mortal Wkly Rep 2012;61(40):816–9.

40. Avery RK, Michaels M. Update on immunizations in solid organ transplant recipients: what clinicians need to know. Am J Transplant 2008;8(1):9–14. http://dx.doi.org/10.1111/j.1600-6143.2007.02051.x.

41. Veroux M, Corona D, Scalia G, et al. Surveillance of human papilloma virus infection and cervical cancer in kidney transplant recipients: preliminary data. Transplant Proc 2009;41(4):1191–4. http://dx.doi.org/10.1016/j.transproceed.2009.03.015.

42. Wong G, Chapman JR, Craig JC. Cancer screening in renal transplant recipients: what is the evidence? Clin J Am Soc Nephrol 2008;3(Suppl 2):S87–100. http://dx.doi.org/10.2215/CJN.03320807.

43. Moyer VA, U.S. Preventive Services Task Force. Screening for cervical cancer: U.S. preventive services task force recommendation statement. Ann Intern Med 2012;156(12):880–91. http://dx.doi.org/10.7326/0003-4819-156-12-201206190-00424 W312.

44. Engels EA, Pfeiffer RM, Fraumeni JF Jr, et al. Spectrum of cancer risk among US solid organ transplant recipients. JAMA 2011;306(17):1891–901. http://dx.doi.org/10.1001/jama.2011.1592.

45. Origoni M, Stefani C, Dell'Antonio G, et al. Cervical human papillomavirus in transplanted Italian women: a long-term prospective follow-up study. J Clin Virol 2011;51(4):250–4. http://dx.doi.org/10.1016/j.jcv.2011.05.017.

Methicillin-Resistant
Staphylococcus aureus Infections

Paul S. Pottinger, MD

KEYWORDS

- MRSA • Methicillin-resistant *Staphylococcus aureus* • Community-acquired MRSA
- Vancomycin • Ceftaroline • Daptomycin • Linezolid

KEY POINTS

- Methicillin-resistant *Staphylococcus aureus* (MRSA) evolved when methicillin-sensitive *Staphylococcus aureus* acquired the *mecA* gene, probably from coagulase-negative staphylococci. MRSA is resistant to all β-lactam antibiotics, except for ceftaroline.
- There are 2 main types of MRSA: hospital-acquired (HA) and community-acquired (CA). CA-MRSA is more common than HA-MRSA, more drug-susceptible, and more likely to present as skin and soft tissue infections (SSTI).
- MRSA SSTI should be suspected if patients present with purulent discharge or abscess. Incision and drainage alone is usually sufficient for cure, although patients with warning signs should also receive a short course of antibiotics.
- Recurrent MRSA SSTI should prompt consideration of decolonization maneuvers; these efforts often fail on first attempt, perhaps because of the many anatomic locations that MRSA may inhabit.
- Treatment of MRSA bloodstream infections includes draining any foci of infection, and infected central lines should be removed. Patients should be carefully assessed for complications, including endocarditis.
- Uncomplicated bacteremia should be treated with 2 weeks of therapy. Complicated bacteremia should be treated for 4 to 6 weeks, and endocarditis for at least 6 weeks. The ideal drug choice for bacteremia remains controversial, but vancomycin is often still appropriate. If patients fail to respond to vancomycin, a change to another agent (daptomycin or linezolid) is warranted, regardless of the vancomycin minimum inhibitory concentration.
- MRSA pneumonia is a highly morbid and mortal infection. Linezolid has not shown superiority over vancomycin in terms of mortality, and it is expensive and potentially toxic, although a modest improvement in short-term clinical outcomes was seen in an industry-sponsored trial, and its dosing is simple. Ceftaroline is not approved by the US Food and Drug Administration for this indication, and it also costs more than vancomycin. Daptomycin should never be used in MRSA pneumonia, because it is inactivated by pulmonary surfactant.
- The number of cases of HA-MRSA seems to be decreasing with good infection prevention techniques in hospitals. CA-MRSA incidence seems to have plateaued. Assiduous use of simple infection control techniques remains the most effective prevention strategy.

Financial Disclosures: None.
1959 Northeast Pacific Street, Box 356130, Courier BB-302, Seattle, WA 98195, USA
E-mail address: abx@uw.edu

Med Clin N Am 97 (2013) 601–619
http://dx.doi.org/10.1016/j.mcna.2013.02.005
0025-7125/13/$ – see front matter © 2013 Elsevier Inc. All rights reserved.

WHAT IS METHICILLIN-RESISTANT *STAPHYLOCOCCUS AUREUS*?

Methicillin-resistant *Staphylococcus aureus* (MRSA) is a species of drug-resistant *Staphylococcus aureus* bacteria.[1] Although methicillin is no longer used in clinical practice (less toxic and more stable drugs such as oxacillin and nafcillin replaced it years ago), the moniker persists.

Where did it come from, and how did it become resistant to methicillin?

Alexander Fleming was working on *S. aureus* in 1928 when he observed inhibition of its growth on media contaminated by *Penicillium* mold.[2] He hypothesized that the mold was secreting an antibacterial chemical, which he called penicillin. When Howard Florey and colleagues[3] subsequently isolated penicillin, and when clinical trials were completed in 1941, the world finally had an effective treatment for deep staphylococcal infections; the antibiotic era had begun in earnest. Although initial production was slow, the precious medication was administered with great effect to infected Allied soldiers during World War II, leading to cures of acute and chronic infected battle wounds which might previously have been fatal.

However, staphylococcal resistance to penicillin was documented within a few years. This resistance happened because, under selective antibiotic pressure, certain strains of *S aureus* began to express penicillinases, enzymes that hydrolyze the lynchpin β-lactam ring of the drug. Although some *S. aureus* strains are still susceptible to penicillin, its usefulness has greatly diminished. Chemists developed a semisynthetic penicillin called methicillin to combat this problem. It was relatively unstable, only available for intravenous (IV) use, and caused an alarming number of cases of interstitial nephritis, but it was resistant to hydrolysis by staphylococcal β-lactamases. It was first deployed in 1959.

Resistance to methicillin was reported in Europe just 2 years later, and then in Boston in 1968.[4] This time, resistance was mediated not by β-lactamases, but by a fundamental change in bacterial cell wall chemistry. Penicillins work by attaching to penicillin-binding proteins, especially penicillin binding protein 2 (PBP-2). PBP-2 is a transpeptidase enzyme that serves the vital function of cross-linking bacterial cell wall precursors into strong, functional walls; they are like the mortar that glues precursor bricks together. Without that mortar, walls cannot form properly, and the cell dies. In MRSA, the *mecA* gene encodes for a mutant gene product called PBP-2A, which is resistant to binding by penicillins and all subsequent β-lactam drugs, including the cephalosporins (with one notable exception, as described later) and carbapenems. The *mecA* gene is located on a transmissible genetic element called the staphylococcal chromosomal cassette (SCC), which has facilitated the acquisition of methicillin resistance by multiple strains of *S. aureus*. Seven major SCC*mec* types have been described. Genetic analysis indicates that they are related to each other and suggests that they probably originated from coagulase-negative staphylococci (eg, *S. epidermidis*).[5] How the SCC*mec* elements entered *S. aureus* is unclear, although the presence of multiple types in MRSA colonizing European swine has led to the theory that swine may have served as a kind of mixing vessel between *S. aureus* and coagulase-negative *Staphylococcus* before transmitting the germs to humans.[6]

The increase of MRSA may be in part a result of our own conquest of other microbes. For example, MRSA itself becomes more drug resistant when patients are treated with antibiotics for other reasons (eg, sinopulmonary infections, urinary tract infections)[7] It is reasonable to suspect that the injudicious use of antibiotics may open up ecological niches in humans that are then colonized by MRSA, although there are many cases in which personal antibiotic exposure is not associated with colonization or infection. In the throat, MRSA may simply be filling the vacuum left by the absence of *S. pneumoniae*. *S. pneumoniae* has been observed to kill MRSA through the elaboration of hydrogen peroxide,[8] and throat MRSA colonization rates have been observed to increase in conjunction with the broad deployment of pneumococcal vaccines.[9,10] This hypothesis remains unproved; if substantiated, it would be a stunning example of an unintended consequence of an otherwise successful public health intervention.

What is the difference between hospital-acquired and community-acquired MRSA?

For the first 20 years after its description, MRSA was something of a clinical oddity: it was found in a small fraction of clinical *S aureus* isolates, and virtually always among patients who had exposure to hospitals. In 1974, only about 2% of *S. aureus* isolates from hospitalized American patients were MRSA; the rest were methicillin-sensitive *S. aureus* (MSSA).[11] Risk factors for hospital-acquired MRSA (HA-MRSA) were understood to include extensive previous antimicrobial exposure, admission to intensive care, presence of an endotracheal tube or central venous catheter, long duration of hospital admission, and poor health care worker compliance with standard hand hygiene practices.[12] MRSA was approached as a rare problem, created in hospitals, spread within hospitals, and seen only in hospitals.

However, in the early 1980s, substantial outbreaks of MRSA infections were reported among patients who had not been recently hospitalized, including injection drug users in Detroit.[13] Spread seemed linked to close contact between patients, and risk factors for infection included incarceration, homelessness, injection drug use, athletics, or living in dormitories or military quarters. In 1999, a report from the Centers for Disease Control (CDC) described 4 previously healthy children with skin infections who were treated empirically with cephalosporins, and later died of culture-proven MRSA, without any identified risk factors for infection.[14]

These cases came to be referred to as community-acquired or community-associated MRSA (CA-MRSA). Genetic analysis of isolates from CA and HA cases reveals molecular differences between the strains beyond their drug susceptibilities. In particular, certain strains of CA-MRSA are notorious for carrying virulence genes on their SCC, including a toxin called Panton-Valentine leukocidin (PVL). This molecule is toxic to host phagocytes, and seems to confer a survival advantage to CA-MRSA even in hosts with normal immune function. Experimental data have raised controversy regarding the role of PVL as a virulence factor,[15] and a recent meta-analysis found that PVL expression was independently associated with skin and soft tissue infections (SSTI) but not necessarily with invasive bloodstream, lung, or musculoskeletal infections.[16] On the other hand, the strain of CA-MRSA that often harbors PVL, called USA300, increased steadily in frequency during the 2000s, and has been shown to cause not only SSTI but also more severe episodes of sepsis when cultured from the bloodstream (**Table 1**).[17]

So, is MRSA worse than MSSA? And is CA-MRSA worse than HA-MRSA?

MRSA and MSSA are more similar than different. Both can present in a variety of ways, ranging from asymptomatic colonization to simple skin abscesses to invasive catastrophes such as necrotizing fasciitis, bacteremia, or pneumonia. Without appropriate treatment, MSSA infections can be as devastating as those caused by MRSA. However, treatment options are more favorable for MSSA. Plus, in some cases, CA-MRSA is not only more drug resistant but also more virulent.[18] Regardless of which

Table 1
Overview of HA-MRSA versus CA-MRSA

	HA-MRSA	CA-MRSA
Risk factors	Health care exposure (current or recent hospitalization, hemodialysis, central venous catheter)	No health care exposure (injection drug use, closely cohorted in jail or dormitories or barracks, athletes, family member infected or colonized)
Common clinical presentations	Bacteremia, Ventilator-associated pneumonia	Asymptomatic colonization, SSTI (especially abscess), orthopedic, bacteremia, pneumonia
Common SCC*mec* type in United States	II	IV
Toxin production	Rare	Common (especially PVL)
Comparative drug resistance	Highly drug resistant	Less drug resistant
Notes	Becoming less common over time, as infection control in hospitals becomes more robust	US incidence stable circa 50% of *S. aureus*. Readily transmitted by contact

gene product(s) are responsible for this virulence, outcomes in deep infections caused by MRSA are often worse than with MSSA. A meta-analysis of 3963 patients with *S. aureus* bacteremia found a pooled mortality odds ratio of 1.93 (95% confidence interval, 1.54–2.42; *P*<.001), meaning roughly 2-fold risk of dying of MRSA bacteremia compared with MSSA.[19]

In terms of comparing implications of CA-MRSA versus HA-MRSA, both are bad. HA strains are comparatively more drug resistant, and CA strains have a propensity for producing more toxins. However, these distinctions may be blurring. In a recent study,[20] outcomes among patients who acquired their infections in the hospital with phenotypic CA-MRSA were similar to those whose infections was caused by phenotypic HA-MRSA: in 384 patients, treatment failure was reported in 23% versus 15%, and 30-day mortality in 16% versus 19%, respectively (no statistically significant differences between groups). Although serious MSSA infections are easier to treat than similar MRSA infections, and although patients with MRSA have increased risk of poor outcomes, all *S. aureus* strains are associated with high morbidity and mortality, and all merit prompt attention and care.

My patients are worried about MRSA. These infections seem bad, but are they actually overblown by the lay media?

Patients should be reassured that there is no need to panic. Whereas approximately 29% of all Americans have asymptomatic nasal colonization with MSSA, the number for MRSA is only 1.5%.[21] The prevalence of MRSA colonization and infection varies substantially by region, and even by patient population within a given city or county. However, the overall numbers of invasive infections are sobering. It is now clear that a dramatic shift has occurred in the epidemiology of MRSA in the United States. Although HA-MRSA infection cases remained essentially steady in the 1990s, CA-MRSA increased astonishingly, from 2% of clinical *S. aureus* isolates in the 1970s to roughly 50% in 1997.[22] The absolute numbers are substantial. Of an estimated 478,000 hospitalizations with a diagnosis of S. aureus infection in US hospitals in 2005, approximately 278,000 were related to either HA-MRSA or CA-MRSA.[23] By a different estimate using the CDC's Active Bacterial Core Surveillance system, in 2005 roughly 94,000 patients developed their first invasive MRSA infection, and approximately 19,000 died.[24] In other nations, MRSA remains extremely rare and limited to HA-MRSA, prompting a "search-and-destroy" approach in response to even a single case. However, as those nations face the development of CA-MRSA, their approach may need to change.[25] In the United States, MRSA is in the community, and seems here to stay, at least for the foreseeable future.

My clinic patient is young, otherwise healthy, and has an abscess on his buttock. This is his first episode. How should I treat skin infections in the age of MRSA?

CA-MRSA has a predilection for the skin, especially the USA300 clone commonly found in the United States. Distinguishing CA-MRSA SSTI from those caused by pyogenic streptococcal species (eg, *Streptococcus pyogenes*) can be challenging without a Gram stain, but there may be helpful clues on presentation. Folliculitis is a common starting point for CA-MRSA infections, and a moist, hot compress may encourage them to drain if applied early enough. However, if drainage is not achieved, lesions may progress to furuncles, carbuncles, and frank abscesses. Significant surrounding cellulitis may complicate these boils, but this is the exception rather than the rule, at least early in the course of illness. Thus, when patients present with uncomplicated, focal, purulent skin infections, suspicion should be high for MRSA, regardless of previous exposure history or classic risk factors.[26] In contrast, simple cellulitis without a focal head may be caused by MRSA, but pyogenic streptococcal species (including *Streptococcus pyogenes*) should move higher on the differential diagnosis (**Table 2**).[27]

Drainage alone is the appropriate treatment of uncomplicated MRSA skin abscesses; antibiotics in addition to drainage are usually unnecessary.[28] This recommendation is based on numerous clinical trials, all of which have yielded essentially the same conclusion. In one example,[29] patients with this syndrome were managed with drainage plus either cephalexin or placebo. However, most were proved to have MRSA, meaning that this was effectively a placebo-versus-placebo study. Even so, 91% of patients in the placebo arm and 84% of those in the cephalexin arm had full resolution of symptoms, presumably because all lesions were drained. Drainage can be performed quickly in the examination room with standard skin preparation, local

Table 2
Features suggestive of SSTI caused by CA-MRSA versus pyogenic streptococci

CA-MRSA	Pyogenic Streptococci

• Furuncle, carbuncle, boil, or abscess
• Unwitnessed "spider bite"
• Recurrent infection
• Common Host Factors:
  ○ No clear risk factors
  ○ Any Age; often adolescents & young adults
  ○ Athletes
  ○ Injection drug users
  ○ Closely cohorted (living in dormitories, barracks, prison)
	• Generalized erythema, sharp borders, no purulence
	• Honey crust of impetigo
	• May also recur if underlying disorder not addressed
	• Common host factors:
	  ○ Any age; impetigo in children, cellulitis in elderly individuals
	  ○ Lymphatic obstruction (eg, postsurgical lymphedema)
	  ○ Tinea pedis, interdigital macerations

anesthesia, and a sterile scalpel or large-gauge needle for smaller lesions. Wounds should be left open and encouraged to drain (with sterile packing material if necessary, changed once or twice daily until drainage has abated). I encourage sending purulent material for Gram stain and culture, but this is optional; because drainage alone is the treatment of choice for uncomplicated infection, confirmation of MRSA and antibiotic resistance testing rarely affects immediate management. However, this information may prove useful in the future, particularly if the infection fails to improve with drainage.

I think my patient has CA-MRSA SSTI, because there is a purulent focus; she is nontoxic, but there is a lot of surrounding erythema and tenderness. I think she needs antibiotics in addition to drainage.

Antibiotics should be considered in addition to drainage for complicated abscesses associated with warning signs (**Box 1**). Many of these patients require at least a brief admission with IV antibiotics to ensure adequate response, and to allow for proper tailoring of step down to oral therapy.

However, initial outpatient management with oral antibiotics can be considered for otherwise healthy patients who have only modest surrounding cellulitis, a nontoxic appearance, and reliable early follow-up plans. In this setting, selection of an oral antibiotic depends on local resistance data, as well as individual patient factors such as allergy history, tolerability, expense, and potential medication interactions. Generally, the most reliable anti-MRSA oral drugs in the United States in 2013 are trimethoprim-sulfamethoxazole (TMP/SMX), doxycycline, minocycline, and linezolid. TMP/SMX and doxycycline often have susceptibility profiles of roughly 90%, versus virtually 100% for linezolid. However, because of its considerable expense, and because it has not been shown to have superior efficacy for this syndrome, linezolid is often a less attractive option than the other two. Clindamycin is less desirable as well, both because of its generally lower susceptibility rates and because of its notorious association with *Clostridium difficile* colitis. However, if the other options are unattractive and local clindamycin resistance patterns are favorable (perhaps >80% susceptible), then it could be considered, provided that an isolate is obtained for testing and that early follow-up is

---

Box 1
Conditions in which antimicrobial therapy is recommended after incision and drainage of an abscess caused by CA-MRSA (adapted from Infectious Diseases Society of America [IDSA] MRSA guidelines)

- Severe or extensive disease (eg, involving multiple sites of infection) or rapid progression in presence of associated cellulitis
- Signs and symptoms of systemic illness
- Associated comorbidities or immunosuppression (diabetes mellitus, human immunodeficiency virus infection/AIDS, neoplasm)
- Extremes of age
- Abscess in area difficult to drain completely (eg, face, hand, genitalia)
- Associated septic phlebitis
- Lack of response to incision and drainage alone

From Liu C, Bayer A, Cosgrove SE, et al. Clinical practice guidelines by the Infectious Diseases Society of America for the treatment of methicillin-resistant *Staphylococcus aureus* infections in adults and children: executive summary. Clin Infect Dis 2011;52(3):285–92.

ensured. Laboratories should test specifically for inducible clindamycin resistance by performing a "D-zone test," because this finding has been associated with clinical failures (**Fig. 1**, **Table 3**).[30]

Regardless of which antibiotic is chosen for outpatient use, the suggested duration is 5 to 10 days, and should be tailored based on individual patient response. Patients who still have considerable signs of inflammation at 10 days of therapy may be failing because of inadequate drainage of the primary lesion or antibiotic resistance, and consultation with an ID specialist is advised.

The patient looks good to go home with oral antibiotics after incision and drainage. Should I give her a dose of vancomycin first?

No reliable evidence supports the practice of administering a single dose of IV antibiotics for those patients who are planning to be discharged on oral medications, and this practice should generally be discouraged.

My patient with suspected MRSA skin infection has one or more warning signs for complicated disease, including a toxic appearance, and I want to admit her. I am comfortable with vancomycin. Is there anything new I should know?

IV therapy is advised for patients admitted with suspected serious MRSA infections, regardless of the source. Vancomycin is an appropriate first-line choice. Its

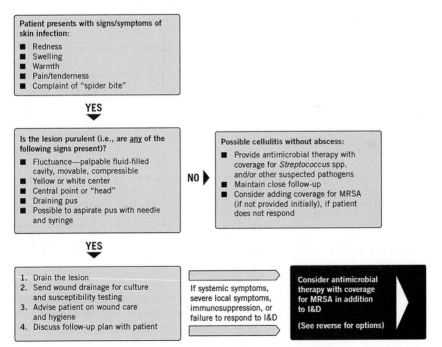

Fig. 1. Outpatient[a] management of CA-MRSA SSTI[b]. [a] For severe infections requiring inpatient management, consider consulting an infectious disease specialist. [b] Visit http://www.cdc.gov/mrsa for more information. I&D, incision and drainage. (*From* Centers for Disease Control. Outpatient Management of MRSA Skin and Soft Tissues Infections. Available at: http://www.cdc.gov/mrsa/treatment/outpatient-management.html.)

Table 3
Options for empirical outpatient antimicrobial treatment of SSTI when MRSA is a consideration[a]

Drug Name	Considerations	Precautions[b]
Clindamycin	FDA-approved to treat serious infections caused by *S aureus* D-zone test should be performed to identify inducible clindamycin resistance in erythromycin-resistant isolates	*Clostridium difficile*-associated disease, although uncommon, may occur more frequently in association with clindamycin compared with other agents
Tetracyclines Doxycycline Minocycline	Doxycycline is FDA-approved to treat *S aureus* skin infections	Not recommended during pregnancy. Not recommended for children younger than 8 y Activity against group A streptococcus, a common cause of cellulitis, unknown
TMP/SMX	Not FDA-approved to treat any staphylococcal infection	May not provide coverage for group A streptococcus, a common cause of cellulitis Not recommended for women in the third trimester of pregnancy Not recommended for infants <2 mo
Rifampin	Use only in combination with other agents	Drug-drug interactions are common
Linezolid	Consultation with an infectious disease specialist is suggested FDA-approved to treat complicated skin infections, including those caused by MRSA	Has been associated with myelosuppression, neuropathy, and lactic acidosis during prolonged therapy

MRSA is resistant to all currently available β-lactam agents (penicillins and cephalosporins) Fluoroquinolones (eg, ciprofloxacin, levofloxacin) and macrolides (erythromycin, clarithromycin, azithromycine) are not optimal for treatment of MRSA SSTIs because resistance is common or may develop rapidly

Role of decolonization
Regimens intended to eliminate MRSA colonization should not be used in patients with active infections. Decolonization regimens may have a role in preventing recurrent infections, but more data are needed to establish their efficacy and to identify optimal regimens for use in community settings. After treating active infections and reinforcing hygiene and appropriate wound care, consider consultation with an infectious disease specialist regarding use of decolonization when there are recurrent infections in an individual patient or members of a household

[a] Data from controlled clinical trials are needed to establish the comparative efficacy of these agents in treating MRSA SSTIs. Patients with signs and symptoms of severe illness should be treated as inpatients.
[b] Consult product labeling for a complete list of potential adverse effects associated with each agent.
From Liu C, Bayer A, Cosgrove SE, et al. Clinical practice guidelines by the Infectious Diseases Society of America for the treatment of methicillin-resistant *Staphylococcus aureus* infections in adults and children: executive summary. Clin Infect Dis 2011;52(3):285–92.

mechanism of action (binding to cell wall precursors, not PBP-2) allows it to remain active even against MRSA. It has been in clinical use since 1958. It is affordable, generally well tolerated, and remains a cornerstone of treatment of MRSA infections. However, it has weaknesses. Over time, some strains of MRSA have shown increasing minimum inhibitory concentrations (MICs) to vancomycin. This "MIC creep" usually happens because of increased cell wall thickness: the more cell wall to target, the more drug required to inhibit growth. Pharmacokinetic modeling indicates that achievement of an area under the curve:MIC ratio of at least 400 should provide the best chance of clinical cure.[31] Achieving that ratio is virtually impossible if the MIC is greater than 2 μg/mL, because the doses of vancomycin required would result in unacceptable risks of side effects, particularly renal toxicity and myelosuppression. This issue is more than academic. Overall, clinical outcomes track negatively with MICs: the higher the MIC, the higher the risk for complications or mortality.[32,33] The implication is that if the vancomycin MIC is greater than 1, then vancomycin should not be used. However, the story is more nuanced. First, recent findings[34] suggest that vancomycin MICs greater than 1.5 are associated with poorer outcomes regardless of the drug chosen. This effect was observed even in patients with MSSA treated appropriately with flucloxacillin, suggesting that increased vancomycin MICs may indicate the presence of yet-undefined virulence factors. Furthermore, many patients with deep MRSA infections treated with vancomycin do well, even if the MIC is later found to be 2 μg/mL.

MICs greater than 2 μg/mL are more alarming. By convention, *S. aureus* with a vancomycin MIC of 4 to 8 μg/mL is called vancomycin intermediate *S. aureus* (VISA). VISA remains rarely detected in the United States, although laboratories face challenges in identifying strains of heteroresistant VISA.[35] Even more alarming (although less common) is vancomycin-resistant MRSA, a term reserved for strains with MICs 16 μg/mL or greater. These strains seem to happen when MRSA acquires the genetic resistance element from vancomycin-resistant *Enterococcus* (VRE), rendering them resistant to vancomycin at any concentration. Regardless of the genetic basis of resistance, isolates with vancomycin MICs greater than 2 μg/mL should not be treated with vancomycin. Alternative treatments are available for these infections, including linezolid, daptomycin, and ceftaroline (described further later).[36]

If vancomycin is selected for SSTI and the patient responds, then no change in therapy is necessary, regardless of vancomycin MIC. On the other hand, if the patient fails to respond, then a change should be considered, especially if the vancomycin MIC is 1 to 2. Vancomycin should not be used if the MIC is known to be greater than 2 (**Box 2**).

My patient's MRSA abscesses keep coming back! Could she be colonized? If so, could I try decolonization?

By definition, MRSA colonization is asymptomatic. Most colonized patients never develop infection, and for that reason, screening is not recommended for the general population. However, many patients who develop MRSA infections are found to be colonized with the same organism at sites distant from the infection, especially the nares. Because nasal colonization with MRSA may be transient, decolonization is not recommended after a first MRSA infection. However, some patients (for reasons that remain unclear) progress from colonization to infection, in the skin or elsewhere, time after time. It may be possible to break the cycle of colonization and infection by attacking MRSA on the surfaces where it dwells, both on the patient's body and in the environment.

Nasal carriage of MRSA has been the focus of attention for many years, and this is the rationale for incorporating topical mupirocin (Bactroban) ointment into decolonization regimens. However, it is now clear that MRSA also readily inhabits other body locations, including the throat, rectum, vagina, and fingernails. It has the ability to remain viable in a wide range of environments, from countertops to beaches[37] to bed bugs.[38]

> **Box 2**
> **Practical advice for the use of vancomycin in treating serious MRSA infections**
>
> - Vancomycin must be dosed IV for MRSA infections (oral vancomycin is not absorbed).
> - Dosage in adults should be based on body weight:
>   - Loading: weight 70 kg or greater: 2 g IV × 1 dose; weight less than 70 kg: 1.5 mg IV × 1 dose
>   - Maintenance: 15 mg/kg (rounded to nearest 250 mg, max 2 gm per dose) IV every 12 hours thereafter; for central nervous system (CNS) infection, dose every 8 hours.
> - Time to check vancomycin trough: before fourth or fifth dose, then weekly thereafter if stable renal function; check more frequently if dynamic renal function.
> - Target trough level: 15 to 20 μg/mL for pneumonia, bacteremia, bone infection, CNS infection; target 10 to 20 μg/mL for SSTI.
>   - If trough is lower than desired level: increase by increment of 250 to 500 mg per dose, and recheck 4 doses later.
>   - If trough higher than desired level: if poor renal function, hold vancomycin and recheck level 24 hours later, then restart at same dose but now at daily interval; if normal renal function, reduce dose by 250 to 500 mg and recheck trough before fourth dose.
> - Peak level: vancomycin peaks should not be checked.

For this reason, multiple attempts at decolonization may be necessary. In one case series, an average of 2 rounds of aggressive decolonization were required to achieve eradication, and some patients needed 10 rounds.[39] Furthermore, that study used oral antibiotics for patients with urinary or rectal carriage. However, the IDSA guidelines do not recommend routine use of oral antibiotics, because of concern that benefits may be outweighed by toxicity and drug resistance. The bottom line: whether decolonization is attempted with a regimen of mupirocin plus chlorhexidine gluconate or chlorinated water, patients should be counseled on diligence, persistence, and attention to detail (**Box 3**).

My hospitalized patient developed a fever unexpectedly 2 days ago. I drew blood cultures, and yesterday the laboratory reported 1 of 2 sets positive for gram-positive cocci in clusters. I anticipated coagulase-negative Stapyhylococcus, but today the report was updated as MRSA. What should I do?

By convention, the discovery of *S. aureus* in a blood culture (either MRSA or MSSA) is taken seriously, even if some bottles are negative. Because MRSA lives on the skin, it can contaminate blood cultures just like coagulase-negative *Staphylococcus*. However, because the consequences of true *S. aureus* bacteremia may be so grave, a workup is recommended. The essential task is to determine whether bacteremia is uncomplicated (and can thus be treated for a minimum of 14 days) or complicated, which requires double, triple, or longer length of therapy (**Box 4**).

Should I add gentamicin for synergy in S. aureus bacteremia?

The practice of adding gentamicin to regimens for *S. aureus* bacteremia stems from that approach in enterococcal endocarditis, in which it is important and well established. However, the benefit of this practice has been insubstantial in uncomplicated *S aureus* bacteremia or native-valve endocarditis. Gentamicin shows synergy *in vitro*

Box 3
Environmental and personal decolonization tips for recurrent MRSA infections

Environmental hygiene: regularly clean high-touch surfaces (eg, counters, door knobs, bath tubs, and toilet seats) with standard household detergents.

Personal hygiene: regular bathing and cleaning of hands with soap and water or an alcohol-based hand gel. Avoid reusing or sharing personal items (disposable razors, linens, and towels) that have contacted infected skin.

Decolonization strategies:

- Nasal decolonization with mupirocin twice daily for 5 to 10 days, plus
- Topical body decolonization regimens with 4% chlorhexidine gluconate for 5 to 14 days (apply to whole body except eyes; allow to dwell for 5 minutes before rinsing off), or
- Dilute bleach baths (1 teaspoon per gallon of water [or 0.75 cup per 0.75 tub or 13 gallons of water]; soak up to the jawline for 15 minutes twice weekly for 3 months).
- Keep fingernails trim, scrub under nails gently with soap and water, avoid picking skin.
- Oral antimicrobial therapy not routinely recommended for decolonization. An oral agent plus rifampin, if the strain is susceptible, may be considered for decolonization if infections recur despite above measures.
- Nasal and topical body decolonization of asymptomatic household contacts may be considered.
- Screening cultures before or after decolonization are not routinely recommended.

Data from Liu C, Bayer A, Cosgrove SE, et al. Clinical practice guidelines by the Infectious Diseases Society of America for the treatment of methicillin-resistant *Staphylococcus aureus* infections in adults and children: executive summary. Clin Infect Dis 2011;52(3):285–92.

Box 4
Management highlights for patients with MRSA bacteremia

- Prompt initiation of antibiotics, regardless of the number of blood culture bottles positive
- MIC testing to vancomycin and at least 1 alternative agent (daptomycin, linezolid, or ceftaroline)
- Consider switching to alternative agent if vancomycin MIC greater than 1, or if failure to improve within 72 hours, or if patient worsens at any time
- Remove central venous catheters
- 2 weeks of therapy if bacteremia is uncomplicated, as defined by:
  - Negative echocardiogram to rule out infective endocarditis, and
  - No indwelling prosthetic material (eg, valves, joints, shunts), and
  - Negative blood cultures within 4 days of antibiotic initiation, and
  - Defervescence within 72 hours of antibiotic initiation, and
  - No evidence of metastatic foci (eg, pulmonary or CNS emboli)
- 4 to 6 weeks of therapy if the above criteria are not met, starting the clock at the patient's first negative blood culture
- Involvement of ID and cardiology if patient rules in for endocarditis. Outcomes are superior for early surgery among those who require valve replacement

and in animal models when added to β-lactams for MSSA endocarditis.[40] However, the benefit of this practice in clinical trials was to shorten bacteremia by an average of 1 day, and no improvement in terms of mortality was shown.[41] Concern over potential renal toxicity prompted a recent trial that found decreased creatinine clearance in 22% of patients who received initial gentamicin (plus nafcillin or vancomycin) versus 8% of patients who received daptomycin only and no gentamicin (P = .005). Gentamicin is not recommended for uncomplicated bacteremia or native-valve endocarditis; for now, in the absence of data regarding gentamicin-free regimens for prosthetic valve infections, and in light of the serious nature of those infections, gentamicin is still endorsed for prosthetic valve endocarditis (plus rifampin and a backbone antibiotic such as vancomycin).

My patient with central-line associated MRSA bacteremia has not cleared his cultures after line removal and a week of IV vancomycin. The vancomycin MIC is 2 μg/mL. What about drugs besides vancomycin for MRSA bacteremia?

Daptomycin (Cubicin) is a lipopeptide antibiotic that attacks the cell membrane (not the outer wall), causing cell death via potassium loss and membrane depolarization. It is approved by the US Food and Drug Administration (FDA) for gram-positive SSTI, *S. aureus* bacteremia, and *S. aureus* right-sided endocarditis. It has also been used off-label for orthopedic infections, with outcomes generally similar to those of patients treated with standard therapy.[42] Because of its chemical structure, daptomycin is inactivated by pulmonary surfactant, and thus is unreliable as a treatment of pneumonia. Therapeutic dose monitoring is neither necessary nor available. Most patients tolerate daptomycin well, although celebrated toxicities include rare instances of rhabdomyolysis in patients also receiving statins,[43] and even more rare cases of pulmonary eosinophilic pneumonia.[44] Daptomycin is officially dosed at 4 mg/kg IV daily for SSTI, and at 6 mg/kg IV daily for bacteremia and endocarditis. However, higher doses may be necessary in cases of bloodstream infection. Perversely, as vancomycin MICs creep up, so too may daptomycin MICs, even although the drugs act on different bacterial targets. In a landmark study of patients with *S aureus* bacteremia (MSSA or MRSA, complicated or uncomplicated), clinical outcomes for patients treated with daptomycin were not inferior to those of patients treated with standard therapy (vancomycin with or without gentamicin for MRSA infections).[45] Of 120 patients in the daptomycin arm, 19 (16%) failed to achieve microbiological cure; 6 of these (32%) developed resistance to daptomycin (MIC ≥2 μg/mL) during treatment. It is not clear whether higher doses of daptomycin may overcome this phenomenon, but it seems to be well tolerated at doses of 10 mg/kg daily,[46] and that dose is recommended by the IDSA for bacteremia that has failed treatment with vancomycin.[1] The duration of bacteremia with MRSA is often longer than that with MSSA, and 7 to 9 days of MRSA bacteremia is common, whether vancomycin or daptomycin is used. Daptomycin is a potent, well-tolerated IV medication with potential benefits in MRSA SSTI and bacteremia; it should never be used in pulmonary infections; and (like any drug) it may fail as a result of resistance acquired during therapy.

My patient has MRSA in a urine culture. Can this be a true pathogen in the urine?

MRSA has been cultivated from virtually every location and fluid in and on the human body; urine is no exception. As with any bacteriuria, contamination of introital flora may contaminate a clean-catch specimen, and the presence of 5 or more squamous epithelial cells per high-powered field should trigger consideration of obtaining a new specimen. However, in the absence of suspicion of contamination, the central question is: does your patient have asymptomatic MRSA bacteriuria or a true ascending urinary tract infection, and if so, is your patient also bacteremic? Concern for the latter possibility has led to the teaching that *S. aureus* in the urine (either MRSA or MSSA) should prompt a workup for bacteremia. But how often are bacteriuric patients also bacteremic?

Satisfactory answers are not readily available. Clearly, bacteremia is often associated with bacteriuria. Among hospitalized patients with *S. aureus* bacteremia (MRSA or MSSA), 24% to 34% also had bacteriuria.[47,48] *S. aureus* in the urine also correlated with a roughly 2-fold increase in complications of bacteremia, including endocarditis, osteomyelitis, septic emboli, or septic shock. In one study, *S. aureus* bacteremic patients who also had bacteriuria were more likely to die of their infection (32% vs 14%; $P = .036$).[47] However, it is less clear how many patients with MRSA in the urine are at risk of developing bacteremia. Given the serious nature of concurrent bacteriuria and bacteremia, it is reasonable to rapidly assess patients with true *S. aureus* bacteriuria (either MSSA or MRSA) and to consider drawing blood cultures, especially in hospitalized patients, those with indwelling urinary catheters or recent urinary surgery, or those at high risk for infective endocarditis.

My patient has culture-proven MRSA pneumonia. What is the best treatment?

MRSA pneumonia is a highly lethal condition, and yet the ideal treatment of MRSA pneumonia remains controversial. Vancomycin has been the treatment of choice for many years, and current recommendations to achieve vancomycin troughs of 15 to 20 μg/mL are based on both experimental data[49] and clinical observations[50] that patients who achieve that level have modestly lower mortality than those whose troughs are higher or lower. However, a meta-analysis of 2 small studies[51] suggested that linezolid (Zyvox) might be superior to vancomycin for MRSA pneumonia. A subsequent larger randomized trial[52] of linezolid versus vancomycin failed to show any significant difference in all-cause mortality at 60 days, although 11% more patients in the linezolid arm achieved clinical improvement.

Linezolid is an oxazolidinone antibiotic which functions by attacking the ribosome, thereby blocking protein synthesis. Its main indications are for nosocomial pneumonia and complicated SSTI. Its spectrum is limited to gram-positive organisms, including MRSA and VRE; like vancomycin, it has no activity against gram-negatives. Linezolid has a reputation for toxicity, including myelosuppression, peripheral neuropathy, optic neuritis, and serotonin syndrome in patients on selective serotonin reuptake inhibiting medications. However, in the pneumonia trial discussed earlier, there was no significant difference in frequency of side effects or toxicities between the linezolid and vancomycin arms. The ease of dosing linezolid, lack of monitoring, and ability to step down to oral dosing are all attractive; cost and potential toxicity are obvious downsides.

What about the new anti-MRSA cephalosporin I have heard about?

Ceftaroline (Teflaro) is a cephalosporin with the unique property of high-level activity against MRSA. It was designed specifically to bind avidly to PBP-2A, and also retains excellent avidity for other PBPs, giving it low MICs for other gram-positives and also a variety of aerobic enteric gram-negatives. It does not possess activity against *Pseudomonas* species, facultative abdominal anaerobes, or atypical respiratory pathogens. It is FDA-approved for the treatment of CA pneumonia and for complicated SSTIs. It is an exciting class of medication, which seems to possess the best attributes of cephalo-sporins (predictable pharmacokinetic/pharmacodynamic qualities) and vancomycin (anti-MRSA activity). It is available only for IV administration, and is dosed every 12 hours. In approval trials, it was generally well tolerated, although minor adverse events included nausea, rash, and subclinical positive direct Coombs tests.[53] Ceftaro-line was found to be clinically noninferior to ceftriaxone in CA pneumonia[54] or to the un-conventional regimen of vancomycin plus aztreonam in cSSTI.[55] It has shown more favorable MICs for *S. pneumoniae* than ceftriaxone and for MRSA than vancomycin. However, the number of patients with MRSA pneumonia in phase 3 trials was insuffi-cient to earn FDA approval for that indication. Similarly, although hopes are high and there is a strong reason to think it will be highly effective, ceftaroline has not yet been approved for MRSA bacteremia. Ceftaroline may be an attractive option for a va-riety of MRSA infections in the future, but its value in MRSA bacteremia and pneumonia remains unproved. It should generally be used only in consultation with ID specialists.

When should I get help from an ID specialist?

This depends on your individual experience, comfort level, and specific patient sit-uation. ID consultation for patients hospitalized with *S. aureus* bacteremia may provide enhanced guideline-directed care (**Box 5**).[56]

Things sound bleak. Are we making any progress with MRSA?

The overall situation with MRSA in the United States is mixed. On the one hand, HA-MRSA infections seem to be decreasing. During 3 years of intensive national surveil-lance, from 2005 to 2008, all HA-MRSA infections decreased by 28%.[57] From 1997 to 2007, the National Healthcare Safety Network reported a decrease in nosocomial MRSA bloodstream infections of nearly 50%.[58] This situation is still unacceptable, but the trend toward improvement is clear; so much so, that CDC has labeled the fight against health care-acquired MRSA infection a winnable battle.[59]

The situation with CA-MRSA is less rosy, and no substantial decrease in CA-MRSA infections has been reported. This situation should not come as a surprise. HA-MRSA can be reduced through a series of evidence-based practices related to health care worker hand hygiene, hospital sanitation, sterile technique during procedures, and so forth. CA-MRSA, on the other hand, is transmitted outside the hospital, and thus outside our direct control. Public health interventions (including information for

---

Box 5
Suggested criteria for infectious diseases consultation for MRSA infection

- Bloodstream infection or endocarditis
- Orthopedic infection
- MRSA isolates with vancomycin MIC greater than 1 μg/mL
- Patients with underlying renal insufficiency
- Patients who develop toxic effects of antibiotics
- Use of IV antibiotics other than vancomycin
- Failure to improve after 3 to 5 days of therapy, or progression of illness after any period of therapy
- Anticipation of outpatient parenteral therapy after discharge

patients and the general public) may drive CA-MRSA rates down over time, but that change will likely happen more slowly.

Why is there no vaccine for MRSA?

There is substantial ongoing effort in development of an MRSA vaccine. Experimental vaccines have yielded intriguing results, including in mouse models.[60,61] However, immunity to S. aureus seems to be complex, as shown by the observation that repeat infections are common. The immune response to MRSA involves both humoral and phagocyte responses, and the best antigenic stimuli remain elusive.[62] A recent human trial yielded impressive antistaphylococcal antibody titers but disappointing results in terms of protection against staphylococcal infection in patients undergoing cardiac surgery; and, perversely, the vaccine was associated with an increased risk of multiorgan system failure compared with placebo (0.9 vs 0.5/100 person-years; $P = .042$).[63] Clearly, there is work to be done in this important area.

I would like to know more about MRSA. What is the single best resource for further reading?

The 2011 IDSA Guidelines[1] are a superb resource. They are freely available online, along with guidelines for treating a variety of other pathogens and infectious syndromes: http://www.idsociety.org/IDSA_Practice_Guidelines.

Where can I find high-quality information to share with my patients about MRSA?

The CDC publishes excellent information online regarding MRSA, for both patients and health care workers: http://www.cdc.gov/mrsa.

REFERENCES

1. Liu C, Bayer A, Cosgrove SE, et al. Clinical practice guidelines by the Infectious Diseases Society of America for the treatment of methicillin-resistant *Staphylococcus aureus* infections in adults and children: executive summary. Clin Infect Dis 2011;52(3):285–92.
2. Fleming A. On the antibacterial action of cultures of a penicillium, with special reference to their use in the isolation of *B. Influenzas*. Br J Exp Pathol 1929;X: 226.
3. Mailer JS, Mason B. Penicillin: medicine's wartime wonder drug and its production at Peoria, Illinois. Available at: http://www.lib.niu.edu/2001/iht810139.html.
4. Barrett FF, McGehee RF, Finland M. Methicillin-resistant *Staphylococcus aureus* at Boston city hospital. N Engl J Med 1968;279:441–8.
5. Tsubakishita S, Kuwahara-Arai K, Sasaki T, et al. Origin and molecular evolution of the determinant of methicillin resistance in staphylococci. Antimicrobial Agents Chemother 2010;54(10):4352–9.
6. Tulinski P, Fluit AC, Wagenaar JA, et al. Methicillin-resistant coagulase-negative staphylococci on pig farms act as a reservoir of heterogeneous SCCmec elements. Appl Environ Microbiol 2011;78(2):299–304.
7. Sun L, Klein EY, Laxminarayan R. Seasonality and temporal correlation between community antibiotic use and resistance in the United States. Clin Infect Dis 2012;55(5):687–94.
8. Selva L, Viana D, Regev-Yochay G, et al. Killing niche competitors by remote-control bacteriophage induction. Proc Natl Acad Sci U S A 2009;106:1234–8.

9. Regev-Yochay G, Dagan R, Raz M, et al. Association between carriage of *Streptococcus pneumoniae* and *Staphylococcus aureus* in children. JAMA 2004;292: 716–20.

10. van Gils EJ, Hak E, Veenhoven RH, et al. Effect of seven-valent pneumococcal conjugate vaccine on *Staphylococcus aureus* colonisation in a randomised controlled trial. PLoS One 2011;6:e20229.

11. Klevens RM, Edwards JR, Tenover FC, et al. Changes in the epidemiology of methicillin-resistant *Staphylococcus aureus* in intensive care units in US hospitals, 1992-2003. Clin Infect Dis 2006;42(3):389–91.

12. Graffunder EM, Venezia RA. Risk factors associated with nosocomial methicillin-resistant *Staphylococcus aureus* (MRSA) infection including previous use of antimicrobials. J Antimicrob Chemother 2002;49:999–1005.

13. Levine DP, Cushing RD, Jui J, et al. Community-acquired methicillin-resistant *Staphylococcus aureus* endocarditis in the Detroit Medical Center. Ann Intern Med 1982;97(3):330–8.

14. Hunt C, Dionne M, Delorme M, et al. Four pediatric deaths from community-acquired methicillin-resistant *Staphylococcus aureus*–Minnesota and North Dakota, 1997-1999. MMWR Morb Mortal Wkly Rep 1999;48(32):707–10.

15. Voyich JM, Otto M, Mathema B, et al. Is Panton-Valentine leukocidin the major virulence determinant in community-associated methicillin-resistant *Staphylococcus aureus* disease? J Infect Dis 2006;194(12):1761–70.

16. Shallcross LJ, Fragaszy E, Johnson AM, et al. The role of the Panton-Valentine leucocidin toxin in staphylococcal disease: a systematic review and meta-analysis. Lancet Infect Dis 2013;13(1):43–54.

17. Kreisel KM, Stine OC, Johnson JK, et al. USA300 methicillin-resistant *Staphylococcus aureus* bacteremia and the risk of severe sepsis: is USA300 methicillin-resistant *Staphylococcus aureus* associated with more severe infections? Diagn Microbiol Infect Dis 2011;70(3):285–90.

18. Chambers HF. Community-associated MRSA–resistance and virulence converge. N Engl J Med 2005;352:1485–7.

19. Cosgrove SE, Sakoulas G, Perencevich EN, et al. Comparison of mortality associated with methicillin-resistant and methicillin-susceptible *Staphylococcus aureus* bacteremia: a meta-analysis. Clin Infect Dis 2003;36(1):53–9.

20. Eells SJ, McKinnell JA, Wang AA, et al. A comparison of clinical outcomes between healthcare-associated infections due to community-associated methicillin-resistant *Staphylococcus aureus* strains and healthcare-associated methicillin-resistant *S. aureus* strains. Epidemiol Infect 2012;1–9.

21. Gorwitz RJ, Kruszon-Moran D, McAllister SK, et al. Changes in the prevalence of nasal colonization with *Staphylococcus aureus* in the United States, 2001-2004. J Infect Dis 2008;197(9):1226–34.

22. Lowy F. *Staphylococcus aureus* infections. N Engl J Med 1998;339:520–32.

23. Klein E, Smith DL, Laxminarayan R. Hospitalizations and deaths caused by methicillin-resistant *Staphylococcus aureus*, United States, 1999-2005. Emerg Infect Dis 2007;13(12):1840–6.

24. Klevens MR, Morrison MA, Nadle J, et al. Invasive methicillin-resistant *Staphylococcus aureus* infections in the United States. JAMA 2007;298(15):1763–71.

25. Holzknecht BJ, Hardardottir H, Haraldsson G, et al. Changing epidemiology of methicillin-resistant *Staphylococcus aureus* in Iceland from 2000 to 2008: a challenge to current guidelines. J Clin Microbiol 2010;48(11):4221–7.

26. Daum RS. Clinical practice. Skin and soft-tissue infections caused by methicillin-resistant *Staphylococcus aureus*. N Engl J Med 2007;357(4):380–90.

27. Jeng A, Beheshti M, Li J, et al. The role of beta-hemolytic streptococci in causing diffuse, nonculturable cellulitis: a prospective investigation. Medicine (Baltimore) 2010;89(4):217–26.

28. Moran GJ, Krishnadasan A, Gorwitz RJ, et al. Methicillin-resistant *S. aureus* infections among patients in the emergency department. N Engl J Med 2006; 355(7):666–74.

29. Rajendran PM, Young D, Maurer T, et al. Randomized, double-blind, placebo-controlled trial of cephalexin for treatment of uncomplicated skin abscesses in a population at risk for community-acquired methicillin-resistant *Staphylococcus aureus* infection. Antimicrobial Agents Chemother 2007;51(11):4044–8.

30. Lewis JS 2nd, Jorgensen JH. Inducible clindamycin resistance in Staphylococci: should clinicians microbiologists be concerned? Clin Infect Dis 2005; 40:280–5.

31. Rybak M, Lomaestro B, Rotschafer JC, et al. Therapeutic monitoring of vancomycin in adult patients: a consensus review of the American Society of Health-System Pharmacists, the Infectious Diseases Society of America, and the Society of Infectious Diseases Pharmacists. Am J Health Syst Pharm 2009;66: 82–98.

32. Howden BP, Ward PB, Charles PG, et al. Treatment outcomes for serious infections caused by methicillin-resistant *Staphylococcus aureus* with reduced vancomycin susceptibility. Clin Infect Dis 2004;38:521–8.

33. Soriano A, Marco F, Martínez JA, et al. Influence of vancomycin minimum inhibitory concentration on the treatment of methicillin-resistant *Staphylococcus aureus* bacteremia. Clin Infect Dis 2008;46(2):193–200.

34. Holmes NE, Turnidge JD, Munckhof WJ, et al. Antibiotic choice may not explain poorer outcomes in patients with *Staphylococcus aureus* bacteremia and high vancomycin minimum inhibitory concentrations. J Infect Dis 2011;204(3):340–7.

35. Khatib R, Jose J, Musta A, et al. Relevance of vancomycin-intermediate susceptibility and heteroresistance in methicillin-resistant *Staphylococcus aureus* bacteraemia. J Antimicrob Chemother 2011;66(7):1594–9.

36. Saravolatz LD, Pawlak J, Johnson LB. In vitro susceptibilities and molecular analysis of vancomycin-intermediate and vancomycin-resistant *Staphylococcus aureus* isolates. Clin Infect Dis 2012;55(4):582–6.

37. Levin-Edens E, Bonilla N, Meschke JS, et al. Survival of environmental and clinical strains of methicillin-resistant *Staphylococcus aureus* in marine and fresh waters. Water Res 2011;45(17):5681–6.

38. Lowe CF, Romney MG. Bedbugs as vectors for drug-resistant bacteria [letter]. Emerg Infect Dis 2011;17(6):1132–4 [serial on the Internet].

39. Buehlmann M, Frei R, Fenner L, et al. Highly effective regimen for decolonization of methicillin-resistant *Staphylococcus aureus* carriers. Infect Control Hosp Epidemiol 2008;29(6):510–6.

40. Sande MA, Courtney KB. Nafcillin-gentamicin synergism in experimental staphylococcal endocarditis. J Lab Clin Med 1976;88:118–24.

41. Korzeniowski O, Sande MA. Combination antimicrobial therapy for *Staphylococcus aureus* endocarditis in patients addicted to parenteral drugs and in non-addicts: a prospective study. Ann Intern Med 1982;97:496–503.

42. Lalani T, Boucher HW, Cosgrove SE, et al. Outcomes with daptomycin versus standard therapy for osteoarticular infections associated with *Staphylococcus aureus* bacteraemia. J Antimicrob Chemother 2008;61(1):177–82.

43. Papadopoulos S, Ball AM, Liewer SE, et al. Rhabdomyolysis during therapy with daptomycin. Clin Infect Dis 2006;42(12):e108–10.

44. Kim PW, Sorbello AF, Wassel RT, et al. Eosinophilic pneumonia in patients treated with daptomycin: review of the literature and US FDA adverse event reporting system reports. Drug Saf 2012;35(6):447–57.

45. Fowler VG Jr, Boucher HW, Corey GR, et al. Daptomycin versus standard therapy for bacteremia and endocarditis caused by *Staphylococcus aureus*. N Engl J Med 2006;355(7):653–65.

46. Besece D, et al. Safety and clinical outcomes of daptomycin at doses ≥10 mg/kg. IDWeek National Meeting [poster abstract 115: 779]. San Diego, October 19, 2012.

47. Perez-Jorge EV, Burdette SD, Markert RJ, et al. *Staphylococcus aureus* bacteremia (SAB) with associated *S. aureus* bacteriuria (SABU) as a predictor of complications and mortality. J Hosp Med 2010;5(4):208–11.

48. Pulcini C, Matta M, Mondain V, et al. Concomitant *Staphylococcus aureus* bacteriuria is associated with complicated *S. aureus* bacteremia. J Infect 2009;59: 240–6.

49. Moise-Broder PA, Forrest A, Birmingham MC, et al. Pharmacodynamics of vancomycin and other antimicrobials in patients with *Staphylococcus aureus* lower respiratory tract infections. Clin Pharm 2004;43(13):925–42.

50. Jeffres MN, Isakow W, Doherty JA, et al. Predictors of mortality for methicillin-resistant *Staphylococcus aureus* health-care-associated pneumonia: specific evaluation of vancomycin pharmacokinetic indices. Chest 2006;130(4):947–55.

51. Wunderink RG, Rello J, Cammarata SK, et al. Linezolid vs vancomycin: analysis of two double-blind studies of patients with methicillin-resistant *Staphylococcus aureus* nosocomial pneumonia. Chest 2003;124:1789–97.

52. Wunderink RG, Niederman MS, Kollef MH, et al. Linezolid in methicillin-resistant *Staphylococcus aureus* nosocomial pneumonia: a randomized, controlled study. Clin Infect Dis 2012;54(5):621–9.

53. Teflaro (ceftaroline fosamil) [prescribing information]. St Louis (MO): Forest Pharmaceuticals; 2011.

54. Rank DR, Friedland HD, Laudano JB. Integrated safety summary of FOCUS 1 and FOCUS 2 trials: phase III randomized, double-blind studies evaluating ceftaroline fosamil for the treatment of patients with community-acquired pneumonia. J Antimicrob Chemother 2011;66(Suppl 3):iii53–9.

55. Friedland HD, O'Neal T, Biek D, et al. CANVAS 1 and 2: analysis of clinical response at day 3 in two phase 3 trials of ceftaroline fosamil versus vancomycin plus aztreonam in treatment of acute bacterial skin and skin structure infections. Antimicrobial Agents Chemother 2012;56(5):2231–6.

56. Jenkins TC, Price CS, Sabel AL, et al. Impact of routine infectious diseases service consultation on the evaluation, management, and outcomes of *Staphylococcus aureus* bacteremia. Clin Infect Dis 2008;46(7):1000–8.

57. Kallen AJ, Mu Y, Bulens S, et al. Health care-associated invasive MRSA infections, 2005-2008. JAMA 2010;304(6):641–8.

58. Burton DC, Edwards JR, Horan TC, et al. Methicillin-resistant *Staphylococcus aureus* central line-associated bloodstream infections in US intensive care units, 1997-2007. JAMA 2009;301(7):727–36.

59. Available at: http://www.cdc.gov/winnablebattles/.

60. Bubeck Wardenburg J, Schneewind O. Vaccine protection against *Staphylococcus aureus* pneumonia. J Exp Med 2008;205(2):287–94.

61. Burnside K, Lembo A, Harrell MI, et al. Vaccination with a UV-irradiated genetically attenuated mutant of *Staphylococcus aureus* provides protection against subsequent systemic infection. J Infect Dis 2012;206(11):1734–44.

62. Spellberg B, Daum R. Development of a vaccine against *Staphylococcus aureus*. Semin Immunopathol 2012;34(2):335–48.

63. Fowler V, Allen K, Moreira E, et al. Efficacy and safety of an investigational *Staphylococcus aureus* vaccine in preventing bacteremia and deep sternal wound infections after cardiothoracic surgery. IDWeek National Meeting [oral abstract 180: LB-1]. San Diego, October 20, 2012.

Influenza

Angelena M. Labella, MD[a],*, Susan E. Merel, MD[b]

KEYWORDS

- Influenza - Pandemic influenza - Viral illnesses - Immunization - Treatment
- Transmission - Chemoprophylaxis

KEY POINTS

- Clinicians should suspect influenza when a patient presents with respiratory symptoms, fever, and systemic symptoms and when influenza virus is circulating in the community.
- Rapid influenza diagnostic tests (RIDTs) can be helpful in confirming the diagnosis, but these are most helpful within 24 hours of symptom onset and have a higher positive predictive value when the prevalence of influenza in the community is high. Reverse transcriptase polymerase chain reaction (RT-PCR) has high sensitivity and specificity but may not be practical in all clinic settings.
- Treatment of influenza is most efficacious within 48 hours of the onset of symptoms. Patients with conditions that predispose them to high-risk complications of influenza and hospitalized patients should be treated regardless of the timing of onset of symptoms. In most cases, oral oseltamivir is the treatment of choice.
- Influenza vaccination is currently recommended for everyone older than 6 months in the United States. Trivalent vaccines are available in several formulations, including a live attenuated nasal spray and an inactivated vaccine in intramuscular and intradermal formulations. The effectiveness of the vaccine in preventing influenza is between 50% and 80% depending on the population; it can be worse in a year in which there is a poor match between vaccine and circulating influenza strains.
- During the 2009 influenza A/H1N1 pandemic, pregnant women and patients with morbid obesity were at high risk for complications including death.
- Although still rare, clinicians should be aware of emerging influenza strains including variant (v) H3N2, which generally requires swine exposure.

Funding Sources: None.
Conflict of Interest: None.
[a] Section of Hospital Medicine, Division of General Medicine, Department of Medicine, New York Presbyterian, Columbia University Medical Center, 177 Fort Washington Avenue, New York, NY 10032, USA; [b] Hospital Medicine Program, Division of General Internal Medicine, Department of Medicine, University of Washington Medical Center, 1959 Northeast Pacific Street, Box 356429, Seattle, WA 98195-6429, USA
* Corresponding author.
E-mail address: aml2250@columbia.edu

Med Clin N Am 97 (2013) 621–645
http://dx.doi.org/10.1016/j.mcna.2013.03.001

medical.theclinics.com

BIOLOGY AND GENETICS OF INFLUENZA
What Are the Different Types of Influenza?

The influenza virus is made up of 8 distinct RNA segments (**Table 1**).[1] These segments each code for a different protein that is essential to the structure and function of the virus. There are 3 genera of influenza viruses: A, B, and C.[2] Influenza A alone has caused pandemic illness, while influenza B and C have caused illness of epidemic proportion only.[3] Influenza A is further subtyped by the glycoproteins on its cell surface: hemagglutinin and neuraminidase. Hemagglutinin, for which there are 16 different molecules, allows the virion (a particle of virus) to anchor to a cell surface, while neuraminidase, for which there are 9 molecules, allows for digestion of host secretions and, later, release of viral particles from the host cell.[4] The influenza virus is named after the types of hemagglutinin and neuraminidase molecules.

How Does the Influenza Virus Change or Mutate Over Time?

Because the influenza virion is made up of 8 independent RNA strands it is subject to genetic changes. The 2 types of genetic changes that have been best described are antigenic drift and antigenic shift or reassortment. Reassortment is when 2 viruses infect the same host cell and then exchange genes during replication (**Fig. 1**). This process results in a new virion that has gene segments from each of its parent virus. This change occurs from viruses specific to one species and can also result in a new virus of interspecies origin. The H1N1 virus that caused the 1918 pandemic was derived from genes (or RNA segments) from human influenza, swine influenza, and avian influenza.[5] The influenza virus can also undergo smaller changes. RNA segments or genes mutate such that the hemagglutinin and neuraminidase molecule do not change their type but only some of their structure. In other words, they are still called by the same number (eg, H1, H2) but may not be recognized by the host's immune system as the same virus. This process is called antigenic drift.

Why Are These Changes Important and How Do They Affect Immunity?

Any antigenic change in the influenza virus, be small changes in the composition of the hemagglutinin molecule or a larger change such as interspecies reassortment, will decrease the likelihood of the host having effective immunity. In addition, the diversity in RNA composition of influenza viruses from year to year makes vaccine development

Table 1		
Eight RNA segments of the influenza genome and corresponding protein and function		
RNA Segment	**Protein**	**Function**
PB2	Transcriptase	Cap binding
PB1	Transcriptase	Cap elongation
PA	Transcriptase	Protease activity
HA	Hemagglutinin	Anchoring to cell
NP	Nuclear protein	RNA binding and transport
NA	Neuraminidase	Release of virus
M1/M2	Matrix proteins	M1, major component of virion; M2, ion channel
NS1/NS2	Nonstructural protein	NS1, RNA transports, translation; NS2, unknown function

Data from Morens DM, Taubenberger JK, Fauci AS. The persistent legacy of the 1918 influenza virus. N Engl J Med 2009;361(3):225–9.

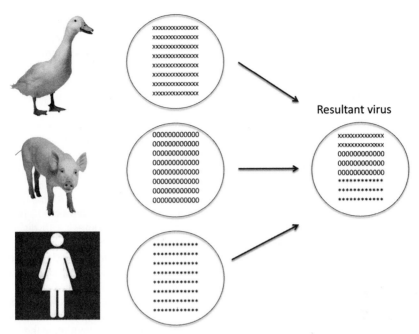

Fig. 1. Illustration of reassortment between 8 RNA segments from duck, pig, and human.

difficult because it becomes more difficult to predict which influenza virus will circulate.

HISTORY OF INFLUENZA
What Types of Influenza Have Affected the World in the Past Century?

The 1918 Influenza A/H1N1 pandemic killed approximately 40 million people worldwide.[6] During the 1918 influenza A/H1N1 pandemic, swine were also dying of a clinical syndrome that seemed akin to human influenza.[7] It was later shown that human anti-influenza antibodies neutralized swine respiratory antigens.[8] This and other experiments suggested that swine influenza had circulated in the human population and originated during the 1918 pandemic.[9] In 1947, the seasonal vaccine failed and it was found that the circulating H1N1 virus had several mutations on the hemagglutinin gene.[10] This incident provides a good example of how antigenic drift can cause public health problems that are similar to those of antigenic shift or reassortment.

In 1957, the H1N1 virus was not recovered from human sputa specimens, but instead, an H2N2 virus was recovered. This new influenza strain had 3 new RNA segments from an avian source along with segments from the 1918 H1N1 virus strain.[11] H1N1 reemerged in 1977 along with the more dominant subtype H3N2. At the same time, it was confirmed that influenza A/H1N1 was circulating in the swine population.[12] In the late 1980s, a new triple reassortment influenza A/H1N1 was circulating in the swine population. This strain had RNA segments from the original 1918 H1N1 strain and segments from the bird influenza.[13] Genetic analysis of strains from the 2009 influenza A/H1N1 pandemic strain showed that they were derived from a new reassortment of 6 gene segments from the known triple reassortment swine virus, and 2 gene segments (neuraminidase and matrix protein) from the 1918 influenza A (H1N1) swine virus lineage.[14]

What Other Variants or Strains of Influenza Are Circulating Now?

Outbreaks of swine-origin influenza in humans are rare; however, the incidence has increased over the past several years. When this occurs the virus is referred to as a variant (v). A hybrid virus of the pandemic 2009 H1N1 virus and the H3N2 virus has recently emerged and is referred to as (v)H3N2.[15] Almost all cases have been in young children who have been exposed to swine in either agriculture or fairs. This strain does not seem to transmit easily from human to human, although there have been documented cases with very close contact.[16,17] If clinicians suspect a case of vH3N2, they should contact their local public health department because a standard RIDT may not rule out the disease. The current vaccine does not protect against vH3N2. vH3N2 strains thus far have been sensitive to the neuraminidase inhibitors but resistant to amantadine and rimantadine.[17]

Since 2003, influenza A/H5N1 has killed over 100 million birds in Asia, Africa, and the Middle East.[18] In 2012, the World Health Organization (WHO) confirmed 610 human infected cases of this virus. Most of these cases had close contact with diseased birds, and 360 of the patients died of their disease.[19] The strain's virulence in humans seems to be partially related to its ability to alter the host's protein synthesis machinery allowing for unrestrained viral replication.[20] The H5N1 virus is, in most cases, neuraminidase inhibitor susceptible, although there have been documented cases of isolates with the N1 neuraminidase mutation.[21] One retrospective study of data mined from clinical records from 12 countries showed a crude survival of 43.5%. Survival was improved greatly with treatment even when started 6 to 8 days after the onset of symptoms.[22]

INFLUENZA A/H1N1 2009 PANDEMIC
What Should Be Known About the 2009 Influenza A/H1N1 Pandemic?

In late March 2009, a novel H1N1 strain was identified in Mexico and found to be of swine origin.[23] In June 2009, the WHO declared the start of this pandemic.[24] This novel strain, often referred to as H1N1pdm09, derives 6 genes from triple reassortment North American swine virus lineages and 2 genes from Eurasian swine virus lineages.[25] Most of the initial patients were between the ages of 13 and 47 years, and only a minority had coexisting conditions.[23] Adults older than 60 years had been disproportionately spared from this disease suggesting that they had cross-over immunity from antigenically similar influenza virus in the past.[26]

What Special Populations Were Disproportionately Affected During the 2009 Influenza A/H1N1 Pandemic?

Although most patients with confirmed H1N1pdm09 disease had an uncomplicated course, severe cases of acute respiratory distress and death were reported and the morbidly obese and pregnant patients seemed to be disproportionately affected.[27] Several observational studies have shown that pregnancy and specifically third trimester pregnancy was a risk factor for more severe H1N1 disease, intensive care unit (ICU) hospitalizations, and morbidity.[28,29] One study showed that pregnant women were 7 times more likely to be hospitalized and 2 times more likely to die than their nonpregnant counterparts.[30] Pregnant women with human immunodeficiency virus (HIV) infection were at an even higher risk of death. Another study showed that while pregnant women constitute only 1% to 2% of the population, this group made up 6% to 9% of patients in ICU.[13]

Morbid obesity was found to be an additional risk factor for severe influenza illness. Morbidly obese patients were found to have a higher likelihood of ICU admissions and death than patients without morbid obesity. The same association was not found with seasonal influenza.[31,32]

INFLUENZA B
How is Influenza B Different from Influenza A?

Influenza B virus is discussed much less than influenza A virus partly because it is the cause of only a minority of seasonal influenza cases each year.[33] The Center for Disease Control and Prevention's (CDC) Morbidity and Mortality Weekly Report (MMWR) showed that influenza B accounted for only 18% of cases from January 2011 to February 2012.[34] In general, the influenza B virus does not undergo the same antigenic changes that result in the pandemics that novel influenza A viruses have caused. In fact, all circulating influenza B viruses are genetically related to 2 distinct lineages.[35] In addition, seals are the only interspecies hosts resulting in less variation and interspecies transmission.[36]

Although it is generally accepted that influenza B causes a disease that is only of intermediate severity, there are certainly cases of fatal influenza B disease each year, especially in the pediatric population.[37] Like influenza A, influenza B is, in most cases, sensitive to the neuraminidase inhibitors. There have been cases of the HY123 mutation in influenza B isolates.[38] Influenza B is resistant to all adamantanes.[39]

MAKING THE DIAGNOSIS OF INFLUENZA
When Should Influenza Be Suspected?

In general, a clinician should suspect influenza when a patient presents with acute onset of fever, cough, and systemic symptoms such as weakness or myalgias between fall and spring. The probability of influenza in an individual patient varies with the prevalence of influenza in the community and with the vaccination status of the patient. It may be more difficult to use vaccination status as a predictor in a year when there is a mismatch between circulating and vaccine strains of influenza.[40] Attempts to develop clinical prediction rules based on symptoms and other aspects of the patient's clinical presentation have been hampered by virus evolution, the wide range of influenza prevalence in different settings, and the possibility of different clinical presentations in different populations such as children and the elderly.[41]

Nationally, influenza-like illness usually hits a peak in January, February, or March. Between 1982 and 2012, influenza activity (as defined by the percentage of respiratory specimens testing positive for influenza virus) has most often peaked in February, followed by January and March.[42] However, this pattern can vary from year to year. Influenza activity peaked twice during the 2009 H1N1 pandemic, once in the spring when the virus first emerged and again in the second week of October.[43] Detailed information about the number of influenza cases in a particular state or community is available from the CDC or from the local health department.

Fever and cough during a local epidemic may be the symptoms that are most predictive of influenza infection, with one study showing a positive predictive value of 79% ($P<.001$) for the diagnosis of seasonal influenza.[44] A systematic review in 2004 concluded that individual symptoms or signs are of limited value in diagnosing influenza. However, rigors, the combination of fever and presentation within 3 days of symptom onset, and sweating were most helpful in making the diagnosis of influenza, with a likelihood ratio of 7.2 for rigors. In the same study, lack of systemic symptoms, lack of cough, and the ability to perform activities of daily living decreased the likelihood of influenza.[45] Two subsequent systematic reviews concluded that independent predictors of influenza varied by patient age and that clinical findings identify patients with influenza-like illness but are not particularly useful for confirming or excluding the diagnosis of influenza.[46,47] **Box 1** provides guidelines from the Infectious Disease Society of America (IDSA) regarding when to suspect influenza.

It may be particularly difficult to make the clinical diagnosis of influenza with certainty in an elderly patient. A study of outpatients older than 60 years in the Netherlands showed a positive predictive value of only 30% for the acute onset of both fever and cough.[48] In a US population of elderly hospitalized patients, the combination of fever, cough, and illness duration of 7 days or less had a positive predictive value of only 53%.[49]

The H1N1 influenza pandemic of 2009 posed particular challenges for clinicians to diagnose disease based on the patients' clinical presentation. More adults infected with H1N1 pandemic influenza in 2009 presented with gastrointestinal symptoms including nausea, vomiting, and diarrhea than had previously been common with seasonal influenza; about 25% of adult patients hospitalized with influenza presented with diarrhea, abdominal pain, or vomiting.[50] Fever may also have been a less prominent part of the initial clinical presentation in hospitalized patients with H1N1pdm09 influenza; 42% of hospitalized patients in one study with laboratory-confirmed H1N1 influenza did not have fever before presentation.[50]

When Should the Test for Influenza Be Performed and What Test Should Be Used?

Diagnostic testing can be helpful in confirming a clinical diagnosis of influenza and should be used when the results will influence clinical decision making or infection control measures (**Box 2**). However, CDC guidelines emphasize that confirmation of diagnostic testing is not required when prescribing antiviral medications and that the decision to administer antivirals should be based on clinical presentation and epidemiologic factors.[51] The IDSA recommends using RT-PCR as the preferred confirmatory test because it is the most sensitive and specific of the options. Furthermore, results are often available within hours. Results of immunofluorescence tests may be available more quickly than results of RT-PCR, but immunofluorescence is

---

Box 1
When to consider the diagnosis of influenza in adults

When influenza viruses are circulating in the community, consider the diagnosis of influenza in the following patient populations:

- Immunocompetent or immunocompromized adults with fever and the acute onset of respiratory symptoms

- Persons with fever and an acute-onset exacerbation of underlying chronic lung disease

- Elderly adults with new or worsening respiratory symptoms (including exacerbation of congestive heart failure) or altered mental status, with or without fever

- Severely ill adults with fever or hypothermia without an alternate explanation

- Adults hospitalized without fever or respiratory symptoms who develop febrile respiratory illness after admission

During any time of year, consider the diagnosis of influenza in patients with acute febrile respiratory symptoms who are epidemiologically linked to an influenza outbreak.

Data from Harper SA, Bradley JS, Englund JA, et al. Seasonal influenza in adults and children—diagnosis, treatment, chemoprophylaxis, and institutional outbreak management: clinical practice guidelines of the Infectious Diseases Society of America. Clin Infect Dis 2009;48(8):1003–32.

Box 2
When to perform a diagnostic test for influenza in adults

During influenza season, consider testing the following populations:

If the patient presents within 5 days of acute febrile respiratory symptoms:

- Outpatient immunocompetent persons of any age who are at high risk of developing complications of influenza

Regardless of when symptoms began:

- Outpatient immunocompromised persons presenting with febrile respiratory symptoms
- Hospitalized persons of any age with fever and respiratory symptoms, including those with a diagnosis of community-acquired pneumonia
- Elderly persons with suspected sepsis or fever of unknown origin
- Persons who develop febrile respiratory symptoms after hospital admission

At any time of the year, consider testing the following populations:

- Health care personnel, residents, or visitors in an institution experiencing an outbreak of influenza, presenting within 5 days of developing febrile respiratory symptoms
  - ○ In investigating a suspected influenza outbreak in an institutional setting, consider testing when there are 2 or more persons with symptoms compatible with influenza, with the onset of symptoms within 2–3 days of each other, *if* the results of testing will change outbreak control strategies in the population *or* the setting includes persons at high risk of influenza complications.
- Persons otherwise linked to an influenza outbreak (eg, travelers who have returned from countries where influenza viruses may be circulating) presenting within 5 days of developing febrile respiratory symptoms

Data from Harper SA, Bradley JS, Englund JA, et al. Seasonal influenza in adults and children–diagnosis, treatment, chemoprophylaxis, and institutional outbreak management: clinical practice guidelines of the Infectious Diseases Society of America. Clin Infect Dis 2009;48(8):1003–32; and Centers for Disease Control. Influenza testing algorithm. Available at: http://www.cdc.gov/flu/professionals/diagnosis/testing_algorithm.htm.

---

less sensitive. Commercially available RIDTs provide results in less than 30 minutes but have decreased sensitivity (generally thought to be 40%–60% in adults, with a range of 10%–80%) compared with RT-PCR or viral culture.[51–54] Although RT-PCR may be the preferred test, it is not available everywhere in a timely manner, and the time it takes to get the results makes it less helpful in an ambulatory setting. Options for diagnostic testing are described further in **Table 2**. Common clinical scenarios and the suggested approach for testing and treatment are described in **Table 3**.

When Should Rapid Influenza Diagnostic Tests (RIDTs) Be Used Given the Test's Low Sensitivity?

Two cost-effectiveness analyses suggest that in patients presenting less than 48 hours after the onset of cough and fever in influenza season, empirical treatment is more cost-effective than approaches involving testing.[44,45] Authors of a systematic review of influenza diagnosis suggest that RIDTs do not add to the cost-effectiveness of treatment when the probability that the patient has influenza is greater than 25% to 30%.[47] In summary, when clinical suspicion for influenza is high and especially if the patient is quite ill, hospitalized, or at high risk for complications of influenza (eg, an immunocompromized or frail elderly patient) RIDTs should be avoided because

Table 2
Diagnostic tests for influenza

Method	Approximate Test Time	Sensitivity	Specificity
1. RT-PCR	Hours	High	Very high
2. Immunofluorescence (direct or indirect antibody staining)	Hours	Moderately high	High
3. Rapid influenza diagnostic tests	<30 min	Low to moderately high	High
4. Viral isolation (standard culture or shell vial culture)	Days	Moderately high	Highest

Listed in the order recommended by the IDSA.
Data from Harper SA, Bradley JS, Englund JA, et al. Seasonal influenza in adults and children–diagnosis, treatment, chemoprophylaxis, and institutional outbreak management: clinical practice guidelines of the Infectious Diseases Society of America. Clin Infect Dis 2009;48(8):1003–32; and Centers for Disease Control. Influenza testing algorithm. http://www.cdc.gov/flu/professionals/diagnosis/testing_algorithm.htm. Accessed May 7, 2013.

of their lower sensitivity. In this situation, one should consider treating empirically and using RT-PCR if it is available and if it would change management (eg, if having strong evidence that the patient's symptoms are caused by influenza would help the patient avoid further testing or treatment of alternative causes, such as antibiotics). Laboratory confirmation of influenza with RT-PCR also may be helpful in making decisions about infection control or prophylaxis for contacts (eg, if the patient is a health care worker or a resident of a long-term care facility).

Whether there is high or low influenza activity in the community at the time of the patient's presentation is helpful in interpreting the results of RIDTs. False-positive and true-negative results are more likely to occur when influenza prevalence in the community is low, such as at the beginning and end of the influenza season. At these times, the negative predictive value of the rapid influenza test is relatively high and may be helpful in excluding influenza. Conversely, when the prevalence of influenza in the community is high, the positive predictive value of the RIDT is also high (although, as discussed above, using an RIDT may not be cost-effective in this setting[51]).

Of note, one study in a laboratory setting comparing 11 commercially available RIDTs, using 23 influenza viruses provided by the CDC, found that while most rapid diagnostic tests detected the viruses at the highest concentrations, many tests did not detect many of the viruses at lower concentrations.[55] These results support current recommendations to collect specimens as early as possible after symptom onset, ideally within 24 to 72 hours after illness onset, when viral concentrations may be higher.

TREATMENT OF INFLUENZA
What Antivirals Are Available and What Are the Advantages and Disadvantages of Each?

Neuraminidase inhibitors block the release of virions from an infected cell so that subsequent cells cannot be infected.[56] The 2 neuraminidase inhibitors that are approved by the Federal Drug Administration (FDA) are oral oseltamivir and inhaled zanamivir. Peramivir is only available for investigational use as are the intravenous formulations of oseltamivir and zanamivir. Oseltamivir is a prodrug that is converted to its active

Table 3
Common outpatient scenarios and suggested approach for diagnosis and treatment

Clinical Scenario	Suggested Approach and Rationale
40-year-old unvaccinated school teacher presenting in January 24 h after acute onset of fever and cough; quite debilitated and unable to perform ADLs	Empiric treatment; consider RT-PCR if available and if it would be helpful in recommending prophylaxis for close contacts
30-year-old man with well-controlled diabetes presenting in November with 4 d of subjective fever and cough	Reassurance and symptomatic treatment of presumed viral upper respiratory tract infection
85-year-old woman residing in a nursing home presenting in January with 48 h of cough and altered mental status without fever	Empiric treatment; consider hospitalization; consider RT-PCR and prophylactic antivirals for close contacts
50-year-old unvaccinated nurse presenting in early October with 5 d of upper respiratory tract symptoms and fever	Consider viral isolation to establish diagnosis if she has had possible exposure to influenza; antivirals unlikely to be helpful
42-year-old oncologist with no medical problems who works in a hospital and takes care of patients who have undergone bone marrow transplant who would like live attenuated intranasal influenza vaccine	Patient is a candidate for LAIV but should not treat patients for 2 wk after vaccine is given
22-year-old asymptomatic woman who lives with her boyfriend who was diagnosed this morning with influenza	Offer patient both influenza vaccine and chemoprophylaxis with oseltamivir
50-year-old man with kidney transplant 7 y previously, presenting with acute onset of nonproductive cough and malaise, which started yesterday. Poor PO intake. Chest radiograph shows normal result	RT-PCR and empirical treatment while waiting for results; consider hospitalization for hydration and close monitoring of renal function
25-year-old woman 1 wk postpartum with 48 h of fever and chills in February	Empiric treatment, RT-PCR and speak with infant's pediatrician

Abbreviations: ADLs, activities of daily living; LAIV, live attenuated intranasal influenza vaccine; PO, Oral.

form in the liver. This drug is generally well tolerated, with some patients experiencing mild nausea,[57] and it has a wide volume of distribution with a half-life of about 6 to 10 hours.[58] In critically ill patients, the solution formulation can be used and given via a nasogastric tube. Zanamivir has poor oral bioavailability and therefore is available as a powder for inhalation use. This drug is generally well tolerated, although bronchospasm can occur.[57] Zanamivir has been shown to reduce length of illness by 1 day when started within 48 hours of symptom onset.[59] Intravenous peramivir has been approved in South Korea and Japan. This formulation differs from other neuraminidase inhibitors in that it binds to multiple sites of the neuraminidase molecule instead of just one (**Tables 3** and **4**).[57]

Inhaled zanamivir was found to cause fatal ventilator failure in a 25-year-old pregnant woman who was found to have severe influenza A requiring ventilator assistance. The patient was given oral oseltamivir and nebulized zanamivir. Over the next several days, the patient was witnessed to have low expiratory tidal volumes, which resolved with a change in the ventilator system. Eventually the patient died of hypoxic respiratory failure thought to be secondary to expiratory filter obstruction by inhaled

Table 4
Treatment options for influenza

Characteristics	Oseltamivir	Zanamivir	Adamantanes
Susceptible influenza types	Most influenza A and B isolates[a]	Influenza A and B isolates	Some influenza A isolates
Available routes of administration	Oral	Inhaled	Oral
Common side effects	Mild nausea	Bronchospasms, headaches	Orthostatic hypotension
Recommended dose	75 mg twice daily × 5 d[b,c]	2 inhalations (10 mg) twice daily × 5 d	not recommended
Contraindications	Hypersensitivity to oseltamivir	Not recommended for patients with COPD and asthma and patients with an allergy to milk[d]	Hypersensitivity to adamantanes
Pregnancy class	C	C	C

[a] Some isolates of influenza and B are not sensitive to oseltamivir.
[b] Some experts agree that in critically ill patients, a dose of 150 mg twice daily should be used for an extended period of time.
[c] Should be renally dosed.
[d] Zanamivir has a lactose carrier.
From CDC - Seasonal influenza (flu) - antiviral medications: summary for clinicians. Available at: http://www.cdc.gov/flu/professionals/antivirals/summary-clinicians.htm. Accessed March 8, 2013.

zanamivir. It is presumed that the obstruction was caused by lactose powder that is part of the Relenza diskhaler product, which should not be reconstituted in liquid.[60]

Another group of anti-influenza drugs is the adamantanes, of which amantadine and rimantadine have been approved by the FDA. These drugs block viral uncoating within the host cell, which is necessary for replication. Influenza B is intrinsically resistant to adamantane therapy.[61] Unfortunately, the adamantanes are also associated with high-level resistance to some influenza A isolates, and studies have shown that adamantane-resistant influenza A is just as pathogenic as its wild-type counterpart.[62] Because of this, there is little role for these drugs in the treatment of influenza and the CDC recommends against their use.[63] **Table 4** provides a summary of treatment options.

Is There a Role for Ribavirin?

Several studies have focused on the role of ribavirin, both the intravenous and the inhaled formulation, and neither showed definitive benefit in clinical trials.[64] Although ribavirin does have *in vitro* activity against influenza, the risks of hemolytic anemia and teratogenicity need to be weighed against the potential benefits.[65]

Should All Patients with Confirmed or Suspected Influenza Be Treated?

Antiviral medications are the most effective when initiated within 48 hours of the onset of symptoms of illness.[59,66] Treatment of influenza not only decreases the duration of illness but also reduces nasal shedding of the virus.[67] Given this fact, all persons who present to care within 48 hours of onset of symptoms of influenza should be offered treatment regardless of comorbidities. The United States Advisory Committee on Immunization Practices (ACIP) and the CDC recommend that all patients who are at higher risk for complications should also receive treatment regardless of the timing of the onset of symptoms (**Box 3**). Patients without conditions that place them at a

---

Box 3
Adults at high risk for complications from influenza

- Adults older than 65 years
- Residents of long-term care institutions, of any age
- Adults who are immunosuppressed (either from immunodeficiencies such as HIV or on immunosuppressive therapy)
- Pregnant or postpartum women (within 2 weeks after delivery)
- People who are morbidly obese (body mass index >40)
- People receiving long-term aspirin therapy
- American Indians/Alaska Natives
- Adults of any age with the following conditions:
  - Chronic pulmonary disease (including asthma, chronic obstructive pulmonary disease, and cystic fibrosis)
  - Hemodynamically significant cardiac disease
  - Hemoglobinopathies including sickle cell disease
  - Chronic metabolic disease including diabetes
  - Any condition that may compromise the handling of respiratory secretions (eg, neuromuscular disease, dementia)
  - Cancer
  - Chronic renal disease

Data from Harper SA, Bradley JS, Englund JA, et al. Seasonal influenza in adults and children–diagnosis, treatment, chemoprophylaxis, and institutional outbreak management: clinical practice guidelines of the Infectious Diseases Society of America. Clin Infect Dis 2009;48(8):1003–32; and Centers for Disease Control. Influenza antiviral medications: summary for clinicians. 2013;888. Available at: http://www.cdc.gov/flu/pdf/professionals/antivirals/antiviral-summary-clinicians.pdf. Accessed November 14, 2012.

---

higher risk for complications should not be offered treatment if they present 48 hours after the onset of symptoms because the risk of potential resistance is higher than the benefit of therapy.[63]

Patients requiring hospitalization secondary to influenza should be treated regardless of the timing of the onset of illness. A recent meta-analysis showed that treatment with neuraminidase inhibitors nonsignificantly reduced mortality in hospitalized patients when compared with patients who did not receive therapy (odds ratio [OR], 0.72; 95% confidence interval [CI], 0.51–1.01).[68] However, there was a significant reduction in mortality when early treatment (less than 48 hours from onset of symptoms) was compared with late treatment (greater than 48 hours from onset of symptoms) (OR, 0.38; 95% CI, 0.27–0.53). In a Canadian study of hospitalized patients with seasonal influenza, 71% received oseltamivir 48 hours after symptoms and there was a statistically significant reduction in death (OR, 0.21; $P = .03$) compared with patients who were untreated.[69] A retrospective study in Thailand showed that any treatment with oseltamivir (regardless of the time of initiation) was associated with increased survival when compared with untreated patients (OR, 0.11; 95% CI, 0.04–0.30).[68]

Some experts think that patients who are critically ill with influenza should be given oseltamivir, 150 mg twice daily, rather than the standard 75 mg twice a day dosage.[52] Higher doses with extended treatment lengths have been shown to decrease the severity of illness in animal models with H5N1.[70] Although there are no randomized controlled trials showing superiority of the higher dose, pharmacokinetic studies have shown that pregnant women seem to metabolize and clear the active form of oseltamivir faster than their nonpregnant counterparts.[58] In contrast, similar studies do not show a need to increase the dose of oseltamivir for morbidly obese patients.[71] The ACIP and CDC recommend a treatment length of 5 days for all patients. Experts agree that this should be extended in the critically ill requiring hospitalization.[52]

During the 2009 influenza A pandemic, the CDC recommended that all pregnant women be treated with oseltamivir if they had suspected or confirmed influenza infection.[72] One study showed that women who were treated within 48 hours of the onset of symptoms were 4 times less likely to require ICU admission or to die. Although oseltamivir is a pregnancy category C drug, most experts think that the benefits to the mother's health outweigh the potential risks to the fetus. Providers should be aware that the postpartum period poses a risk of more severe disease.[72,73] It seems that immediately postpartum immunologic function is not normal and takes weeks to months to return to baseline.

Should the Elderly Population Be Treated Differently for Influenza?

All patients older than 65 years are considered to be at high risk for complications of influenza and should be treated with antivirals.[74] Pharmacokinetic studies of oseltamivir have shown a slightly increased exposure-to-dose ratio in elderly patients because of age-related decline in renal function, but dose adjustment is not thought to be necessarily based on age alone.[75] Safety and adverse effect profile of oseltamivir in the elderly is thought to be similar to that in younger adults. In one placebo-controlled study of frail elderly residents of nursing facilities with a mean age of about 80 years treated with oseltamivir for prophylaxis, rates of gastrointestinal symptoms such as nausea and vomiting were similar in the 2 groups, with headache being the only symptom that was more common in the treatment group than in the placebo group.[76] **Table 5** provides a list of patient examples of who to treat.

What Should Be Done if the Patient Does Not Respond to Oseltamivir?

During the 2009 H1N1 pandemic, approximately 1% to 1.5% of the strains were neuraminidase resistant, overwhelmingly because of an H275Y amino acid substitution of the neuraminidase gene.[77] Ultradeep sequencing of isolates from nasopharyngeal swabs of persons who were untreated from a household outbreak showed minor populations of viruses with the H275Y mutation. Transmission of this mutated virus was found, suggesting some fitness advantage of this strain over the wild type.[77] Resistance to neuraminidase inhibitors arises when the neuraminidase gene mutates such that the inhibitor can no longer recognize the receptor site. Mutations result in various degrees of resistance to the different available neuraminidase inhibitors. Thus far, most mutations of the influenza A/H1 strains that result in high-level resistance to oseltamivir still confer adequate susceptibility to zanamivir.[78] Neuraminidase inhibitor resistance should be considered when one is failing oseltamivir therapy and gastrointestinal absorption of that drug can be relied upon. Neuraminidase inhibitor resistance can be tested by plaque assay, neuraminidase inhibition assays, and neuraminidase gene sequencing.

When Should a Patient Be Treated for Concomitant Bacterial Pneumonia?

Bacterial pneumonia is a well-known complication of both seasonal and pandemic influenza. During the 2009 H1N1 pandemic, it was estimated that 29% of fatal cases were complicated by a secondary bacterial pneumonia.[79] Although bacterial

Table 5
Vaccine formulations and recommended populations

Type	Administration	Indications	Contraindications
"Regular" trivalent inactivated	Intramuscular	Children and adults older than 6 mo, including healthy adults, adults with chronic medical conditions and pregnant women	See below[a]
Intradermal trivalent inactivated	Intradermal	Adults aged 18 through 64 y	See below[a]
"High-dose" trivalent inactivated	Intramuscular	Adults older than 65 y	See below[a]
Live attenuated	Intranasal	Healthy, nonpregnant children and adults aged 2–49 y	Egg allergy of any severity; chronic illness including heart disease, kidney disease, and lung disease including asthma; caregivers for severely immunocompromised persons[a,b]

[a] Contraindications to all of the above vaccines include severe egg allergy, severe past reaction to influenza vaccine, current moderate to severe illness with fever, a history of Guillain-Barré syndrome within 6 weeks of receipt of the influenza vaccine in the past.[110]
[b] According to the CDC, persons in close contact with patients who are so immunocompromised that they require care in a protected environment such as a bone marrow transplant unit should not receive the LAIV. Close contacts of other immunocompromised patients such as health care personnel in neonatal intensive care units, oncology clinics, and HIV clinics may receive LAIV.
Data from Anon. Prevention and control of influenza with vaccines: Recommendations of the Advisory Committee on Immunization Practices (ACIP) — United States, 2012–13 influenza season. Available at: http://www.cdc.gov/mmwr/preview/mmwrhtml/mm6132a3.htm. Accessed December 30, 2012; and Anon. CDC - Seasonal influenza (flu) - vaccination: summary for clinicians. Available at: http://www.cdc.gov/flu/professionals/vaccination/vax-summary.htm. Accessed December 30, 2012.

pneumonia caused by *Staphylococcus aureus* is widely publicized, the most common causative pathogen is *Streptococcus pneumoniae*. In general, patients who can be treated as an outpatient with suspected secondary bacterial pneumonia should be treated with age-appropriate antibiotic coverage for community-acquired pneumonia. It is not necessary to treat *S aureus* infection in this situation. Patients who are critically ill or who have a strong history of *S aureus* infections or those with necrotizing pneumonia should be broadly covered with intravenous antibiotics including coverage for methicillin-resistant *S aureus* pneumonia.[80]

TRANSMISSION AND PREVENTION OF INFLUENZA
How is Influenza Transmitted?

Influenza is transmitted between individuals through large-particle respiratory droplets; transmission is primarily related to close contact (probably within 1 m) with an infected person, but infection may also occur through surfaces contaminated with respiratory droplets. Adults are generally considered infectious from the day before symptom onset until 5 to 10 days after the first symptoms appear. There is a more prolonged period of viral shedding in children and immunocompromized patients, and one study of an elderly cohort of patients hospitalized for pneumonia also showed prolonged influenza viral shedding in this population; severely immunocompromized patients may shed virus for weeks or months.[81,82]

What Types of Vaccines Are Available and What Are the Guidelines for Vaccination Against Influenza?

Since 2010, the ACIP has recommended annual influenza vaccines for everyone older than 6 months in the United States.[83] Previously, the CDC only recommended that higher risk populations and health care workers be vaccinated. This newer recommendation is meant to streamline the vaccination process and improve protection of the community against influenza. Also, vaccination of everyone may prevent complications among higher risk populations; for example, one large Medicare database study showed a correlation between increased rates of influenza vaccination in children and a decreased rate of hospitalizations for pneumonia and influenza in older adults, with no significant association with vaccination rates among the older patients themselves. Because vaccination is more efficacious in children than in the elderly, vaccinating children may actually be an important way to prevent complications among the elderly.[84]

There are 2 types of influenza vaccine: trivalent inactivated vaccine (TIV) (available in standard and high-dose formulations for intramuscular administration and in a standard formulation for intradermal administration) and the live attenuated intranasal influenza vaccine (LAIV), which is available as a nasal spray. Currently, both vaccines are trivalent, meaning that they contain influenza A H1N1, A H3N2, and influenza B viral antigens. A quadrivalent LAIV, which includes a second influenza B virus lineage, is expected to be available for the 2013–2014 influenza season. There are several important contraindications to receiving the LAIV including pregnancy, chronic illness, and egg allergy of any severity. Among healthy nonpregnant individuals aged 2 through 49 years, there is no official recommendation for either the LAIV or the TIV and either is reasonable.[83]

The High dose TIV (known as "Fluzone High Dose") was introduced in the 2009–2010 influenza season and is approved for use in people 65 years and older. Clinical trials have suggested that elderly patients do have higher antibody levels after immunization with the high-dose vaccine as opposed to the standard dose TIV; however, it is not clear whether this confers greater protection against influenza. The safety profile of the 2 vaccines is thought to be similar, although adverse events such as pain and swelling at the injection site and malaise were more frequent in patients receiving the high-dose TIV. A study to compare the effectiveness of low- and high-dose TIV in preventing illness in the elderly is expected to be completed in 2014–2015. The CDC and ACIP are not expressing a preference for the low- or high-dose vaccine in the elderly population at this time.[85] The "Fluzone Intradermal" vaccine was first made available in the 2011–2012 flu season and has been shown to provide an immune response similar to the standard intramuscular TIV. This vaccine requires 40% less antigen than the standard TIV, so more doses of vaccine can be made from the same amount of antigen and may be more acceptable to individuals with a needle phobia.[86]

All currently available influenza vaccines are prepared by inoculating virus into chicken eggs. People who report serious reactions to eggs, such as angioedema or respiratory distress, or who require emergency medical care after egg exposure are more likely to have a serious systemic reaction to the influenza vaccine and should be referred to an allergy specialist before administering influenza vaccine. According to the ACIP guidelines, people who developed hives after egg exposure without more severe symptoms can be vaccinated with TIV and observed for at least 30 minutes for signs of a reaction.[83]

Guidelines or expert recommendations are available regarding vaccination in special populations such as patients who have undergone solid organ transplant and other immunocompromized populations. Experts have reviewed available data on the safety and efficacy of vaccines before and after solid organ transplant, and vaccination with TIV 3 months or later after transplantation is strongly recommended in this population. The level of seroprotection is generally reduced in patients who underwent solid organ as compared with the general population, and this may vary depending on the transplant and immunosuppressive regimen, with patients who underwent lung transplant having lower response rates and recipients of kidney transplant generally having very good seroprotection rates.[87] There are theoretical concerns about T-cell responses to influenza vaccines causing early allograft rejection, and some case reports and small case series support this but elevated rates of rejection or allograft dysfunction in immunized patients have not been seen.[88] The optimal timing of the first yearly immunization after transplant is not known, but guidelines suggest immunizing 3 to 6 months after transplant. Close contacts of patients who have undergone transplant should also be immunized.[87] Experts also recommend immunization with TIV for patients with autoimmune diseases such as rheumatoid arthritis and lupus, and there is no evidence that the degree of disease activity at the time of vaccination affects the efficacy or safety of the vaccine.[89] However, patients taking rituximab for rheumatologic disease or hematologic malignancy have little or no protective response to influenza vaccine because of B-cell depletion.[90,91] A meta-analysis of studies of influenza vaccination in patients who are immunocompromised because of HIV infection, malignancy, respiratory disease with glucocorticoid use, autoimmune disease on immunosuppression, or solid organ or hematological transplant concluded that vaccination does decrease the risk of influenza-like illness in these populations. There is limited evidence supporting a transient increase in viremia and a decrease in the percentage of CD4+ cells in patients who test HIV positive after influenza vaccination, but no evidence of worsening of clinical HIV related to influenza vaccination.

Updated vaccine guidelines, including detailed dosing information and guidelines for vaccination in children and people with egg allergies, are issued yearly by the CDC through the ACIP and are published in MMWR; the guidelines for the 2012–2013 influenza season were published in August of 2012.[82]

How Effective Is Influenza Vaccination in Preventing Illness?

Influenza vaccine effectiveness varies with patient age and immune status as well as with the match between circulating and vaccine strains in a particular year. The effectiveness of influenza vaccine in preventing laboratory-confirmed symptomatic influenza is estimated at 50% to 80% depending on the population studied.[92,93] A randomized controlled trial of the efficacy of TIV in healthy adults aged 18 to 64 years during the 2006–2007 influenza season in the Czech republic and Finland found an efficacy of about 60%.[94] Vaccine effectiveness is probably reduced in patients with chronic illness and in the elderly, with one study conducted during a season of poor antigenic match and circulating strains finding a vaccine effectiveness of only 36% in patients with high-risk medical conditions such as chronic lung, heart, or kidney disease.[95]

Who Should Receive Chemoprophylaxis?

Chemoprophylaxis against influenza should not be used as a substitute for vaccination. Antivirals should be used judiciously to avoid contributing unnecessarily to the development of resistance and to preserve available supplies. Chemoprophylaxis is only recommended in patients who present within 48 hours of exposure to an infected person, are at high risk of developing complications from influenza (see **Box 3**), and have not been vaccinated, have been vaccinated within the past 2 weeks, or are severely immunosuppressed and may not have responded appropriately to the vaccine. Vaccination should be administered along with chemoprophylaxis if the patient has no strong contraindications. Patients should be treated for a total of 7 days. Institutionalized patients can be treated for up to 2 weeks to control further outbreaks.[63] One study showed that daily oseltamivir, when given to patients who underwent either stem cell transplant or solid organ transplant in the past year, may reduce the incidence of PCR-confirmed influenza.[96]

What is the Role of Nonpharmacologic Methods in the Prevention of Transmission of Influenza?

Clinicians should implement proven strategies to prevent transmission of influenza and other respiratory viruses in the health care setting. The most effective single measure is vaccination of all health care workers. Effective strategies to improve vaccination rates among health care workers include mandating vaccines for all workers without contraindications, providing vaccine without cost, and improving access by making vaccines available at the site during work hours.[97] Mandatory vaccination of health care workers has been shown to dramatically increase the percentage of health care workers who are vaccinated, but these policies are controversial.[98] Health care workers who develop fever and respiratory symptoms should be excluded from work until at least 24 hours after they no longer have a fever; those wishing to return to work before respiratory symptoms have resolved should be evaluated by occupational health to determine whether they can safely be in contact with patients and at minimum should wear a mask until symptoms resolve. More stringent criteria should apply to workers caring for severely immunocompromized patients such as patients who underwent hematopoietic stem cell transplant, and organizations should develop guidelines according to CDC recommendations. Clinicians should advocate within their organizations for sick leave policies for health care workers that are flexible and allow providers with suspected or confirmed influenza to stay home as appropriate. Facemasks, droplet precautions, and hand hygiene are also important parts of the prevention strategy in the health care setting.[97] In the community, facemasks and hand hygiene may also be helpful in preventing transmission in households, although compliance is an issue. In a cluster randomized trial in Hong Kong, hand washing and facemasks seemed to prevent influenza transmission if started within 36 hours of symptom onset, with an adjusted odds ratio of 0.33, 95% CI 0.13–0.87.[99]

COMPLICATIONS OF INFLUENZA
What Are Some Infectious Complications of Influenza?

Myocarditis is a rare but potentially life-threatening complication of both influenza A and influenza B. A recent study showed that among patients with influenza-related myocarditis, most of these patients have fulminant disease. In addition, the number of patients with myocarditis seems to be increased during periods of pandemic influenza A.[100]

What Are Some Noninfectious Complications of Influenza?

Influenza has been associated with various neuropsychiatric adverse events (NPAE) including encephalitis, loss or depressed level of consciousness, delirium, convulsion, and hallucinations. For sometime, these symptoms were thought be caused by oseltamivir; however, newer studies have shown a more distinct association with inflammation caused by the virus and not the treatment.[101,102] In addition, treatment with oseltamivir seems to have decreased the incidence of NPAE. Interestingly, a large observational study showed that influenza infections are associated with transient Parkinson's symptoms but does not predispose one to Parkinson disease.[103]

There may be some association between thrombotic events and influenza infection, although data remains conflicting.[104] Several studies have shown that the influenza vaccine has decreased the incidence of deep venous thrombosis.[105]

FUTURE DIRECTIONS IN RESEARCH AND POLICY

Studies have suggested that patients are not well educated about the risks and benefits of influenza vaccination and antiviral treatment; in one study, 37% of patients in an internal medicine clinic thought that the influenza vaccine could cause influenza and 63% were unaware that antiviral medication is ineffective against bacteria.[106] There are likely important racial and economic disparities in vaccination and appropriate use of antiviral medication as well. Among Medicare beneficiaries, white patients are more likely to be vaccinated than African American or Hispanic patients; this should be a target for further research and public health efforts.[107]

In a recent article, Poland and Jacobson[108,109] argue that clinicians, scientist, and the public alike need to help to end the antivaccinationist's campaign. The investigators suggest that the funding of studies to address the concerns about vaccines, the improvement of vaccine monitoring programs, and the education of both clinicians and the public will help to accelerate this effort.

REFERENCES

1. Morens DM, Taubenberger JK, Fauci AS. The persistent legacy of the 1918 influenza virus. N Engl J Med 2009;361(3):225–9. Available at: http://www.pubmedcentral.nih.gov/articlerender.fcgi?artid=2749954&tool=pmcentrez&rendertype=abstract. Accessed December 22, 2012.
2. Watts G. A/H1N1 influenza virus: the basics. BMJ 2009;339:b3046. Available at: http://www.ncbi.nlm.nih.gov/pubmed/19633037. Accessed December 23, 2012.
3. Rambaut A, Pybus OG, Nelson MI, et al. The genomic and epidemiological dynamics of human influenza A virus. Nature 2008;453(7195):615–9. Available at: http://www.nature.com.ezproxy.cul.columbia.edu/nature/journal/v453/n7195/full/nature06945.html. Accessed November 2, 2012.
4. Watts G. A/H1N1 influenza virus: the basics. BMJ 2009;339(2):b3046. Available at: http://www.bmj.com.ezproxy.cul.columbia.edu/content/339/bmj.b3046?view=long&pmid=19633037. Accessed December 4, 2012.
5. Garten RJ, Davis CT, Russell CA, et al. Antigenic and genetic characteristics of swine-origin 2009 A(H1N1) influenza viruses circulating in humans. Science 2009;325(5937):197–201. Available at: http://www.ncbi.nlm.nih.gov/pmc/articles/PMC3250984. Accessed November 6, 2012.
6. Oxford JS. Influenza A pandemics of the 20th century with special reference to 1918: virology, pathology and epidemiology. Rev Med Virol 2000;10(2):119–33. Available at: http://www.ncbi.nlm.nih.gov/pubmed/10713598. Accessed December 23, 2012.
7. Zimmer SM, Burke DS. Historical perspective–emergence of influenza A (H1N1) viruses. N Engl J Med 2009;361(3):279–85. Available at: http://www.ncbi.nlm.nih.gov/pubmed/19564632. Accessed December 4, 2012.

8. Shope RE. The Incidence of neutralizing antibodies for swine influenza virus in the sera of human beings of different ages. J Exp Med 1936;63(5): 669–84. Available at: http://www.pubmedcentral.nih.gov/articlerender.fcgi?artid=2133359&tool=pmcentrez&rendertype=abstract. Accessed December 23, 2012.

9. Nakajima K, Nobusawa E, Nakajima S. Genetic relatedness between A/Swine/Iowa/15/30(H1N1) and human influenza viruses. Virology 1984;139(1):194–8. Available at: http://www.ncbi.nlm.nih.gov/pubmed/6495656. Accessed December 23, 2012.

10. Kilbourne ED, Smith C, Brett I, et al. The total influenza vaccine failure of 1947 revisited: major intrasubtypic antigenic change can explain failure of vaccine in a post-World War II epidemic. Proc Natl Acad Sci U S A 2002;99(16): 10748–52. Available at: http://www.pubmedcentral.nih.gov/articlerender.fcgi?artid=125033&tool=pmcentrez&rendertype=abstract. Accessed December 23, 2012.

11. Scholtissek C, Rohde W, Von Hoyningen V, et al. On the origin of the human influenza virus subtypes H2N2 and H3N2. Virology 1978;87(1):13–20. Available at: http://www.ncbi.nlm.nih.gov/pubmed/664248. Accessed December 23, 2012.

12. Finkelman BS, Viboud C, Koelle K, et al. Global patterns in seasonal activity of influenza A/H3N2, A/H1N1, and B from 1997 to 2005: viral coexistence and latitudinal gradients. PLoS One 2007;2(12):e1296. Available at: http://www.pubmedcentral.nih.gov/articlerender.fcgi?artid=2117904&tool=pmcentrez&rendertype=abstract. Accessed November 6, 2012.

13. Jain S, Kamimoto L, Bramley AM, et al. Hospitalized patients with 2009 H1N1 influenza in the United States, April-June 2009. N Engl J Med 2009;361(20): 1935–44. Available at: http://www.ncbi.nlm.nih.gov/pubmed/19815859. Accessed November 23, 2012.

14. Shinde V, Bridges CB, Uyeki TM, et al. Triple-reassortant swine influenza A (H1) in humans in the United States, 2005-2009. N Engl J Med 2009;360(25): 2616–25. Available at: http://www.ncbi.nlm.nih.gov/pubmed/19423871. Accessed December 22, 2012.

15. Wong KK, Greenbaum A, Moll ME, et al. Outbreak of influenza A (H3N2) variant virus infection among attendees of an agricultural fair, Pennsylvania, USA, 2011. Emerg Infect Dis 2012;18(12):1937–44. Available at: http://www.ncbi.nlm.nih.gov/pubmed/23171635. Accessed December 23, 2012.

16. Centers for Disease Control and Prevention (CDC). Influenza A (H3N2) variant virus-related hospitalizations: Ohio, 2012. MMWR Morb Mortal Wkly Rep 2012; 61:764–7. Available at: http://www.ncbi.nlm.nih.gov/pubmed/23013722. Accessed December 23, 2012.

17. Centers for Disease Control and Prevention (CDC). Update: influenza A (H3N2)v transmission and guidelines - five states, 2011. MMWR Morb Mortal Wkly Rep 2012;60(51–52):1741–4. Available at: http://www.ncbi.nlm.nih.gov/pubmed/22217624. Accessed December 23, 2012.

18. Dolin R. Influenza–interpandemic as well as pandemic disease. N Engl J Med 2005;353(24):2535–7. Available at: http://www.ncbi.nlm.nih.gov/pubmed/16354889. Accessed December 22, 2012.

19. Anon. Cumulative number of confirmed human cases of avian influenza A(H5N1) reported to WHO. WHO. Available at: http://www.who.int/influenza/human_animal_interface/H5N1_cumulative_table_archives/en/. Accessed December 29, 2012.

20. Abdel-Ghafar AN, Chotpitayasunondh T, Gao Z, et al. Update on avian influenza A (H5N1) virus infection in humans. N Engl J Med 2008;358(3):261–73. Available at: http://www.ncbi.nlm.nih.gov/pubmed/18199865. Accessed December 29, 2012.

21. De Jong MD, Tran TT, Truong HK, et al. Oseltamivir resistance during treatment of influenza A (H5N1) infection. N Engl J Med 2005;353(25):2667–72. Available at: http://www.ncbi.nlm.nih.gov/pubmed/16371632. Accessed November 20, 2012.

22. Adisasmito W, Chan PK, Lee N, et al. Effectiveness of antiviral treatment in human influenza A(H5N1) infections: analysis of a Global Patient Registry. J Infect Dis 2010;202(8):1154–60. Available at: http://www.ncbi.nlm.nih.gov/pubmed/20831384. Accessed November 19, 2012.

23. Perez-Padilla R, De la Rosa-Zamboni D, Ponce de Leon S, et al. Pneumonia and respiratory failure from swine-origin influenza A (H1N1) in Mexico. N Engl J Med 2009;361(7):680–9. Available at: http://www.ncbi.nlm.nih.gov/pubmed/19564631. Accessed November 14, 2012.

24. Dawood FS, Jain S, Finelli L, et al. Emergence of a novel swine-origin influenza A (H1N1) virus in humans. N Engl J Med 2009;360(25):2605–15. Available at: http://www.ncbi.nlm.nih.gov/pubmed/19423869. Accessed November 6, 2012.

25. Smith GJ, Vijaykrishna D, Bahl J, et al. Origins and evolutionary genomics of the 2009 swine-origin H1N1 influenza A epidemic. Nature 2009;459(7250):1122–5. Available at: http://www.ncbi.nlm.nih.gov/pubmed/19516283. Accessed November 2, 2012.

26. Hancock K, Veguilla V, Lu X, et al. Cross-reactive antibody responses to the 2009 pandemic H1N1 influenza virus. N Engl J Med 2009;361(20):1945–52. Available at: http://www.ncbi.nlm.nih.gov/pubmed/19745214. Accessed December 31, 2012.

27. Domínguez-Cherit G, Namendys-Silva SA, De la Torre A, et al. H1N1 influenza pandemic of 2009 compared with other influenza pandemics: epidemiology, diagnosis, management, pulmonary complications, and outcomes. Curr Infect Dis Rep 2010;12(3):204–10. Available at: http://www.ncbi.nlm.nih.gov/pubmed/21308531. Accessed December 23, 2012.

28. Dolan GP, Myles PR, Brett SJ, et al. The comparative clinical course of pregnant and non-pregnant women hospitalised with influenza A(H1N1)pdm09 infection. PLoS One 2012;7(8):e41638. Available at: http://www.pubmedcentral.nih.gov/articlerender.fcgi?artid=3411676&tool=pmcentrez&rendertype=abstract. Accessed December 23, 2012.

29. Hansen C, Desai S, Bredfeldt C, et al. A large, population-based study of 2009 pandemic influenza A virus subtype H1N1 infection diagnosis during pregnancy and outcomes for mothers and neonates. J Infect Dis 2012;206(8):1260–8. Available at: http://www.ncbi.nlm.nih.gov/pubmed/22859826. Accessed December 23, 2012.

30. Van Kerkhove MD, Vandemaele KA, Shinde V, et al. Risk factors for severe outcomes following 2009 influenza A (H1N1) infection: a global pooled analysis. PLoS Med 2011;8(7):e1001053. Available at: http://www.pubmedcentral.nih.gov/articlerender.fcgi?artid=3130021&tool=pmcentrez&rendertype=abstract. Accessed November 14, 2012.

31. Hanslik T, Boelle PY, Flahault A. Preliminary estimation of risk factors for admission to intensive care units and for death in patients infected with A(H1N1)2009 influenza virus, France, 2009-2010. PLoS Curr 2010;2:RRN1150. Available at: http://www.pubmedcentral.nih.gov/articlerender.fcgi?artid=2836028&tool=pmcentrez&rendertype=abstract. Accessed December 23, 2012.

32. Greenbaum BD, Li OT, Poon LL, et al. Viral reassortment as an information exchange between viral segments. Proc Natl Acad Sci U S A 2012;109(9):3341–6.

33. Centers for Disease Control and Prevention (CDC). Estimates of deaths associated with seasonal influenza — United States, 1976-2007. MMWR Morb Mortal Wkly Rep 2010;59(33):1057–62. Available at: http://www.ncbi.nlm.nih.gov/pubmed/20798667. Accessed December 23, 2012.

34. Anon. Update: influenza activity — United States, October 2, 2011–February 11, 2012. Available at: http://www.cdc.gov.ezproxy.cul.columbia.edu/mmwr/preview/mmwrhtml/mm6107a3.htm#fig1. Accessed December 10, 2012.

35. Rota PA, Wallis TR, Harmon MW, et al. Cocirculation of two distinct evolutionary lineages of influenza type B virus since 1983. Virology 1990;175(1):59–68. Available at: http://www.ncbi.nlm.nih.gov/pubmed/2309452. Accessed December 23, 2012.

36. Osterhaus AD. Influenza B virus in seals. Science 2000;288(5468):1051–3. Available at: http://www.sciencemag.org/content/288/5468/1051.full. Accessed November 11, 2012.

37. Paddock CD, Liu L, Denison AM, et al. Myocardial injury and bacterial pneumonia contribute to the pathogenesis of fatal influenza B virus infection. J Infect Dis 2012;205(6):895–905. Available at: http://jid.oxfordjournals.org.ezproxy.cul.columbia.edu/content/205/6/895.full. Accessed December 10, 2012.

38. Higgins RR, Beniprashad M, Chong-King E, et al. Recovery of influenza B virus with the H273Y point mutation in the neuraminidase active site from a human patient. J Clin Microbiol 2012;50(7):2500–2. Available at: http://www.ncbi.nlm.nih.gov/pubmed/22535992. Accessed November 14, 2012.

39. Hurt AC, Holien JK, Parker MW, et al. Oseltamivir resistance and the H274Y neuraminidase mutation in seasonal, pandemic and highly pathogenic influenza viruses. Drugs 2009;69(18):2523–31. Available at: http://www.ncbi.nlm.nih.gov/pubmed/19943705. Accessed December 29, 2012.

40. Barry MA. A 29-year-old woman with flu-like symptoms review of influenza diagnosis and treatment. JAMA 2010;304(6):671–8.

41. Woolpert T, Brodine S, Lemus H, et al. Determination of clinical and demographic predictors of laboratory-confirmed influenza with subtype analysis. BMC Infect Dis 2012;12(1):129. Available at: http://www.pubmedcentral.nih.gov/articlerender.fcgi?artid=3407722&tool=pmcentrez&rendertype=abstract. Accessed November 9, 2012.

42. Centers for Disease Control. The flu season. Available at: http://www.cdc.gov/flu/about/season/flu-season.htm. Accessed May 7, 2013.

43. Centers for Disease Control. Updated CDC Estimates of 2009 H1N1 influenza cases, Hospitalizations and deaths in the United States, April 2009-April 10, 2010. Available at: http://www.cdc.gov/h1n1flu/estimates_2009_h1n1.htm. Accessed November 9, 2012.

44. Monto AS, Gravenstein S, Elliott M, et al. Clinical signs and symptoms predicting influenza infection. Arch Intern Med 2000;160(21):3243–7. Available at: http://www.ncbi.nlm.nih.gov/pubmed/11088084. Accessed May 7, 2013.

45. Ebell M, White L, Casault T. A systematic review of the history and physical examination to diagnose influenza. J Am Board Fam Pract 2004;1–5. Available at: http://www.jabfm.com/content/17/1/1.short. Accessed November 8, 2012.

46. Woolpert T, Brodine S, Lemus H, et al. Determination of clinical and demographic predictors of laboratory-confirmed influenza with subtype analysis. BMC Infect Dis 2012;12(1):129.

47. Call SA, Vollenweider MA, Hornung CA, et al. Does this patient have influenza? JAMA 2005;293(8):987–97.
48. Govaert TM, Dinant GJ, Aretz K, et al. The predictive value of influenza symptomatology in elderly people. Fam Pract 1998;15(1):16–22. Available at: http://www.ncbi.nlm.nih.gov/pubmed/9527293. Accessed May 7, 2013.
49. Walsh E, Cox C, Falsey A. Clinical features of influenza A virus infection in older hospitalized persons. J Am Geriatr Soc 2002. Available at: http://onlinelibrary.wiley.com/doi/10.1046/j.1532-5415.2002.50404.x/full. Accessed November 9, 2012.
50. Writing Committee of the WHO Consultation on Clinical Aspects of Pandemic (H1N1) 2009. Clinical aspects of pandemic 2009 influenza. N Engl J Med 2010;362:1708–19.
51. Centers for Disease Control. Guidance for clinicians on the use of rapid influenza diagnostic tests. Available at: http://www.cdc.gov/flu/pdf/professionals/diagnosis/clinician_guidance_ridt.pdf. Accessed November 14, 2012.
52. Harper SA, Bradley JS, Englund JA, et al. Seasonal influenza in adults and children–diagnosis, treatment, chemoprophylaxis, and institutional outbreak management: clinical practice guidelines of the Infectious Diseases Society of America. Clin Infect Dis 2009;48(8):1003–32. Available at: http://www.ncbi.nlm.nih.gov/pubmed/19281331. Accessed October 26, 2012.
53. Rothberg M, He S, Rose D. Management of influenza symptoms in healthy adults: cost-effectiveness of rapid testing and antiviral therapy. J Gen Intern Med 2003;18(10). Available at: http://archpedi.ama-assn.org/cgi/reprint/159/11/1055.pdf. Accessed November 14, 2012.
54. Smith KJ, Roberts MS. Cost-effectiveness of newer treatment strategies for influenza. Am J Med 2002;113(4):300–7. Available at: http://www.ncbi.nlm.nih.gov/pubmed/12361816. Accessed May 7, 2013.
55. Centers for Disease Control. Evaluation of 11 commercially available rapid influenza diagnostic tests–United States, 2011-2012. MMWR Morb Mortal Wkly Rep 2012;61(43):2008–10.
56. Baz M, Abed Y, Papenburg J, et al. Emergence of oseltamivir-resistant pandemic H1N1 virus during prophylaxis. N Engl J Med 2009;361(23):2296–7. Available at: http://www.ncbi.nlm.nih.gov/pubmed/19907034. Accessed December 6, 2012.
57. Ison MG. Antivirals and resistance: influenza virus. Curr Opin Virol 2011;1(6):563–73. Available at: http://www.ncbi.nlm.nih.gov/pubmed/22440914. Accessed December 10, 2012.
58. Beigi RH, Han K, Venkataramanan R, et al. Pharmacokinetics of oseltamivir among pregnant and nonpregnant women. Am J Obstet Gynecol 2011;204(6 Suppl 1):S84–8. Available at: http://www.pubmedcentral.nih.gov/articlerender.fcgi?artid=3111757&tool=pmcentrez&rendertype=abstract. Accessed December 19, 2012.
59. Hayden FG, Osterhaus AD, Treanor JJ, et al. Efficacy and safety of the neuraminidase inhibitor zanamivir in the treatment of influenzavirus infections. GG167 Influenza Study Group. N Engl J Med 1997;337(13):874–80. Available at: http://www.ncbi.nlm.nih.gov/pubmed/9302301. Accessed December 24, 2012.
60. Steel HM, Peppercorn AF. Fatal respiratory events caused by zanamivir nebulization. Clin Infect Dis 2010;51(1):121. Available at: http://cid.oxfordjournals.org.ezproxy.cul.columbia.edu/content/51/1/121.1.full. Accessed December 10, 2012.
61. Pinto LH, Lamb RA. The M2 proton channels of influenza A and B viruses. J Biol Chem 2006;281(14):8997–9000. Available at: http://www.ncbi.nlm.nih.gov/pubmed/16407184. Accessed November 11, 2012.

62. Abed Y, Goyette N, Boivin G. Generation and characterization of recombinant influenza A (H1N1) viruses harboring amantadine resistance mutations. Antimicrobial Agents Chemother 2005;49(2):556–9. Available at: http://aac.asm.org. ezproxy.cul.columbia.edu/content/49/2/556.abstract?ijkey=c0bfb3bca36aed 1da778a0527398811e3ba56635&keytype2=tf_ipsecsha. Accessed December 24, 2012.

63. Fiore AE, Fry A, Shay D, et al. Antiviral agents for the treatment and chemoprophylaxis of influenza — recommendations of the Advisory Committee on Immunization Practices (ACIP). MMWR Recomm Rep 2011;60(1):1–24. Available at: http://www.ncbi.nlm.nih.gov/pubmed/21248682. Accessed November 16, 2012.

64. Chan-Tack KM, Murray JS, Birnkrant DB. Use of ribavirin to treat influenza. N Engl J Med 2009;361(17):1713–4. Available at: http://www.ncbi.nlm.nih.gov/pubmed/19846864. Accessed November 16, 2012.

65. Graci JD, Cameron CE. Mechanisms of action of ribavirin against distinct viruses. Rev Med Virol 2006;16(1):37–48. Available at: http://www.ncbi.nlm.nih. gov/pubmed/16287208. Accessed December 19, 2012.

66. Monto AS, Fleming DM, Henry D, et al. Efficacy and safety of the neuraminidase inhibitor zanamivirin the treatment of influenza A and B virus infections. J Infect Dis 1999;180(2):254–61. Available at: http://www.ncbi.nlm.nih.gov/pubmed/10395837. Accessed December 31, 2012.

67. Leekha S, Zitterkopf NL, Espy MJ, et al. Duration of influenza A virus shedding in hospitalized patients and implications for infection control. Infect Control Hosp Epidemiol 2007;28(9):1071–6. Available at: http://www.ncbi.nlm.nih.gov/pubmed/17932829. Accessed November 8, 2012.

68. Hanshaoworakul W, Simmerman JM, Narueponjirakul U, et al. Severe human influenza infections in Thailand: oseltamivir treatment and risk factors for fatal outcome. PLoS One 2009;4(6):e6051. Available at: http://www.pubmedcentral. nih.gov/articlerender.fcgi?artid=2699035&tool=pmcentrez&rendertype= abstract. Accessed November 15, 2012.

69. McGeer A, Green KA, Plevneshi A, et al. Antiviral therapy and outcomes of influenza requiring hospitalization in Ontario, Canada. Clin Infect Dis 2007;45(12): 1568–75. Available at: http://cid.oxfordjournals.org.ezproxy.cul.columbia.edu/content/45/12/1568.full. Accessed November 2, 2012.

70. Yen HL, Monto AS, Webster RG, et al. Virulence may determine the necessary duration and dosage of oseltamivir treatment for highly pathogenic A/Vietnam/1203/04 influenza virus in mice. J Infect Dis 2005;192(4):665–72. Available at: http://jid.oxfordjournals.org.ezproxy.cul.columbia.edu/content/192/4/665.full. Accessed December 19, 2012.

71. Thorne-Humphrey LM, Goralski KB, Slayter KL, et al. Oseltamivir pharmacokinetics in morbid obesity (OPTIMO trial). J Antimicrob Chemother 2011;66(9): 2083–91. Available at: http://www.ncbi.nlm.nih.gov/pubmed/21700623. Accessed December 19, 2012.

72. Anon. CDC H1N1 flu. Updated interim recommendations for obstetric health care providers related to use of antiviral medications in the treatment and prevention of influenza for the 2009-2010 season. Available at: http://www.cdc.gov/H1N1flu/pregnancy/antiviral_messages.htm. Accessed December 30, 2012.

73. Centers for Disease Control and Prevention (CDC). Maternal and infant outcomes among severely ill pregnant and postpartum women with 2009 pandemic influenza A (H1N1)–United States, April 2009-August 2010. MMWR Morb Mortal Wkly Rep 2011;60(35):1193–6. Available at: http://www.ncbi.nlm.nih.gov/pubmed/21900872. Accessed December 30, 2012.

74. Harper SA, Bradley JS, Englund JA, et al. Seasonal influenza in adults and children–diagnosis, treatment, chemoprophylaxis, and institutional outbreak management: clinical practice guidelines of the Infectious Diseases Society of America. Clin Infect Dis 2009;48(8):1003–32.
75. Smith JR, Rayner CR, Donner B, et al. Oseltamivir in seasonal, pandemic, and avian influenza: a comprehensive review of 10-years clinical experience. Adv Ther 2011;28(11):927–59. Available at: http://www.ncbi.nlm.nih.gov/pubmed/22057727. Accessed October 30, 2012.
76. Peters P, Gravenstein S. Long-term use of oseltamivir for the prophylaxis of influenza in a vaccinated frail older population. J Am Geriatr Soc 2001;49:1025–31. Available at: http://onlinelibrary.wiley.com/doi/10.1046/j.1532-5415.2001.49204.x/full. Accessed November 15, 2012.
77. Ghedin E, Holmes EC, Depasse JV, et al. Presence of oseltamivir-resistant pandemic A/H1N1 minor variants before drug therapy with subsequent selection and transmission. J Infect Dis 2012;206(10):1504–11. Available at: http://www.ncbi.nlm.nih.gov/pubmed/22966122. Accessed December 10, 2012.
78. Hurt AC, Hardie K, Wilson NJ, et al. Community transmission of oseltamivir-resistant A(H1N1)pdm09 influenza. N Engl J Med 2011;365(26):2541–2. Available at: http://www.ncbi.nlm.nih.gov/pubmed/22204735. Accessed December 29, 2012.
79. Van der Sluijs KF, Van der Poll T, Lutter R, et al. Bench-to-bedside review: bacterial pneumonia with influenza - pathogenesis and clinical implications. Crit Care 2010;14(2):219. Available at: http://www.ncbi.nlm.nih.gov/pmc/articles/PMC2887122/?report=abstract. Accessed December 19, 2012.
80. Hayashi Y, Vaska VL, Baba H, et al. Influenza-associated bacterial pathogens in patients with 2009 influenza A (H1N1) infection: impact of community-associated methicillin-resistant *Staphylococcus aureus* in Queensland, Australia. Intern Med J 2012;42(7):755–60. Available at: http://www.ncbi.nlm.nih.gov/pubmed/21981384. Accessed December 19, 2012.
81. Leekha S, Zitterkopf NL, Espy MJ, et al. Duration of influenza A virus shedding in hospitalized patients and implications for infection control. Infect Control Hosp Epidemiol 2007;28(9):1071–6.
82. Anon. CDC - Seasonal influenza (flu) - ACIP recommendations: introduction and biology of influenza. Available at: http://www.cdc.gov/flu/professionals/acip/clinical.htm#signs. Accessed December 30, 2012.
83. Anon. Prevention and control of influenza with vaccines: recommendations of the Advisory Committee on Immunization Practices (ACIP) — United States, 2012–13 influenza season. Available at: http://www.cdc.gov/mmwr/preview/mmwrhtml/mm6132a3.htm. Accessed December 30, 2012.
84. Cohen SA, Chui KK, Naumova EN. Influenza vaccination in young children reduces influenza-associated hospitalizations in older adults, 2002-2006. J Am Geriatr Soc 2011;59(2):327–32. Available at: http://www.pubmedcentral.nih.gov/articlerender.fcgi?artid=3111961&tool=pmcentrez&rendertype=abstract. Accessed November 15, 2012.
85. Anon. CDC - Seasonal influenza (flu) - Q & A: Fluzone high-dose seasonal influenza vaccine. Available at: http://www.cdc.gov/flu/protect/vaccine/qa_fluzone.htm. Accessed December 30, 2012.
86. Anon. CDC - Seasonal influenza (flu) - Q & A: intradermal influenza vaccination. Available at: http://www.cdc.gov/flu/protect/vaccine/qa_intradermal-vaccine.htm. Accessed December 30, 2012.

87. Kumar D, Blumberg EA, Danziger-Isakov L, et al. Influenza vaccination in the organ transplant recipient: review and summary recommendations. Am J Transplant 2011;11(10):2020–30. Available at: http://www.ncbi.nlm.nih.gov/pubmed/21957936. Accessed December 30, 2012.

88. Avery RK. Influenza vaccines in the setting of solid-organ transplantation: are they safe? Curr Opin Infect Dis 2012;25(4):464–8. Available at: http://www.ncbi.nlm.nih.gov/pubmed/22710319. Accessed November 8, 2012.

89. Bijl M, Agmon-Levin N, Dayer JM, et al. Vaccination of patients with autoimmune inflammatory rheumatic diseases requires careful benefit-risk assessment. Autoimmun Rev 2012;11(8):572–6. Available at: http://www.ncbi.nlm.nih.gov/pubmed/22037116. Accessed November 15, 2012.

90. Eisenberg RA, Jawad AF, Boyer J, et al. Rituximab-treated patients have a poor response to influenza vaccination. J Clin Immunol 2012. Available at: http://www.ncbi.nlm.nih.gov/pubmed/23064976. Accessed November 13, 2012.

91. Yri OE, Torfoss D, Hungnes O, et al. Rituximab blocks protective serologic response to influenza A (H1N1) 2009 vaccination in lymphoma patients during or within 6 months after treatment. Blood 2011;118(26):6769–71. Available at: http://www.ncbi.nlm.nih.gov/pubmed/22058114. Accessed December 2, 2012.

92. Nicholson KG, Wood JM, Zambon M. Influenza. Lancet 2003;362(9397): 1733–45. Available at: http://www.ncbi.nlm.nih.gov/pubmed/14643124. Accessed December 12, 2012.

93. Anon. CDC - Seasonal influenza (flu) - flu vaccine effectiveness. Available at: http://www.cdc.gov/flu/professionals/vaccination/effectivenessqa.htm. Accessed December 30, 2012.

94. Beran J, Vesikari T, Wertzova V, et al. Efficacy of inactivated split-virus influenza vaccine against culture-confirmed influenza in healthy adults: a prospective, randomized, placebo-controlled trial. J Infect Dis 2009;200(12):1861–9. Available at: http://www.ncbi.nlm.nih.gov/pubmed/19909082. Accessed December 13, 2012.

95. Herrera GA, Iwane MK, Cortese M, et al. Influenza vaccine effectiveness among 50-64-year-old persons during a season of poor antigenic match between vaccine and circulating influenza virus strains: Colorado, United States, 2003-2004. Vaccine 2007;25(1):154–60. Available at: http://www.ncbi.nlm.nih.gov/pubmed/17064823. Accessed December 13, 2012.

96. Ison MG, Szakaly P, Shapira MY, et al. Efficacy and safety of oral oseltamivir for influenza prophylaxis in transplant recipients. Antivir Ther 2012;17(6):955–64. Available at: http://www.ncbi.nlm.nih.gov/pubmed/22728756. Accessed December 23, 2012.

97. Anon. CDC - Seasonal influenza (flu) - prevention strategies for seasonal influenza in healthcare settings. Available at: http://www.cdc.gov/flu/professionals/infectioncontrol/healthcaresettings.htm. Accessed December 30, 2012.

98. Derber CJ, Shankaran S. Health-care worker vaccination for influenza: strategies and controversies. Curr Infect Dis Rep 2012;14(6):627–32. Available at: http://www.ncbi.nlm.nih.gov/pubmed/22941054. Accessed December 18, 2012.

99. Cowling BJ, Chan KH, Fang VJ, et al. Facemasks and hand hygiene to prevent influenza transmission in households: a cluster randomized trial. Ann Intern Med 2009;151(7):437–46. Available at: http://www.ncbi.nlm.nih.gov/pubmed/19652172. Accessed December 17, 2012.

100. Ukimura A, Ooi Y, Kanzaki Y, et al. A national survey on myocarditis associated with influenza H1N1pdm2009 in the pandemic and postpandemic season in Japan. J Infect Chemother 2012. Available at: http://www.ncbi.nlm.nih.gov/pubmed/23089894. Accessed December 31, 2012.

101. Toovey S, Prinssen EP, Rayner CR, et al. Post-marketing assessment of neuro-psychiatric adverse events in influenza patients treated with oseltamivir: an updated review. Adv Ther 2012;29(10):826–48. Available at: http://www.ncbi.nlm.nih.gov/pubmed/23054689. Accessed November 15, 2012.
102. Nakamura K, Schwartz BS, Lindegårdh N, et al. Possible neuropsychiatric reaction to high-dose oseltamivir during acute 2009 H1N1 influenza A infection. Clin Infect Dis 2010;50(7):e47–9. Available at: http://www.ncbi.nlm.nih.gov/pubmed/20192728. Accessed December 30, 2012.
103. Toovey S, Jick SS, Meier CR. Parkinson's disease or Parkinson symptoms following seasonal influenza. Influenza Other Respi Viruses 2011;5(5):328–33. Available at: http://www.ncbi.nlm.nih.gov/pubmed/21668692. Accessed December 30, 2012.
104. Bunce PE, High SM, Nadjafi M, et al. Pandemic H1N1 influenza infection and vascular thrombosis. Clin Infect Dis 2011;52(2):e14–7. Available at: http://www.ncbi.nlm.nih.gov/pubmed/21288835. Accessed December 30, 2012.
105. Zhu T, Carcaillon L, Martinez I, et al. Association of influenza vaccination with reduced risk of venous thromboembolism. Thromb Haemost 2009;102(6):1259–64. Available at: http://www.ncbi.nlm.nih.gov/pubmed/19967159. Accessed December 30, 2012.
106. Gaglia MA, Cook RL, Kraemer KL, et al. Patient knowledge and attitudes about antiviral medication and vaccination for influenza in an internal medicine clinic. Clin Infect Dis 2007;45(9):1182–8. Available at: http://www.ncbi.nlm.nih.gov/pubmed/17918080. Accessed November 14, 2012.
107. Hebert P, Frick K. The causes of racial and ethnic differences in influenza vaccination rates among elderly Medicare beneficiaries. Health Serv Res 2005;40(2). Available at: http://onlinelibrary.wiley.com/doi/10.1111/j.1475-6773.2005.0e371.x/full. Accessed November 8, 2012.
108. Poland GA, Jacobson RM. The age-old struggle against the antivaccinationists. N Engl J Med 2011;364(2):97–9.
109. Anon. CDC - Seasonal influenza (flu) - antiviral medications: summary for clinicians. Available at: http://www.cdc.gov/flu/professionals/antivirals/summary-clinicians.htm. Accessed December 30, 2012.
110. Centers for Disease Control. Influenza vaccination: a summary for clinicians. Available at: http://www.cdc.gov/flu/professionals/vaccination/vax-summary.htm. Accessed November 15, 2012.

Pneumococcus

Samuel Y. Ash, MD[a],*, John V.L. Sheffield, MD[b]

KEYWORDS

- Pneumococcus • *Streptococcus pneumoniae* • Bacterial pneumonia
- Invasive pneumococcal disease • Bacterial illnesses • Antibiotic resistance
- Immunization • Treatment

KEY POINTS

- The peak incidence of pneumococcal illness occurs in the very young and in the elderly. Human immunodeficiency virus and asplenia are also key risk factors.
- The virulence of a particular pneumococcal organism depends on the serotype of its capsule.
- Pneumococcus is the most common cause of pneumonia in hospitalized patients and may be the most common bacterial cause in the outpatient setting as well.
- Despite advances in antibiotics and critical care, pneumococcal bacteremia remains a mortal and morbid disease, particularly for those patients with septic shock.
- Although the rate of change of pneumococcal antibiotic resistance has slowed, it continues to increase.
- Selective pressure by immunization may be resulting in an increase in pneumococcal disease caused by serotypes not included in the vaccines as well as the antimicrobial resistance of those serotypes.
- The Advisory Committee on Immunization Practices now recommends that patients with immunocompromising conditions, functional or anatomic asplenia, cerebrospinal fluid leaks, or cochlear implants who have not previously received pneumococcal conjugate vaccine 13 (PCV13) or 23 valent polysaccharide vaccine (PPSV23) be given PCV13 first followed by PPSV23 8 weeks later.

OVERVIEW

Streptococcus pneumoniae is one of the most common bacterial pathogens encountered in medicine.[1] First isolated in 1881 by Louis Pasteur, pneumococcus, as it is commonly known, continues to be an important cause of mortality and

Funding Sources: None.
Conflict of Interest: None.
[a] Department of Medicine, University of Washington Medical Center, 1959 Northeast Pacific Street, Box 356421, Seattle, WA 98195, USA; [b] Division of General Internal Medicine, Department of Medicine, Harborview Medical Center, University of Washington, 325 Ninth Avenue, Box 359782, Seattle, WA 98104, USA
* Corresponding author.
E-mail address: samash@uw.edu

morbidity in all age groups, from children to the elderly, both in the United States and worldwide.[2]

EPIDEMIOLOGY

The rates of infection with S pneumoniae vary widely depending on how infection is defined. In general, invasive pneumococcal disease is defined as an infection confirmed by the isolation of S pneumoniae from what is normally a sterile site, such as in the case of meningitis or bacteremia. Noninvasive disease thus includes all other clinical S pneumoniae infections from nonsterile sites such as pneumonia and the respiratory tract. Rates of colonization include patients from whom S pneumoniae is isolated, but who do not have clinical disease. The most recent estimate of invasive disease in the United States is 12.9 cases per 100,000 population per year, and the estimated death rate caused by invasive S pneumoniae infections is 1.3 per 100,000 population per year.[3]

Noninvasive infection rates are more difficult to quantify, in part because of the high rates of colonization by S pneumoniae in both healthy and sick individuals.[4,5] Colonization in ill patients poses a particularly challenging problem because it is may be unclear whether, for example, a patient's underlying pneumonia is caused by S pneumoniae or whether there is another pathogen present and S pneumoniae is isolated as an innocent bystander from the patient's upper respiratory tract. S pneumoniae has been isolated from the nasopharynx of as many as 24% of patients with pneumonia, and even experts have, in the same year, offered estimates of the rates of pneumonia directly attributable to S pneumoniae infection that range from 31.6 to 500 cases per 100,000 population per year.[6,7]

RISK FACTORS

Perhaps easier to discern than the overall rates of infection with S pneumoniae are the risk factors for both invasive and noninvasive disease. Although outbreaks were common in the past and still happen occasionally, such as a well-known occurrence at an overcrowded jail in 1994, most infections with S pneumoniae are sporadic.[8] The peak incidence of pneumococcal infections occurs in young children and in the elderly, with the current estimates for incidence of invasive disease being 31.4 cases per 100,000 per year in patients less than the age of 1 year and 37.0 cases per 100,000 per year in patients older than 65 years.[2,9] Young patients, especially those younger than 2 years, are at particular risk because of their lack of immunoglobulin (Ig) G2.[10] Other risk factors include hypogammaglobulinemia, complement deficiency (especially deficiency of C3b), asplenia, nephrotic syndrome (caused by the loss of serum complement and IgG), diabetes, alcoholism, cirrhosis, and nonhematologic malignancies.[10] There are also associations between S pneumoniae infections and chronic obstructive pulmonary disease, heart failure, cerebral vascular disease, epilepsy, dementia, cigarette smoke, recent hospitalization and institutionalization, and human immunodeficiency virus (HIV).[11,12]

As risk factors, both HIV and asplenia warrant particular attention. With regard to HIV, the rate of pneumococcal pneumonia is 5.5 to 17.6 times higher in patients with acquired immunodeficiency syndrome (AIDS), and in one study the rate of pneumococcal bacteremia in patients with AIDS was 9.4 per 1000 population per year, compared with 0.07 per 1000 population per year in patients aged 20 to 55 years.[12] The clinical presentation of pneumococcal pneumonia is similar in patients with HIV to those without HIV, although blood cultures may be more sensitive in patients with HIV compared with patients who are not infected with HIV. Also, patients with HIV are more likely to be neutropenic and less likely to have a significant leukocytosis.[12] The treatment of patients with HIV and *S pneumoniae* infections is similar to that of patients not infected with HIV, and although some studies show the case fatality rate to be lower in patients with HIV (11% vs 18.5%) others have shown it to be similar at around 15%.[12,13] Patients with asplenia, either functional or anatomic, who have pneumococcal infections are at high risk for mortality from overwhelming sepsis.[14]

PATHOGENESIS AND STRUCTURE

The mechanisms by which *S pneumoniae* cause disease are primarily related to its surface components, most notably its polysaccharide capsule and its cell wall.[15] The capsule's primary physiologic role is to protect the bacterium from phagocytosis by polymorphonuclear leukocytes. The capsule does not elicit any inflammatory response, but its chemical composition and size are the primary determinants of *S pneumoniae*'s virulence.[16] The importance of the capsule is underscored by the protection provided by anticapsular antibodies, and that the virulence of a particular pneumococcal organism depends on the serotype of its capsule.[15] For instance, serotype 3 *S pneumoniae* is very virulent, whereas serotype 37 lacks clinically significant virulence in humans.[16,17]

Although the capsule is the primary determinant of *S pneumoniae*'s virulence, it is the cell wall that provokes a host's immune response. The cell wall is responsible for the recruitment of leukocytes to the site of infection; it also induces the production of cytokines and initiates the procoagulant cascade.[15] In addition, changes in penicillin-binding proteins in the cell wall result in resistance to penicillin and other β-lactam antibiotics.[18]

The other surface components implicated in pneumococcal disease are the surface proteins, which are, for the most part, unidentified. One known surface protein is worth particular mention: pneumolysin. Pneumolysin is an intracellular protein and is released when *S pneumoniae* is lysed by, for instance, certain antibiotics. It is active in pore formation and is cytotoxic to nearly every cell in the lung.[15,19]

The frequent colonization of otherwise healthy patients with *S pneumoniae* suggests that, although it has numerous pathogenic components, in many instances these are not sufficient to result in a clinical infection. Infection may require a preceding event such as a viral illness.[15] This is borne out not only by in vitro data that show that viruses and cytokines enhance pneumococcal adherence but also by epidemiologic data that show peak rates of pneumococcal infection during the winter and early spring when viral infections such as influenza are also more prevalent.[20–23]

PNEUMONIA

As might be anticipated given its name, *S pneumoniae* is a frequent cause of pneumonia, especially community-acquired pneumonia. Because of the limitations in diagnosis noted earlier, the incidence of pneumococcal pneumonia is likely higher than indicated by retrospective studies. Regardless, it is the most common identified cause of community-acquired pneumonia in hospitalized patients as well as those admitted to intensive care units, and it may be the most common overall cause of pneumonia in the community setting.[24–27]

The classic clinical presentation of pneumococcal pneumonia involves the sudden onset of rigors followed by a cough productive of rusty sputum. Other frequent symptoms include chest pain as well as occasional nausea, vomiting, and diarrhea.[28] Less common is pneumococcal pneumonia associated fulminant diarrhea, known as croupous colitis.[29]

Making a diagnosis of pneumonia specifically caused by S pneumoniae can be challenging, as previously mentioned. The radiologic manifestations of pneumococcal pneumonia vary. A review of the chest radiograph patterns of 40 patients with pneumococcal pneumonia, 13 of whom were bacteremic, revealed that 12 of them had lobar opacity, 12 had a patchy bronchopneumonic pattern, 9 had interstitial changes, and 7 had a mixed pattern.[30] These patterns of opacity may be further modified by underlying disease such as emphysema. Hospitalized patients may more commonly have a bronchopneumonic pattern than the classic lobar pattern, with 61% presenting with the former compared with 39% with the latter.[14,31] S pneumoniae rarely causes cavitation or a true necrotizing pulmonary infection.[32,33]

The role of sputum collection in diagnosis of pneumococcal pneumonia is also fraught because its accuracy depends largely on how it is obtained and the criteria by which it is evaluated.[34] Its usefulness is further limited by patients' frequent inability to produce a specimen of sufficient quality and by the administration of antibiotics before it is obtained.[24,35] In one study, a good-quality sputum specimen could only be obtained in 14.4% of patients with community-acquired pneumonia.[36] Although older studies showed the sensitivity of sputum culture to be 40% to 50%, more recent data suggest that, if a good-quality sputum sample can be obtained in a patient who has not received antibiotics, then the sputum Gram stain and culture may be up to 80% to 93% sensitive respectively.[37–39] However, the Infectious Disease Society of America (IDSA) only recommends sputum Gram stain and culture in patients with community-acquired pneumonia who are admitted to the intensive care unit, who have failed outpatient therapy, or who have any of the following: cavitary infiltrates seen on imaging, a history of active alcohol abuse, severe obstructive or structural lung disease, a positive Legionella or pneumococcal urinary antigen test, or a pleural effusion.[40] Blood cultures should also be part of the routine evaluation of such patients.

Because of the challenges involved in making a firm diagnosis of pneumococcal pneumonia, other diagnostic strategies have been developed. The most commonly used is the pneumococcal urinary antigen, which has a sensitivity of 70.5% in hospitalized patients with community-acquired pneumonia, and, when patients with non-pneumococcal pneumonia are used as the control group, a specificity of 96%.[41] However, it should be noted that, in certain populations such as children, the specificity may be lower (less than 70% in some cases) because of high rates of nasopharyngeal colonization.[42]

Once a diagnosis of pneumococcal pneumonia is made, the treatment depends in large part on the severity of illness. Because only 12% to 30% of cases of pneumococcal bacteremia are the result of nosocomial infections, empiric therapy for suspected pneumococcal pneumonia should typically be based on guidelines for community-acquired disease (**Table 1**).[14] The decision as to what level of care is appropriate, outpatient versus inpatient, and inpatient versus intensive care unit, should be based both on objective scoring systems such as the confusion, uremia, respiratory rate, low blood pressure, age 65 years or younger (CURB-65) criteria, and prognostic models like the Pneumonia Severity Index, as well as physician determination of subjective factors. Patients with a CURB-65 score greater than or equal to 2 should usually be hospitalized.[40]

BACTEREMIA

Pneumococcal bacteremia is a highly morbid and mortal disease. In at least one study done during the preantibiotic era, 36.7% of patients with pneumococcal pneumonia became bacteremic and 77.5% of those bacteremic patients died as a result of their

Table 1
Empiric antibiotic therapy for community-acquired pneumonia

Outpatient Treatment	
Previously healthy and no use of antimicrobials in prior 3 mo	Macrolide or doxycycline for 5–7 d
Presence of medical comorbidities or recent use of antimicrobials	Respiratory fluoroquinolone (moxifloxacin, gemifloxacin, or levofloxacin) or a β-lactam plus a macrolide for 5–7 d
In regions with high level of macrolide-resistant S pneumoniae	Consider respiratory fluoroquinolone for 5–7 d
Inpatients, not in intensive care units	Respiratory fluoroquinolone or a β-lactam plus a macrolide
Inpatients, in intensive care units	A β-lactam plus either azithromycin or a respiratory fluoroquinolone if bacteremic therapy for 10–14 d
Special scenarios	See IDSA guidelines for recommendations regarding concern for pseudomonal or methicillin-resistant Staphylococcus aureus infections

Data from Mandell LA, Wunderink RG, Anzueto A, et al. Infectious Diseases Society of America/ American Thoracic Society consensus guidelines on the management of community-acquired pneumonia in adults. Clin Infect Dis 2007;44(Suppl 2):S27–72.

infection.[43] It is with bacteremic patients that antibiotics have made the most profound difference in outcomes, and have dramatically improved outcomes; estimates of mortality for patients with pneumococcal bacteremia now range from 7% to 30%.[44–46]

As might be expected, the highest mortality is seen in patients with pneumococcal bacteremia who are seriously ill. In our cohort from Harborview Medical Center in Seattle, WA, from 1992 to 2000, the mortality was only 1.2% for patients with mild disease, who were treated exclusively outside the intensive care unit (ICU) on the medicine wards.[47] In contrast, patients whose pneumococcal infections are serious enough to warrant admission to the ICU have mortalities from 36% to nearly 80%.[44,46]

With regard to the treatment of these critically ill patients, intensive care does not seem to have a significant impact on their mortality, but for certain clinical scenarios it may be beneficial.[44] Based on our own observations at Harborview, patients with pneumococcal bacteremia admitted to the ICU for acute respiratory failure requiring mechanical ventilation had significantly better survival in the 1990s compared with the 1970s (mortality, 55% vs 81%; P<.05). However, Harborview patients in septic shock requiring vasopressors fared no better in the 1990s than in the 1970s (mortality, 86% vs 93%; nonsignificant).[47] Moreover, even with 40 years of improvements in critical care, the latter group, patients with pneumococcal bacteremia in septic shock, had a mortality similar to that in Austrian and Gold's[45] original cohort from the 1950s at Kings County Hospital in Brooklyn (NY). Thus, our observational data suggest that advances in ICU care have improved outcomes for patients with pneumococcal bacteremia and respiratory failure, but outcomes for patients in septic shock remain poor.

OTHER INFECTIONS

As mentioned earlier, S pneumoniae is one of the most common bacterial causes of human disease.[1] As such, it causes a wide range of infectious syndromes, from the aforementioned pneumonia and bacteremia to otitis media, meningitis, endocarditis, pericarditis, osteomyelitis, septic arthritis, and even brain abscesses. Although many of these syndromes are uncommon, pneumococcus can cause a suppurative infection nearly anywhere in the body.[48] Given their relative frequency, 2 types of pneumococcal infection warrant particular mention.

The first is otitis media. S pneumoniae is the most common bacterial cause of otitis media in children, and is responsible for 28% to 55% of cases.[49] Because of this, as of 2001, the cost of otitis media caused by S pneumoniae in the United States was between 2 billion and 5.3 billion dollars.[49]

Although less common than pneumococcal otitis media, meningitis caused by S pneumoniae is a more mortal and morbid disease. A recent meta-analysis found that, despite antibiotics and other advanced interventions, the mortality in pneumococcal meningitis remains 34.9% to 44.2%.[50] One question that has arisen in the treatment of meningitis in general, including pneumococcal meningitis, is what role, if any, steroids play as an adjuvant therapeutic. In the aforementioned meta-analysis, the lower mortality (34.9%) was in patients who received adjuvant steroid therapy and the higher rate (44.2%) was seen in those who did not There is some thought that steroids may be particularly beneficial in patients with pneumococcal meningitis compared with other forms of infectious meningitis, because the studies that have shown the greatest benefit for steroids have tended to have a predominance of cases of meningitis caused by S pneumoniae.[50,51] However, the greatest concern for potential complications of antibiotic-resistant pneumococcal infections has been primarily in the setting of meningitis, and it was the emergence of penicillin-resistant and cefotaxime-resistant S pneumoniae isolates resulting in meningitis treatment failures that prompted the addition of vancomycin to the empiric treatment of community-acquired meningitis.[52,53] However, steroids may accentuate the problem of resistant disease because they may decrease the permeability of the blood-brain barrier to vancomycin, theoretically increasing the risk of treatment failures in the setting of resistant infections.[51,54,55] In addition, glucocorticoids may potentiate the effects of ischemia on neurons, resulting in more tissue damage in the setting of infection.[51,56] Thus, in the era of antibiotic resistance, the use of steroids in pneumococcal meningitis, although recommended, remains an open question.

ANTIMICROBIAL RESISTANCE

Early in the antibiotic era, all S pneumoniae were sensitive to penicillin. The first reported decreases in susceptibility to penicillin and other antibiotics were in Australia and New Guinea in the 1960s, followed by South Africa in the 1970s and ultimately throughout the remainder of Africa, Asia, Europe, and the rest of the world.[57,58] During the late 1980s and 1990s the rates of reported resistance climbed rapidly. Examination of isolates from several large, mostly urban, hospitals between 1987 and 1992 showed a 60-fold increase in high-level penicillin resistance, and by 1998 the overall rate of penicillin resistance was between 24% and 29%. Perhaps more concerning was that as many of 14% of isolates were resistant to 3 or more classes of antibiotics.[57,59,60]

However, in the early 2000s, that trend of increasing resistance rates changed. Data from a large longitudinal study that included 39,495 isolates collected between 2000 and 2004 showed that the rates of S pneumoniae resistance to a variety of antibiotics plateaued and may even have decreased during that time frame. For instance, the rate of high-level resistance to penicillin decreased from 26.3% in year 1 of the study to 16.5% in year 4. This decline in high-level resistance was accompanied by an increase in intermediate resistance from 12.5% to 20.0%, but the overall rate of penicillin non-susceptibility during the study period remained stable, and declined slightly from

38.8% to 36.5%. The rates of resistance to other classes of antibiotics, such as macrolides and quinolones, were also stable during that time frame at 27.5% to 30.7% and 0.8% to 1.1% respectively, and the rate of resistance to trimethoprim-sulfamethoxazole decreased from 33.9% to 24.1%. Less heartening was that the rate of resistance to multiple classes of antibiotics, although stable, was 30% across the 4 years of the study, and 8% of the isolates were resistant to 5 classes of antibiotics.[61]

Although these recent data are reassuring, the rates of resistance tell only part of the story. First, as with rates of pneumococcal infections, the rates of drug-resistant *S pneumoniae* vary depending on the definitions used for susceptible and nonsusceptible, and differ more when the terms intermediate resistance and high-level resistance are used.

Before 2008, the Clinical and Laboratory Standards Institute (CLSI) *S pneumoniae* minimum inhibitory concentration (MIC) breakpoints for β-lactam/penicillin susceptibility were selected primarily based on their implications for the treatment of meningitis. However, the penetration of penicillin into the in the cerebrospinal fluid (CSF) is significantly less than into the alveoli, middle ear, and sinuses, where the concentrations of penicillin approach those reached in the blood. Therefore, in 2008 the CLSI revised its MIC breakpoints, dramatically changing the percentage of *S pneumoniae* isolates with nonmeningitic penicillin MICs in the susceptible range.[62] A comparison between the new and old breakpoints is given in **Table 2**.

Because of this change in definitions, it can be difficult to compare rates of resistance reported before and after 2008. What is perhaps more helpful is to track the relative rates of isolates with various penicillin MICs. Analysis of data from The Surveillance Network (TSN), an electronic database of quantitative and qualitative susceptibility data from North American Laboratories, from 1996 to 2008 shows generally stable rates of penicillin MICs during that period (**Fig. 1**).[62]

The most recent data available for antibiotic susceptibility in the United States come from the US Centers for Disease Control and Prevention (CDC) reference laboratory testing of 3446 isolates in 2010 and from the SENTRY Antimicrobial Surveillance Program. Based on the 2011 CLSI breakpoints (which are the same as those from 2008), the CDC data show rates of pneumococcal penicillin susceptibility, intermediate resistance, and resistance in the United States to be 89.4%, 5.5%, and 5.1% respectively (**Table 3**).[3] The SENTRY data tell a slightly different story. Defined by breakpoint, they

Table 2
Comparison of concentration breakpoints (MICs) for β-lactam/penicillin susceptibility

	MIC (μg/mL)		
	Susceptible	Intermediate	Resistant
Before 2008			
Meningitis or nonmeningitis, any route of administration	≤0.06	0.12–1	≥2
After 2008			
For meningitis, intravenous administration	≤0.06	None	≥0.12
For nonmeningitis, intravenous administration	≤2	4	≥8
For nonmeningitis, oral administration	≤0.06	0.12–1	≥2

Data from Mera RM, Miller LA, Amrine-Madsen H, et al. Impact of new Clinical Laboratory Standards Institute *Streptococcus pneumoniae* penicillin susceptibility testing breakpoints on reported resistance changes over time. Microb Drug Resist 2011;17(1):47–52.

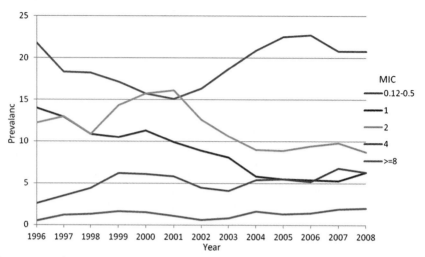

Fig. 1. Rates of penicillin MICs (µg/mL) among isolates from the TSN database from 1996 to 2008. (*Data from* Mera RM, Miller LA, Amrine-Madsen H, et al. Impact of new Clinical Laboratory Standards Institute *Streptococcus pneumoniae* penicillin susceptibility testing breakpoints on reported resistance changes over time. Microb Drug Resist 2011;17(1):47–52.)

show a decrease in penicillin susceptibility at 0.06 µg/mL for 71.6% in 1998 to 56.3% in 2011, and at 2 µg/mL from 96.8% in 1998 to 85.2% in 2011 (**Fig. 2**, **Table 4**).[63] Thus, although the rate of change of antibiotic resistance has not been as great as was observed in the late 1980s and early 1990s, the overall trend continues to be worrisome.

Although the changes in CLSI breakpoints, and the stabilization of the rate of change in MIC, may be reassuring, resistant pneumococcal infections persist. The true question is: what are the clinical implications of these resistant infections for patients? Austrian and Gold[45] wrote in their classic article on *S pneumoniae* in 1964, that at that time, "no well-documented case of therapeutic failure as a result of pneumococcal resistance [had] ever been reported." However, this is no longer the case.

Table 3
Rates of *S pneumoniae* resistance in 2010

Antibiotic	Susceptible (%)	Intermediate (%)	Resistant (%)
Penicillin	89.4	5.5	5.1
Cefotaxime	91.4	6.8	1.8
Erythromycin	73.8	0.5	25.7
Trimethoprim/sulfa	77.6	6.7	15.7
Tetracycline	84.9	0.6	14.5
Levofloxacin	99.7	0	0.3
Vancomycin	100	0	0

Based on 2011 definitions.
Data from CDC - ABCs: 2010 Strep pneumoniae Surveillance Report - Active Bacterial Core surveillance. Available at: http://www.cdc.gov/abcs/reports-findings/survreports/spneu10.html. Accessed March 18, 2013.

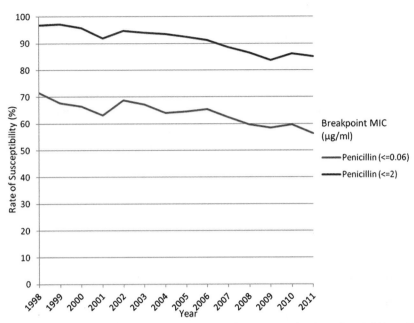

Fig. 2. Rates of *S pneumoniae* susceptibility from the SENTRY database from 1998 to 2011 for varying MICs. (*Data from* Jones RN, Sader HS, Mendes RE, et al. Update on antimicrobial susceptibility trends among *Streptococcus pneumoniae* in the United States: report of ceftaroline activity from the SENTRY Antimicrobial Surveillance Program (1998–2011). Diagn Microbiol Infect Dis 2013;75(1):107–9.)

Pneumococcal resistance is most clinically relevant in meningitis. As previously mentioned, penicillin does not penetrate the CSF well, and there have been many documented treatment failures and poor clinical outcomes attributed to resistant disease.[58,60] Treatment failures related to resistance to cephalosporins have also been reported, prompting the addition of vancomycin to the recommended empiric therapy for pneumococcal meningitis.[52,64]

The implications of resistant infections outside the central nervous system are less clear. In general, resistant isolates of *S pneumoniae* do not seem to be any more or less virulent than susceptible isolates.[64] Treatment failures have been reported when using oral β-lactam antibiotics for the treatment of otitis media, and this may, in part, be because of the low penetration of oral antibiotics into the middle ear relative to the MIC of resistant *S pneumoniae*. However, 50% to 60% of acute otitis media spontaneously resolves, and a stepwise approach to treatment that uses β-lactam antibiotics, specifically amoxicillin, as first-line therapy in uncomplicated otitis media continues to be recommended.[64,65] Although there have been a few reports of β-lactam treatment failure for pneumococcal pneumonia, in general, it seems that pneumococcal pneumonia and bacteremia clinical outcomes may not be affected by resistant disease.[64,66,67] This may be because of the previously mentioned good penetration that β-lactams have into the lungs as well as the frequent use of intravenous antibiotics in these syndromes, and is reflected in the continued recommendations by the IDSA to use β-lactams as part of first-line therapy for hospitalized patients with community-acquired pneumonia.[40,62,64] However, a more recent review did find a small detrimental outcome associated with patients who had penicillin-nonsusceptible *S pneumoniae* in

Table 4
Rates of *S pneumoniae* susceptibility from the SENTRY database from 1998–2011

Year	Penicillin (≤0.06)	Penicillin (≤2)	Amoxicillin/ Clavulanate (≤2)	Ceftriaxone (≤1)	Erythromycin (≤0.25)	Clindamycin (≤0.25)	Tetracycline (≤2)	Trimethoprim/ Sulfamethoxazole (≤0.5)	Levofloxacin (≤2)	Ciprofloxacin (≤4)
					% Susceptible by Agent (MIC Breakpoint in µg/mL)					
1998	71.6	96.8	97.1	97.0	82.2	96.2	88.8	73.8	99.8	2.2
1999	67.6	97.1	96.6	97.0	76.5	92.9	84.5	66.5	99.1	1.5
2000	66.5	95.7	93.4	95.0	74.3	92.3	83.6	67.3	99.3	3.8
2001	63.1	91.9	91.8	94.1	70.6	91.4	83.2	62.9	99.6	2.7
2002	68.7	94.7	93.8	97.4	74.1	92.4	86.7	70.1	98.7	2.8
2003	67.1	94.0	93.2	98.1	72.3	89.9	83.9	69.4	99.2	4.9
2004	64.0	93.5	90.9	97.3	70.5	89.4	86.2	67.1	99.2	1.7
2005	64.6	92.5	89.8	95.9	67.7	87.9	82.9	70.4	99.1	3.0
2006	65.4	91.2	89.4	96.6	67.2	83.7	80.0	72.0	99.1	3.7
2007	62.4	88.6	86.1	93.2	67.4	82.5	78.3	71.2	99.7	2.8
2008	59.6	86.5	83.5	91.3	63.2	80.0	77.3	67.1	99.4	4.0
2009	58.5	83.8	82.2	87.2	60.6	78.9	75.2	65.4	99.2	3.3
2010	59.7	86.1	83.9	90.4	60.4	79.6	76.9	67.9	99.7	2.2
2011	56.3	85.2	81.1	88.3	55.2	78.2	74.1	65.2	98.8	3.5

Data from Jones RN, Sader HS, Mendes RE, et al. Update on antimicrobial susceptibility trends among *Streptococcus pneumoniae* in the United States: report of ceftaroline activity from the SENTRY Antimicrobial Surveillance Program (1998–2011). Diagn Microbiol Infect Dis 2013;75(1):107–9.

the setting of pneumonia (odds ratio 1.31, 95% confidence intervals [CIs] 1.08–1.59).[68] Also, there is significant concern regarding the clinical impact of resistance to other classes of antibiotics, most notably macrolides and fluoroquinolones.[69]

Mechanistically, β-lactam resistance is the result of changes in 1 or more of the penicillin-binding proteins in the bacterial cell wall that results in decreased affinity for penicillin and other β-lactam antibiotics.[58] In contrast, acrolide resistance is expressed as one of 2 phenotypes. The first is called the M phenotype and is the result of an efflux pump associated with the *mef*(A) gene that pumps macrolides out of the cell. The second is called the MLS_B phenotype and is caused by the *erm*(B) gene, which alters the macrolide-binding site through methylation.[69–71] Unlike the recent trends in penicillin resistance, the percentage of *S pneumoniae* isolates resistant to macrolides continues to be high: greater than 25% at the last estimate in the United States (see **Tables 3** and **4**), and, as of the mid-2000s, was still increasing.[3,72] Macrolide resistance may also result in clinical failure.[73–75]

S pneumoniae resistance to fluoroquinolones has also been reported, and, as with β-lactam resistance, increased rapidly during the 1990s.[76] Fluoroquinolone resistance results from mutations that alter *S pneumoniae*'s topoisomerases, and the rates of resistance vary depending on the specific agent used. Newer fluoroquinolones, often referred to as the respiratory fluoroquinolones, such as moxifloxacin, gemifloxacin, and high-dose levofloxacin, are associated with less resistance than, for example, ciprofloxacin; hence the recommendation for the use of fluoroquinolones in community-acquired pneumonia (see **Table 1**).[40,76] Although the current rates of resistance to the newer fluoroquinolones remains low at the moment (see **Table 4**), based on genetic similarities observed between levofloxacin-nonsusceptible *S pneumoniae* and widespread pneumococcal clones, there is the potential for a rapid increase in pneumococcal fluoroquinolone resistance, especially with the ongoing wide use of fluoroquinolone antibiotics.[69,77] Also, as with macrolide resistance, fluoroquinolone resistance may also result in clinical failure of therapy for pneumococcal infections.[77,78]

Risk factors for the development of an infection with fluoroquinolone-resistant *S pneumoniae* include prior fluoroquinolone use, old age, and certain geographic areas.[76,79–81] Risk factors for infection with β-lactam–resistant organisms include young and old age, recent prior β-lactam or macrolide use, alcoholism, medical comorbidities, immunosuppression, and exposure to a child in a day care center.[82–86]

Geographic variation is seen with both β-lactam and macrolide resistance. For instance, in the United States, rates of both penicillin and erythromycin resistance are highest in the southeast and south-central regions of the country, and lowest in the northwest.[61] In addition, the MLS_B phenotype of macrolide resistance is more common in several European countries, whereas, in the United States, the M phenotype predominates.[70] These differences are likely caused, in part, by differences in antibiotic usage between regions, and stem from the varying prevalences of resistant clones. The mechanisms by which these clones spread have potentially significant epidemiologic and clinical impact, particularly when they become multidrug resistant. Multidrug resistance in particular likely spreads via genetic material carried by a small number of predominant clones, as shown by the global distribution of certain clones such as Spain[23F]-1.[81,87]

The worldwide spread of multidrug-resistant *S pneumoniae* has prompted a desire to find new antibiotics that may be active against these infections. Chief among these is vancomycin. As of 2011, no pneumococcal isolates had been found to be nonsusceptible to vancomycin.[3,63] Other options include linezolid, for which resistant isolates have also not been found and which compares well with third-generation cephalosporins in the clinical treatment of pneumococcal bacteremia in particular, and tigecycline, which has in vitro activity against penicillin-nonsusceptible *S pneumoniae*.[63,88,89] At the moment *S pneumoniae* isolates also seem to be nearly uniformly susceptible to ceftaroline (99.1%–100% depending on breakpoint criteria), which has been shown in small studies to be effective in the treatment of community-acquired pneumonia and for the treatment of multidrug-resistant pneumococcus.[63,90,91]

VACCINATION

The persistently high morbidity and mortality of pneumococcal infections and the ongoing increase in rates of pneumococcal resistance to multiple classes of antimicrobial therapy emphasize the importance of preventing infection in the first place. Although a variety of strategies, such as prophylactic antibiotics, have been and continue to be used to reduce the number of infections, the most widespread and clinically applicable to the general population is vaccination.[92,93]

The first pneumococcal vaccine was licensed in the United States in 1977 and was based on work done by Austrian and colleagues[94] and others in the 1950s–1980s.[95] Two types of pneumococcal vaccines are currently in widespread clinical use. The first to be developed were the polysaccharide vaccines. The current polysaccharide vaccine in clinical use was introduced in 1983 and contains purified polysaccharide antigen from the 23 capsular serotypes that are most commonly responsible for invasive pneumococcal disease in the developed world.[95,96] Because it includes 23 polysaccharide antigens, the 23 valent polysaccharide vaccine (PPSV23) has the clinical benefit of covering approximately 90% of disease-causing isolates.[97,98] It has been shown to be 44% effective for the prevention of pneumococcal bacteremia in older adults, may be effective against both bacteremic and nonbacteremic disease in both middle-aged and older adults, and is 60% to 70% effective in preventing invasive pneumococcal disease overall.[95,99,100] Part of the reason for this low rate of effectiveness may be because PPSV23 does not prevent mucosal colonization with *S pneumoniae*. In addition, although more than 80% of healthy adults who receive the polysaccharide vaccine develop antibodies against the serotypes contained in the vaccine, because PPSV23 induces T-cell–independent B-cell responses its administration may result in a poor vaccine response in immunocompromised and immunosuppressed patients, elderly patients, patients with renal failure, patients with hematologic malignancies, and patients less than the age of 2 years.[95,96,101]

The desire for a more effective vaccine, particularly one that would potentially be more helpful to the aforementioned at-risk populations, led to the development of the pneumococcal conjugate vaccines, the first of which, PCV7, was licensed in the United States in 2000.[102] PCV7 contains 7 serotypes of purified capsular polysaccharide antigen (4, 9V, 14, 19F, 23F, 18C, and 6B) conjugated to a nontoxic variant of diphtheria toxin called CRM_{197}, and, because it stimulates a T-cell–dependent response, it is more immunogenic, especially in young children.[95,96] PCV7 has been very successful. It has been shown to decrease rates of invasive pneumococcal disease in children caused by vaccine serotypes by 78% to 97%, and by all serotypes, including those not in the vaccine, by 50% to 89%.[95,103,104] It has also dramatically reduced the incidence of pneumococcal meningitis in both children and adults as well as the rates of invasive pneumococcal disease in adults in general.[103,105] This latter effect is likely caused by herd immunity, partially related to PCV7's effectiveness by decreasing the nasopharyngeal carriage of *S pneumoniae* in young children, who are frequently the source of infections in adults.[96]

Despite all of their perceived benefits, questions regarding the pneumococcal vaccines remain. As mentioned earlier, because of the manner in which it stimulates an immune response, there are concerns regarding the immunogenicity of PSV23 in certain at-risk populations. In addition, it is possible that the effectiveness data for polysaccharide vaccines in general may be driven by larger, earlier studies such as Austrian and colleagues[94] work with gold miners, or by case control and cohort studies.[101] A recent meta-analysis by Huss and colleagues[106] showed that pneumococcal polysaccharide vaccines may be beneficial in decreasing the rates of presumptive pneumococcal pneumonia (relative risk [RR] 0.64, CI 0.43–0.96) and pneumonia from all causes (RR 0.73, CI 0.56–0.94), but not pneumococcal bacteremia (RR 0.90, CI 0.46–1.77), pneumococcal bronchitis (RR 0.76, CI 0.76–1.12), death from pneumococcal infection (RR 0.93, CI 0.29–3.05), death from pneumonia (RR 0.88, CI 0.62–1.25), or death from all causes (RR 0.97, CI 0.87–1.09).

The conjugate vaccines are more effective than PSV23, but PCV7 only contains 7 of the more than 90 known serotypes.[9] Thus, although it has resulted in a decrease in the rates of disease attributed to those serotypes, nonvaccine serotypes such as 11, 15, and 19A have become more prevalent.[71,107] For instance, between 1998 and 2003, in patients infected with HIV, invasive pneumococcal disease caused by serotypes in PCV7 decreased by 62%, but invasive pneumococcal disease caused by nonvaccine serotypes increased by 44%.[108]

An additional concern regarding PCV7 in particular has been its effect on the rates of antibiotic resistance in serotypes not contained within the vaccine. A nonvaccine serotype of particular interest is 19A, which has become more prominent as a cause of invasive pneumococcal disease and now is responsible for 8.2% to 28.3% of invasive pneumococcal disease.[71,109] Not only has serotype 19A become a more common cause of invasive pneumococcal disease, but it also has become increasingly antibiotic resistant.[71,96,109,110] Hampton and colleagues[110] found that, in patients aged 5 to 64 years, using an MIC of greater than or equal to 4, 6.6% of serotype 19A isolates collected between 1998 and 1999 were nonsusceptible to penicillin; by 2007 to

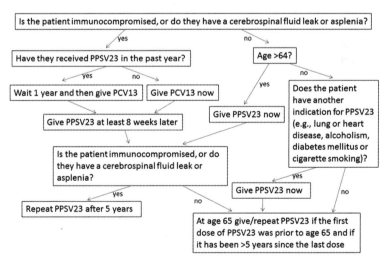

Fig. 3. ACIP recommendations for prevention of invasive pneumococcal disease among adults using PCV13 and PCV23. (*From* Centers for Disease Control and Prevention (CDC). Use of 13-valent pneumococcal conjugate vaccine and 23-valent pneumococcal polysaccharide vaccine for adults with immunocompromising conditions: recommendations of the Advisory Committee on Immunization Practices (ACIP). MMWR Morb Mortal Wkly Rep 2012;61:816–9.)

2008 that rate had increased to 77.8%. Perhaps even more concerning are the data from the Asian Network for Surveillance of Resistant Pathogens (ANSORP) study data from 2008 to 2009, which showed 86.0% and 79.8% of serotype 19A isolates to be erythromycin and multidrug-resistant respectively.[71]

One potential way to combat the increase in both serotypes not contained in PCV7, and resistant serotypes not contained in PCV7 in particular, is the expansion of the number of serotypes contained in the vaccine. In 2010, an expanded conjugate vaccine, PCV13, which contains the same 7 serotypes as PCV7 plus serotypes 1, 3, 5, 6A, 7F, and 19A, as well as CRM_{17}, was licensed for use in children, and in 2011 it was licensed for use in adults older than 50 years.[95,102] Whether this expanded vaccine will simply result in other serotypes gaining a more prominent, and perhaps a more resistant, role remains unclear. This possibility is of particular concern in immunocompromised patients in whom only 50% of invasive pneumococcal disease was caused by serotypes contained in PCV13 in 2010.[102] Because an additional 21% of invasive pulmonary disease in those patients is caused by serotypes contained in PPSV23, the Advisory Committee on Immunization Practices (ACIP) now recommends that patients aged 19 years and older with immunocompromising conditions, functional or anatomic asplenia, CSF leaks, or cochlear implants who have not previously received PCV13 or PPSV23 be given PCV13 first followed by PPSV23 8 weeks later (**Fig. 3**).[102]

SUMMARY

Although great progress has been made both in the prevention and treatment of *S pneumoniae*, it continues to be a significant cause of morbidity and mortality worldwide. As with other bacteria, pneumococcal antibiotic resistance continues to be of great and growing concern, and although conjugate vaccines in particular have been beneficial in reducing the rates of invasive pneumococcal disease, *S pneumoniae*'s ability to adapt to selective pressure is an ongoing clinical challenge.

REFERENCES

1. Musher DM. Infections caused by *Streptococcus pneumoniae*: clinical spectrum, pathogenesis, immunity, and treatment. Clin Infect Dis 1992;14(4):801–7.
2. Burman LA, Norrby R, Trollfors B. Invasive pneumococcal infections: incidence, predisposing factors, and prognosis. Rev Infect Dis 1985;7(2):133–42.
3. CDC - ABCs: 2010 *Streptococcus pneumoniae* surveillance report - active bacterial core surveillance. Available at: http://www.cdc.gov/abcs/reports-findings/survreports/spneu10.html. Accessed November 4, 2012.
4. Dowling JN, Sheehe PR, Feldman HA. Pharyngeal pneumococcal acquisitions in "normal" families: a longitudinal study. J Infect Dis 1971;124(1):9–17.
5. Hendley JO, Sande MA, Stewart PM, et al. Spread of *Streptococcus pneumoniae* in families. I. Carriage rates and distribution of types. J Infect Dis 1975; 132(1):55–61.
6. Austrian R. Some observations on the pneumococcus and on the current status of pneumococcal disease and its prevention. Rev Infect Dis 1981;3(Suppl): S1–17.
7. Broome CV, Facklam RR. Epidemiology of clinically significant isolates of *Streptococcus pneumoniae* in the United States. Rev Infect Dis 1981;3(2):277–81.
8. Hoge CW, Reichler MR, Dominguez EA, et al. An epidemic of pneumococcal disease in an overcrowded, inadequately ventilated jail. N Engl J Med 1994; 331(10):643–8.

9. CDC - Surveillance of pneumococcal - Chapter 11-Vaccine preventable diseases. Available at: http://www.cdc.gov/vaccines/pubs/surv-manual/chpt11-pneumo.html. Accessed November 14, 2012.

10. Janoff EN, Rubins JB. Invasive pneumococcal disease in the immunocompromised host. Microb Drug Resist 1997;3(3):215–32.

11. Lipsky BA, Boyko EJ, Inui TS, et al. Risk factors for acquiring pneumococcal infections. Arch Intern Med 1986;146(11):2179–85.

12. Janoff EN, Breiman RF, Daley CL, et al. Pneumococcal disease during HIV infection. Epidemiologic, clinical, and immunologic perspectives. Ann Intern Med 1992;117(4):314–24.

13. Redd SC, Rutherford GW 3rd, Sande MA, et al. The role of human immunodeficiency virus infection in pneumococcal bacteremia in San Francisco residents. J Infect Dis 1990;162(5):1012–7.

14. Marrie TJ. Pneumococcal pneumonia: epidemiology and clinical features. Semin Respir Infect 1999;14(3):227–36.

15. Tuomanen EI, Austrian R, Masure HR. Pathogenesis of pneumococcal infection. N Engl J Med 1995;332(19):1280–4.

16. Knecht JC, Schiffman G, Austrian R. Some biological properties of pneumococcus type 37 and the chemistry of its capsular polysaccharide. J Exp Med 1970;132(3):475–87.

17. Austrian R. Some aspects of the pneumococcal carrier state. J Antimicrob Chemother 1986;18(Suppl A):35–45.

18. Hakenbeck R, Briese T, Chalkley L, et al. Antigenic variation of penicillin-binding proteins from penicillin-resistant clinical strains of *Streptococcus pneumoniae*. J Infect Dis 1991;164(2):313–9.

19. Boulnois GJ, Paton JC, Mitchell TJ, et al. Structure and function of pneumolysin, the multifunctional, thiol-activated toxin of *Streptococcus pneumoniae*. Mol Microbiol 1991;5(11):2611–6.

20. Trampuz A, Widmer AF, Fluckiger U, et al. Changes in the epidemiology of pneumococcal bacteremia in a Swiss university hospital during a 15-year period, 1986-2000. Mayo Clin Proc 2004;79(5):604–12.

21. Cundell DR, Weiser JN, Shen J, et al. Relationship between colonial morphology and adherence of *Streptococcus pneumoniae*. Infect Immun 1995;63(3):757–61.

22. Håkansson A, Kidd A, Wadell G, et al. Adenovirus infection enhances in vitro adherence of *Streptococcus pneumoniae*. Infect Immun 1994;62(7):2707–14.

23. Ginsberg J, Mohebbi MH, Patel RS, et al. Detecting influenza epidemics using search engine query data. Nature 2009;457(7232):1012–4.

24. Bartlett JG, Mundy LM. Community-acquired pneumonia. N Engl J Med 1995;333(24):1618–24.

25. Fang GD, Fine M, Orloff J, et al. New and emerging etiologies for community-acquired pneumonia with implications for therapy. A prospective multicenter study of 359 cases. Medicine (Baltimore) 1990;69(5):307–16.

26. Bochud PY, Moser F, Erard P, et al. Community-acquired pneumonia. A prospective outpatient study. Medicine (Baltimore) 2001;80(2):75–87.

27. File TM. Community-acquired pneumonia. Lancet 2003;362(9400):1991–2001.

28. Heffron R. Pneumonia: with special reference to pneumococcus lobar pneumonia. Cambridge (MA): Harvard University Press; 1979.

29. del Rio C, McGowan JE Jr. Severe diarrhea in pneumococcal bacteremia: croupous colitis. JAMA 1987;257(2):189.

30. Kantor HG. The many radiologic facies of pneumococcal pneumonia. AJR Am J Roentgenol 1981;137(6):1213–20.

31. Ort S, Ryan JL, Barden G, et al. Pneumococcal pneumonia in hospitalized patients. Clinical and radiological presentations. JAMA 1983;249(2):214–8.
32. Leatherman JW, Iber C, Davies SF. Cavitation in bacteremic pneumococcal pneumonia. Causal role of mixed infection with anaerobic bacteria. Am Rev Respir Dis 1984;129(2):317–21.
33. Isaacs RD. Necrotizing pneumonia in bacteraemic pneumococcal infection. Br J Dis Chest 1986;80(3):295–6.
34. Rein M, Gwaltney J, O'Brien W, et al. Accuracy of Gram's stain in identifying pneumococci in sputum. JAMA 1978;239(25):2671–3.
35. Marrie TJ. Community-acquired pneumonia. Clin Infect Dis 1994;18(4):501–13 [quiz: 514–5].
36. García-Vázquez E, Marcos MA, Mensa J, et al. Assessment of the usefulness of sputum culture for diagnosis of community-acquired pneumonia using the PORT predictive scoring system. Arch Intern Med 2004;164(16):1807–11.
37. Musher DM, Montoya R, Wanahita A. Diagnostic value of microscopic examination of Gram-stained sputum and sputum cultures in patients with bacteremic pneumococcal pneumonia. Clin Infect Dis 2004;39(2):165–9.
38. Lentino JR, Lucks DA. Nonvalue of sputum culture in the management of lower respiratory tract infections. J Clin Microbiol 1987;25(5):758–62.
39. Barrett-Connor E. The nonvalue of sputum culture in the diagnosis of pneumococcal pneumonia. Am Rev Respir Dis 1971;103(6):845–8.
40. Mandell LA, Wunderink RG, Anzueto A, et al. Infectious Diseases Society of America/American Thoracic Society consensus guidelines on the management of community-acquired pneumonia in adults. Clin Infect Dis 2007;44(Suppl 2): S27–72.
41. Sordé R, Falcó V, Lowak M, et al. Current and potential usefulness of pneumococcal urinary antigen detection in hospitalized patients with community-acquired pneumonia to guide antimicrobial therapy. Arch Intern Med 2011; 171(2):166–72.
42. Dowell SF, Garman RL, Liu G, et al. Evaluation of Binax NOW, an assay for the detection of pneumococcal antigen in urine samples, performed among pediatric patients. Clin Infect Dis 2001;32(5):824–5.
43. Tilghman R, Finland M. Clinical significance of bacteremia in pneumococcic pneumonia. Arch Intern Med 1937;59(4):602–19.
44. Hook EW 3rd, Horton CA, Schaberg DR. Failure of intensive care unit support to influence mortality from pneumococcal bacteremia. JAMA 1983;249(8):1055–7.
45. Austrian R, Gold J. Pneumococcal bacteremia with especial reference to bacteremic pneumococcal pneumonia. Ann Intern Med 1964;60:759–76.
46. Ortqvist A, Grepe A, Julander I, et al. Bacteremic pneumococcal pneumonia in Sweden: clinical course and outcome and comparison with non-bacteremic pneumococcal and mycoplasmal pneumonias. Scand J Infect Dis 1988;20(2):163–71.
47. Sheffield JV, Chu L, Root R. Pneumococcal bacteremia a Harborview Medical Center: impact of intensive care unit support. New Orleans (LA): Clinical Infectious Diseases; 1997. p. 438.
48. Taylor SN, Sanders CV. Unusual manifestations of invasive pneumococcal infection. Am J Med 1999;107(1A):12S–27S.
49. Eskola J, Kilpi T, Palmu A, et al. Efficacy of a pneumococcal conjugate vaccine against acute otitis media. N Engl J Med 2001;344(6):403–9.
50. Vardakas KZ, Matthaiou DK, Falagas ME. Adjunctive dexamethasone therapy for bacterial meningitis in adults: a meta-analysis of randomized controlled trials. Eur J Neurol 2009;16(6):662–73.

51. de Gans J, van de Beek D. Dexamethasone in adults with bacterial meningitis. N Engl J Med 2002;347(20):1549–56.

52. Tunkel AR, Hartman BJ, Kaplan SL, et al. Practice guidelines for the management of bacterial meningitis. Clin Infect Dis 2004;39(9):1267–84.

53. Cunha BA. Clinical relevance of penicillin-resistant *Streptococcus pneumoniae*. Semin Respir Infect 2002;17(3):204–14.

54. Coyle PK. Glucocorticoids in central nervous system bacterial infection. Arch Neurol 1999;56(7):796–801.

55. Viladrich PF, Gudiol F, Liñares J, et al. Evaluation of vancomycin for therapy of adult pneumococcal meningitis. Antimicrob Agents Chemother 1991;35(12):2467–72.

56. Sapolsky RM, Pulsinelli WA. Glucocorticoids potentiate ischemic injury to neurons: therapeutic implications. Science 1985;229(4720):1397–400.

57. Jernigan DB, Cetron MS, Breiman RF. Minimizing the impact of drug-resistant *Streptococcus pneumoniae* (DRSP). A strategy from the DRSP Working Group. JAMA 1996;275(3):206–9.

58. Gold HS, Moellering RC Jr. Antimicrobial-drug resistance. N Engl J Med 1996; 335(19):1445–53.

59. Whitney CG, Farley MM, Hadler J, et al. Increasing prevalence of multidrug-resistant *Streptococcus pneumoniae* in the United States. N Engl J Med 2000; 343(26):1917–24.

60. Doern GV, Brueggemann AB, Huynh H, et al. Antimicrobial resistance with *Streptococcus pneumoniae* in the United States, 1997 98. Emerg Infect Dis 1999;5(6):757–65.

61. Jenkins SG, Brown SD, Farrell DJ. Trends in antibacterial resistance among *Streptococcus pneumoniae* isolated in the USA: update from PROTEKT US Years 1-4. Ann Clin Microbiol Antimicrob 2008;7:1.

62. Mera RM, Miller LA, Amrine-Madsen H, et al. Impact of new Clinical Laboratory Standards Institute *Streptococcus pneumoniae* penicillin susceptibility testing breakpoints on reported resistance changes over time. Microb Drug Resist 2011;17(1):47–52.

63. Jones RN, Sader HS, Mendes RE, et al. Update on antimicrobial susceptibility trends among *Streptococcus pneumoniae* in the United States: report of ceftaroline activity from the SENTRY Antimicrobial Surveillance Program (1998-2011). Diagn Microbiol Infect Dis 2013;75(1):107–9.

64. Friedland IR, McCracken GH Jr. Management of infections caused by antibiotic-resistant *Streptococcus pneumoniae*. N Engl J Med 1994;331(6):377–82.

65. Takata GS, Chan LS, Shekelle P, et al. Evidence assessment of management of acute otitis media: I. The role of antibiotics in treatment of uncomplicated acute otitis media. Pediatrics 2001;108(2):239–47.

66. Pallares R, Gudiol F, Liñares J, et al. Risk factors and response to antibiotic therapy in adults with bacteremic pneumonia caused by penicillin-resistant pneumococci. N Engl J Med 1987;317(1):18–22.

67. Feldman C, Kallenbach JM, Miller SD, et al. Community-acquired pneumonia due to penicillin-resistant pneumococci. N Engl J Med 1985;313(10):615–7.

68. Tleyjeh IM, Tlaygeh HM, Hejal R, et al. The impact of penicillin resistance on short-term mortality in hospitalized adults with pneumococcal pneumonia: a systematic review and meta-analysis. Clin Infect Dis 2006;42(6):788–97.

69. Rivera AM, Boucher HW. Current concepts in antimicrobial therapy against select gram-positive organisms: methicillin-resistant *Staphylococcus aureus*, penicillin-resistant pneumococci, and vancomycin-resistant enterococci. Mayo Clin Proc 2011;86(12):1230–43.

70. Hyde TB, Gay K, Stephens DS, et al. Macrolide resistance among invasive *Streptococcus pneumoniae* isolates. JAMA 2001;286(15):1857–62.

71. Kim SH, Song JH, Chung DR, et al. Changing trends in antimicrobial resistance and serotypes of streptococcus pneumoniae isolates in Asian Countries: an Asian Network for Surveillance of Resistant Pathogens (ANSORP) Study. Antimicrob Agents Chemother 2012;56(3):1418–26.

72. Pérez-Trallero E, García-de-la-Fuente C, García-Rey C, et al. Geographical and ecological analysis of resistance, coresistance, and coupled resistance to antimicrobials in respiratory pathogenic bacteria in Spain. Antimicrob Agents Chemother 2005;49(5):1965–72.

73. Musher DM, Dowell ME, Shortridge VD, et al. Emergence of macrolide resistance during treatment of pneumococcal pneumonia. N Engl J Med 2002; 346(8):630–1.

74. Kelley MA, Weber DJ, Gilligan P, et al. Breakthrough pneumococcal bacteremia in patients being treated with azithromycin and clarithromycin. Clin Infect Dis 2000;31(4):1008–11.

75. Lonks JR, Garau J, Gomez L, et al. Failure of macrolide antibiotic treatment in patients with bacteremia due to erythromycin-resistant *Streptococcus pneumoniae*. Clin Infect Dis 2002;35(5):556–64.

76. Chen DK, McGeer A, de Azavedo JC, et al. Decreased susceptibility of *Streptococcus pneumoniae* to fluoroquinolones in Canada. Canadian Bacterial Surveillance Network. N Engl J Med 1999;341(4):233–9.

77. Fuller JD, Low DE. A review of *Streptococcus pneumoniae* infection treatment failures associated with fluoroquinolone resistance. Clin Infect Dis 2005;41(1): 118–21.

78. Davidson R, Cavalcanti R, Brunton JL, et al. Resistance to levofloxacin and failure of treatment of pneumococcal pneumonia. N Engl J Med 2002;346(10): 747–50.

79. Anderson KB, Tan JS, File TM Jr, et al. Emergence of levofloxacin-resistant pneumococci in immunocompromised adults after therapy for community-acquired pneumonia. Clin Infect Dis 2003;37(3):376–81.

80. Ho PL, Tse WS, Tsang KW, et al. Risk factors for acquisition of levofloxacin-resistant *Streptococcus pneumoniae*: a case-control study. Clin Infect Dis 2001;32(5):701–7.

81. Ho PL, Yung RW, Tsang DN, et al. Increasing resistance of *Streptococcus pneumoniae* to fluoroquinolones: results of a Hong Kong multicentre study in 2000. J Antimicrob Chemother 2001;48(5):659–65.

82. Yu VL, Chiou CC, Feldman C, et al. An international prospective study of pneumococcal bacteremia: correlation with in vitro resistance, antibiotics administered, and clinical outcome. Clin Infect Dis 2003;37(2):230–7.

83. Ruhe JJ, Hasbun R. *Streptococcus pneumoniae* bacteremia: duration of previous antibiotic use and association with penicillin resistance. Clin Infect Dis 2003; 36(9):1132–8.

84. Campbell GD Jr, Silberman R. Drug-resistant *Streptococcus pneumoniae*. Clin Infect Dis 1998;26(5):1188–95.

85. Clavo-Sánchez AJ, Girón-González JA, López-Prieto D, et al. Multivariate analysis of risk factors for infection due to penicillin-resistant and multidrug-resistant *Streptococcus pneumoniae*: a multicenter study. Clin Infect Dis 1997;24(6): 1052–9.

86. Vanderkooi OG, Low DE, Green K, et al. Predicting antimicrobial resistance in invasive pneumococcal infections. Clin Infect Dis 2005;40(9):1288–97.

87. Reinert RR, Jacobs MR, Appelbaum PC, et al. Relationship between the Original Multiply Resistant South African Isolates of *Streptococcus pneumoniae* from 1977 to 1978 and Contemporary International Resistant Clones. J Clin Microbiol 2005;43(12):6035–41.

88. San Pedro GS, Cammarata SK, Oliphant TH, et al. Linezolid versus ceftriaxone/cefpodoxime in patients hospitalized for the treatment of *Streptococcus pneumoniae* pneumonia. Scand J Infect Dis 2002;34(10):720–8.

89. Fritsche TR, Sader HS, Stilwell MG, et al. Antimicrobial activity of tigecycline tested against organisms causing community-acquired respiratory tract infection and nosocomial pneumonia. Diagn Microbiol Infect Dis 2005;52(3): 187–93.

90. File TM Jr, Low DE, Eckburg PB, et al. Integrated analysis of FOCUS 1 and FOCUS 2: randomized, doubled-blinded, multicenter phase 3 trials of the efficacy and safety of ceftaroline fosamil versus ceftriaxone in patients with community-acquired pneumonia. Clin Infect Dis 2010;51(12):1395–405.

91. Saravolatz LD, Stein GE, Johnson LB. Ceftaroline: a novel cephalosporin with activity against methicillin-resistant *Staphylococcus aureus*. Clin Infect Dis 2011;52(9):1156–63.

92. Robinson KA, Baughman W, Rothrock G, et al. Epidemiology of invasive *Streptococcus pneumoniae* infections in the United States, 1995-1998: opportunities for prevention in the conjugate vaccine era. JAMA 2001;285(13):1729–35.

93. Hirst C, Owusu-Ofori S. Prophylactic antibiotics for preventing pneumococcal infection in children with sickle cell disease. Cochrane Database Syst Rev 2012;(9):CD003427.

94. Austrian R, Douglas RM, Schiffman G, et al. Prevention of pneumococcal pneumonia by vaccination. Trans Assoc Am Physicians 1976;89:184–94.

95. CDC - Pinkbook: pneumococcal disease chapter - epidemiology of vaccine-preventable diseases. Available at: http://www.cdc.gov/vaccines/pubs/pinkbook/pneumo.html. Accessed November 14, 2012.

96. van der Poll T, Opal SM. Pathogenesis, treatment, and prevention of pneumococcal pneumonia. Lancet 2009;374(9700):1543–56.

97. Plouffe JF, Breiman RF, Facklam RR. Bacteremia with *Streptococcus pneumoniae*. Implications for therapy and prevention. Franklin County Pneumonia Study Group. JAMA 1996;275(3):194–8.

98. Broome CV, Facklam RR, Allen JR, et al. From the center for disease control. Epidemiology of pneumococcal serotypes in the United States, 1978–1979. J Infect Dis 1980;141(1):119–23.

99. Jackson LA, Neuzil KM, Yu O, et al. Effectiveness of pneumococcal polysaccharide vaccine in older adults. N Engl J Med 2003;348(18):1747–55.

100. Vila-Corcoles A, Salsench E, Rodriguez-Blanco T, et al. Clinical effectiveness of 23-valent pneumococcal polysaccharide vaccine against pneumonia in middle-aged and older adults: a matched case-control study. Vaccine 2009;27(10): 1504–10.

101. Fine MJ, Smith MA, Carson CA, et al. Efficacy of pneumococcal vaccination in adults. A meta-analysis of randomized controlled trials. Arch Intern Med 1994; 154(23):2666–77.

102. Centers for Disease Control and Prevention (CDC). Use of 13-valent pneumococcal conjugate vaccine and 23-valent pneumococcal polysaccharide vaccine for adults with immunocompromising conditions: recommendations of the Advisory Committee on Immunization Practices (ACIP). MMWR Morb Mortal Wkly Rep 2012;61:816–9.

103. Whitney CG, Farley MM, Hadler J, et al. Decline in invasive pneumococcal disease after the introduction of protein-polysaccharide conjugate vaccine. N Engl J Med 2003;348(18):1737–46.

104. Centers for Disease Control and Prevention (CDC). Invasive pneumococcal disease in children 5 years after conjugate vaccine introduction–eight states, 1998-2005. MMWR Morb Mortal Wkly Rep 2008;57(6):144–8.

105. Hsu HE, Shutt KA, Moore MR, et al. Effect of pneumococcal conjugate vaccine on pneumococcal meningitis. N Engl J Med 2009;360(3):244–56.

106. Huss A, Scott P, Stuck AE, et al. Efficacy of pneumococcal vaccination in adults: a meta-analysis. CMAJ 2009;180(1):48–58.

107. Musher DM. Pneumococcal vaccine–direct and indirect ("herd") effects. N Engl J Med 2006;354(14):1522–4.

108. Flannery B, Heffernan RT, Harrison LH, et al. Changes in invasive pneumococcal disease among HIV-infected adults living in the era of childhood pneumococcal immunization. Ann Intern Med 2006;144(1):1–9.

109. Pichichero ME, Casey JR. Emergence of a multiresistant serotype 19A pneumococcal strain not included in the 7-valent conjugate vaccine as an otopathogen in children. JAMA 2007;298(15):1772–8.

110. Hampton LM, Farley MM, Schaffner W, et al. Prevention of antibiotic-nonsusceptible *Streptococcus pneumoniae* with conjugate vaccines. J Infect Dis 2012;205(3):401–11.

Complications of Antibiotic Therapy

Jenny Wright, MD[a,b,*], Douglas S. Paauw, MD, MACP[b]

KEYWORDS

- Antibiotics • Side effects • Drug interactions • Drug-induced lupus

KEY POINTS

- Macrolides and quinolones are associated with QT prolongation.
- Amoxicillin/clavulanate is probably the most common antibiotic to cause drug-induced liver disease.
- Trimethoprim/sulfamethoxazole is associated with many important side effects including agranulocytosis, hemolytic anemia, hyperkalemia, and the highest risk for cutaneous allergy. It also is the cause of severe drug interactions with warfarin and methotrexate.
- Quinolones have several unique side effects including tendonitis and tendon rupture, as well as retinal detatchment. Quinolones are also an important cause of delirium and hallucinations in elderly patients.

INTRODUCTION

Antibiotics can be life-saving, and help in treating many infectious diseases. Antibiotics also pose the risk of predisposing patients to superinfections, and can have serious direct toxicities and side effects. Antibiotics are also common causes of drug interactions that can cause other prescribed medications to increase to dangerously high levels, creating severe problems. Knowing the risk of drug interactions and understanding direct toxicities of antibiotics help physicians make wise choices in their use by allowing an appropriate assessment of risk versus benefit and making selections that are less risky for patients.

ANTIBIOTIC COMPLICATIONS BY SYSTEM
Hematologic

There are many potential hematologic complications of antibiotic therapy. Perhaps the best known are immune hemolytic anemia (IHA), the most common offenders being

Funding Sources: None.
Conflict of Interest: None.
[a] General Internal Medicine Center, University of Washington Medical Center, 4245 Roosevelt Way Northeast, Box 354760, Seattle, WA 98105, USA; [b] Department of Medicine, University of Washington School of Medicine, Box 356420, Seattle, WA 98105, USA
* Corresponding author.
E-mail address: sonic@uw.edu

Med Clin N Am 97 (2013) 667–679
http://dx.doi.org/10.1016/j.mcna.2013.02.006
0025-7125/13/$ – see front matter Published by Elsevier Inc.

medical.theclinics.com

cefotetan, ceftriaxone, piperacillin, and, less commonly, other β-lactamase inhibitors.[1] In cases of drug-induced IHA, a history of previous exposure to the drug is common, the time course of development of the anemia is helpful in making the diagnosis, and treatment is primarily withdrawal of the drug. That said, it is often difficult to differentiate between a drug-induced IHA and an idiopathic autoimmune hemolytic anemia, direct antiglobulin testing being positive in both cases.

Antibiotics can also result in anemia by other mechanisms. Sulfonamides, nitrofurantoin, and dapsone can precipitate a hemolytic anemia in patients with glucose-6-phosphate dehydrogenase (G6PD) deficiency. G6PD deficiency is the most common erythrocyte enzyme deficiency, and can be caused by various mutations on the X chromosome. It is particularly common among people of African descent. Because of the high frequency of the mutation coupled with the common use of trimethoprim/sulfamethoxazole (TMP/SMX) and dapsone in patients with human immunodeficiency virus (HIV) disease, many physicians providing care to HIV-positive patients will screen for this mutation. Aplastic anemia is a well-known potential adverse effect of chloramphenicol, now rarely used, but it can also occur with sulfonamides, albeit with a much lower frequency.[2] Isoniazid can cause an isolated/pure red cell aplasia.

Isolated thrombocytopenia is also a known potential side effect of antimicrobial therapy. Agents implicated include linezolid and TMP/SMX; less commonly reported are piperacillin and vancomycin.[3] Patients requiring prolonged treatment with linezolid (>2 weeks) should be monitored for development of thrombocytopenia and, though less common, anemia.

Another hematologic side effect seen in long-term antibiotic therapy is agranulocytosis. Historically this was a concern with prolonged nafcillin therapy; now that there are agents with more favorable dosing schedules, this medication is rarely used for a prolonged period. Other agents associated with this very rare but concerning complication include dapsone, TMP/SMX, β-lactams, and erythromycin.[4–6]

Cardiac

Multiple antibiotics are associated with QT prolongation and, in turn, an increased risk of sudden cardiac death attributed to torsades de pointes. It should be noted that the risk in the general population is low. For example, in a recent study assessing risk of sudden cardiac death in patients on azithromycin there were 47 additional cardiovascular deaths per 1 million antibiotic courses[7]; however, both drug-drug interactions and patient factors such as baseline cardiovascular disease/risk factors can increase the risk further.

Antimicrobials associated with QT prolongation include macrolides and quinolones, antifungal azole agents, and pentamidine. The macrolides clarithromycin and erythromycin have historically been reported to be the antibiotics most highly associated with torsades de pointes, although recent publications have also implicated azithromycin.[7,8] This class of antibiotics likely increases risk based on 2 mechanisms, a direct effect of potassium channels and inhibition of cytochrome P450 enzymes leading to increased levels of other QT-prolonging medications, the latter less so with azithromycin. Quinolones are another class of very commonly prescribed antibiotics associated with QT prolongation. Cardiac fatalities have led to the withdrawal of some quinolones (most notably gatifloxacin) from the market. These medications primarily appear to result in QT prolongation owing to effects on potassium channels, and less so because of drug-drug interactions. Risk of QT prolongation is highest with moxifloxacin.[9]

When prescribing antibiotics that carry an increased risk of QT prolongation, it is important to be mindful of additional risk factors that may amplify this otherwise small risk. Such factors include: (1) drug-drug interactions, for example prescription of erythromycin and diltiazem, which results in elevated erythromycin levels; (2) additive effect of being on multiple QT-prolonging medications, other common culprits being methadone and antipsychotic agents; and (3) patient factors resulting in an increased inherent cardiac risk, including cardiomyopathy, electrolyte abnormalities, or renal failure leading to increased drug levels.

Respiratory

Overall pulmonary complications of antibiotic therapy are rare. Nitrofurantoin is an antibiotic used for treatment of both acute cystitis and prevention of recurrent cystitis. It can rarely be associated with pulmonary toxicity, occurring in less than 1% of patients on nitrofurantoin. The most common pulmonary reaction is an acute pulmonary toxicity, likely a hypersensitivity reaction. Within a month of starting therapy, patients present with systemic manifestations, including fever and rash, and pulmonary symptoms, including cough and dyspnea. Evaluation will frequently reveal eosinophilia and bilateral infiltrates on chest radiography.[10] Patients typically recover quickly with discontinuation of the drug, and should not be rechallenged with this medication in the future. Less common is a chronic nitrofurantoin pulmonary toxicity, which presents insidiously with cough and dyspnea in patients on chronic, daily nitrofurantoin, sometimes years after starting therapy. Laboratory evaluation may reveal a positive antinuclear antibody (ANA) test, and lung computed tomography will reveal a pattern consistent with pulmonary fibrosis, bilateral ground-glass opacifications, and contraction bronchiectasis. The mainstay of treatment is withdrawal of the drug. Fibrosis may be irreversible, although there are reports of slow improvement.[10] The role of corticosteroids is debated.

An even less commonly reported complication of long-term nitrofurantoin use is immune-mediated concomitant pulmonary and liver disease. It is recommended that patients with chronic pulmonary toxicity be screened for concomitant liver disease.

Gastrointestinal

Patients treated with antibiotics frequently develop diarrhea and although *Clostridium difficile* is obviously of great concern, the majority of cases will not be attributable to this infection. In general, antibiotic-associated diarrhea may occur in 10% to 25% of patients treated with amoxicillin-clavulanate, 15% to 20% of patients treated with cefixime, 5% to 10% of those treated with amoxicillin, and 2% to 5% of patients treated with other cephalosporins, fluoroquinolones, macrolides, and tetracycline.[11] Although it is difficult to clinically differentiate between *C difficile* infection and non–*C difficile* antibiotic-associated diarrhea, characteristics of non–*C difficile* diarrhea may include patient history of antibiotic-associated diarrhea, more moderate severity of diarrhea, and an otherwise benign physical examination, for example a normal abdominal examination and normal vital signs.

Judicious use of antibiotics is likely the best form of prevention, although clearly at times antibiotic use cannot be avoided. There is limited evidence that use of probiotics may be beneficial in the prevention of antibiotic-associated diarrhea, although studies have used a variety of probiotic preparations including bacteria and yeast. At present, both the optimal probiotic formulation and the correct dosing remain unclear.[12]

Nausea is a symptom frequently encountered in practice for which it is often difficult to identify a specific cause, although it should be noted that there are some antibiotics for which this is a very common side effect, including erythromycin (25%), metronidazole (12%), TMP/SMX (>10%), fluoroquinolones (2%–8%), and, to a lesser extent, amino-penicillins (eg, amoxicillin) and third-generation and fourth-generation cephalosporins.[13] The temporal relationship of the side effect (nausea) with initiation of antibiotic therapy will often be the best hint that this is the origin.

A less common gastrointestinal side effect of antibiotic therapy is pill esophagitis, associated primarily with doxycycline. Symptoms include substernal chest pain and odynophagia.[14] This side effect can be prevented by having the patient take the medication with a full glass of water and avoid lying down for at least 30 minutes after taking the medication.

Hepatobiliary

Several antibiotics have notable liver toxicities. As discussed elsewhere in this article, nitrofurantoin and minocycline have reported hepatic toxicities. Other agents known to cause drug-induced liver injury (DILI) are amoxicillin/clavulanic acid, sulfonamides, macrolides, and quinolones, in addition to several antituberculosis agents, most notably isoniazid. Amoxicillin/clavulanate may be the most common antibiotic implicated in DILI, and the risk seems to be increased in older patients. DILI remains a rare side effect; overall, the estimated frequency reported in studies is low, for example, 1.7 per 10,000 treatment courses.[15] Estimates regarding the frequency of liver injury for sulfonamides are also somewhat low; the frequency in cases resulting in hospitalization has been estimated to be 4.8 per million patients treated.[16] Ceftriaxone can cause biliary sludge and can trigger acalculous cholecystitis; this is much more common with prolonged courses of the drug, such as in the treatment of endocarditis or osteomyelitis.

Renal

Antibiotics can be nephrotoxic by way of several mechanisms. In the inpatient setting antibiotics such as intravenous aminoglycosides, amphotericin, colistin, and vancomycin can result in kidney injury. In the case of vancomycin it remains debatable as to what degree the nephrotoxicity is due to the medication itself rather than patient factors that independently increase the risk of acute kidney injury, such as hypotension.[17] It should also be noted that the risk is higher when vancomycin is dosed to maintain high trough levels; again this is fraught with confounders, given these are typically sicker patients overall.

Allergic interstitial nephritis (AIN) is a hypersensitivity reaction rather than a direct nephrotoxic side effect of a drug. In keeping with this, AIN is most commonly seen with the antibiotics most commonly associated with hypersensitivity reactions, such as β-lactams and sulfonamides; other agents implicated include quinolones, most commonly ciprofloxacin, erythromycin, vancomycin, and minocycline. In addition to renal manifestations, patients may present with systemic symptoms such as fever and rash, which is most common with the β-lactam antibiotics and sulfonamides. The classic laboratory finding of eosinophiluria is in fact not as good a screening test as is commonly believed; the sensitivity is likely only 67%, although the specificity is 87%.[18] Definitive diagnosis is made by kidney biopsy. Treatment involves withdrawal of the offending agent. It is unclear whether corticosteroid therapy is of benefit.

Electrolyte Abnormalities

Hyperkalemia is a common side effect of TMP/SMX therapy. Because of direct effects of the medication on the distal renal tubules, serum potassium is increased in approximately 20% of patients. These interactions are of well-documented clinical significance. Studies have found that patients on renin-angiotensin blocking antihypertensives who are prescribed TMP/SMX have a 7-fold increased risk of hospitalization for hyperkalemia compared with patients on the same antihypertensives prescribed amoxicillin.[19] Similarly, risk of hospitalization for hyperkalemia was increased 12-fold in patients on chronic spironolactone prescribed TMP/SMX in comparison with amoxicillin.[20] For this reason, caution should be exercised when prescribing this antibiotic to patients with a predisposition to hyperkalemia resulting from renal disease or other medications such as spironolactone, angiotensin-converting enzyme inhibitors, or angiotensin receptor blockers. Elderly patients are at greatest risk for this complication.

Aminoglycosides are rarely used in outpatient practice, but are well known for their nephrotoxic side effects. An aminoglycoside occasionally used in the outpatient setting of management of drug-resistant tuberculosis infection is capreomycin, given by intramuscular injection. This agent is associated with frequent hypokalemia.[21]

Hypokalemia is also associated with penicillin and antistaphylococcal penicillins such as nafcillin and dicloxacillin, although the clinical implications of this in outpatient practice are negligible. This side effect has been reported in the setting of large-dose parenteral therapy.[22]

Genitourinary

Vulvovaginal candidiasis is a common complication of antibiotic therapy. Studies indicate that up to one-quarter of women treated with a short course of oral antibiotics develops symptomatic vulvovaginal candidiasis.[23,24] Median onset in one of the larger studies was 5 days, based on enrollment criteria that would be 5 to 7 days after starting antibiotic therapy.[24] Women with a history or vulvovaginal candidiasis after antibiotic treatment were, not surprisingly, at higher risk of developing this complication again. Women frequently use probiotics in various oral and vaginal preparations to prevent this complication, although there are no strong data to support this.[25,26]

Rheumatologic

Drug-induced lupus is characterized by development of symptoms of idiopathic systemic lupus erythematosus (SLE) in the setting of exposure to a medication and with resolution of the symptoms with discontinuation of the medication. Several antibiotics are associated with drug-induced lupus, most notably minocycline, with an estimated incidence of 5 cases per 10,000 prescriptions.[27] Other antibiotics associated with drug-induced lupus are isoniazid and nitrofurantoin. In the case of minocycline, patients are frequently young women; otherwise, drug-induced lupus tends to occur in older patients with equal frequency in both genders, quite unlike idiopathic SLE. This complication typically occurs after patients have been on the offending drug for a prolonged period; longer duration of therapy and higher cumulative dose of the medication are both risk factors in its development.

Minocycline-induced lupus typically presents with arthralgias, myalgias, fatigue, and fever, and is unique in its association with hepatic manifestations. Less commonly, it is associated with cutaneous manifestations and rarely with pleuritis or pericarditis. Patients will typically have elevated inflammatory markers, namely erythrocyte sedimentation rate and, again somewhat unique to minocycline-induced lupus, an elevated C-reactive protein and transaminitis. A positive ANA test is typical, though not required to make the diagnosis of drug-induced lupus. Although antihistone antibody is present in more than 90% of cases overall, it is only present in the minority of the minocycline-associated cases.[27] Other laboratory findings commonly found in minocycline-induced lupus is a positive perinuclear antineutrophil cytoplasmic antibody, present in 67% to 100% of patients, and anti-Smith antibodies, present in approximately 40% of patients.[27]

Dermatologic

The most common dermatologic adverse reaction associated with antibiotic therapy is a drug-induced exanthem, a "drug rash." The classic description is a maculopapular eruption, particularly prominent on the trunk, symmetric in distribution overall. Unlike viral exanthems, these drug-induced rashes are typically pruritic. The most common antibiotics implicated are penicillins including aminopenicillins (eg, amoxicillin), antistaphlyococcal penicillins (eg, dicloxacillin), and the antipseudomonal penicillins (eg, piperacillin), in addition to sulfonamides (eg, TMP/SMX). The rash typically starts within 7 to 14 days of initiation of therapy. A population at particularly high risk of developing adverse cutaneous reactions to antibiotics is patients with HIV disease; up to 40% of HIV-positive patients on TMP/SMX will develop a cutaneous adverse reaction.[28] Management, in all patient populations, involves removal of the offending agents. If needed, oral antihistamines and topical steroids can be prescribed for associated pruritus.

Should a patient with a drug rash have significant systemic symptoms, such as fever and abdominal pain, Drug Rash with Eosinophilia and Systemic Symptoms (DRESS) should be considered. This rare, poorly understood, but life-threatening drug reaction has mortality rates of up to 10%.[29] A recent review found antibiotics implicated to include minocycline, dapsone, vancomycin, and sulfonamides, although nonantibiotic pharmacologic agents such as allopurinol and anticonvulsants are more common causes.[29] Presentation is typically 2 to 6 weeks after drug therapy is initiated, symptoms typically including a diffuse morbilliform rash, hypereosinophilia, lymphadenopathy, and, frequently, hepatitis, although other organ systems can also be affected. Management includes withdrawal of the offending agent. Patients are also frequently treated with corticosteroids, although treatment recommendations remain an area of active investigation.

Another important life-threatening dermatologic complication of antibiotic therapy is Steve Johnson syndrome (SJS) and toxic epidermal necrolysis (TEN), conditions of similar pathophysiology, differing mainly according to the extent of skin involvement. SJS is defined as involving less than 10% and TEN greater than 30% of body surface area, with an overlap syndrome in patients falling between these two levels. Mortality is high, at 5% for SJS and 30% for TEN. Patients are typically relatively young, 20 to 40 years old.[30] These are rare diseases most commonly caused by medications; antibiotics implicated include sulfonamides and β-lactams. These conditions are thought to represent hypersensitivity reactions. A typical patient will frequently develop systemic symptoms such as fever and malaise, even before onset of a painful blistering rash. Nikolsky's sign (lateral pressure resulting in shearing of the skin) is present, though not pathognomonic. Treatment involves removal of the offending agent and supportive care, with patients often requiring intensive care in settings such as a burn unit.

Penicillins and TMP/SMX are the most common antibiotics associated with drug-induced urticaria, another hypersensitivity reaction. These hives manifest quickly, within minutes to hours, and can be life-threatening if associated with angioedema or anaphylaxis. Should patients have a history of life-threatening penicillin hypersensitivity reactions, caution is advised when prescribing cephalosporins, as approximately 10% will have cross-reactivity, which in the case of a life-threatening reaction would rarely outweigh the benefit.[31] Although structurally similar to cephalosporins and penicillins, cross-reactivity with carbapenems (imipenem and meropenem) and monobactams (aztreoman) does not occur; therefore, these antibiotics can be safely used in patients with a history of hypersensitivity reactions to penicillin.[6]

Fixed drug eruptions are likely underdiagnosed cutaneous drug reactions, which present as well-demarcated erythematous patches with a predilection for the face, lips, genitalia, or buttocks. On the first exposure they typically occur 1 to 2 weeks after the antibiotic is started; subsequent exposures will result in the eruption occurring within days, in the same location. Antibiotics implicated include sulfonamides (TMP/SMX), tetracyclines, metronidazole, ampicillin, and dapsone.[28] Use of the offending agent should be avoided in the future.

Photosensitivity is common and is associated with many antibiotic agents, including doxycycline and ciprofloxacin. Doxycycline is one of the most common offenders, studies reporting rates of up to 20%.[32] This figure is of particular interest because doxycycline is frequently prescribed for malaria prophylaxis to patients traveling to sunny locations. Use of sunscreen should be advised.

Neurologic

Peripheral neuropathy can be a manifestation of toxicity to several antibiotic agents including isoniazid, metronidazole, and nitrofurantoin. In the case of isoniazid, typically used to treat latent tuberculosis, peripheral neuropathy can be prevented by concomitant administration of vitamin B_6, pyridoxine. Metronidazole-associated and nitrofurantoin-associated neuropathy is seen in patients on long-term therapy; in ambulatory medicine nitrofurantoin is often used daily for prevention of urinary tract infections, and patients with recurrent C difficile infection may receive multiple courses of metronidazole. These patients need to be monitored for signs or symptoms of neurotoxicity and, if noted, the medication should be discontinued. Metronidazole-induced peripheral neuropathy is predominantly a sensory neuropathy that usually improves once therapy is stopped. It is more common with longer courses of therapy. Metronidazole has also been rarely a cause of reversible optic neuritis and cerebellar disease.

Ciprofloxacin and imipenem are both known to carry an increased risk of seizure in patients predisposed to seizure, such as patients with a history of seizures, or at risk of accumulating high levels of the drug in their system, such as those with renal failure.[33] In neither case is this clearly a class effect; neither fluoroquinolones such as levofloxacin nor carbapenems such as meropenem seem to carry a significant risk.

Delirium is frequently multifactorial and common in the setting of infection, therefore teasing out if antibiotics are deliriogenic can be challenging. However, fluoroquinolones, ciprofloxacin more so than levofloxacin, have frequently been implicated in drug-induced delirium[34,35]; this does not preclude their use in the elderly, although this is something providers should be aware of.

Drug Fever

Parenteral therapy with β-lactams (penicillins and cephalosporins) is associated with drug-induced fever, as is therapy with several other antibiotics including sulfonamides. Diagnosis requires that infectious causes are ruled out. Laboratory abnormalities frequently noted in the case of drug fever include mild transaminitis, possibly eosinophilia; clinically patients are often noted to appear well and not to have the expected tachycardia associated with fever.[6] Regarding the discussion on drug-induced lupus, fever can be an adverse effect associated with minocycline use. Fever is also seen in other drug-related syndromes such as DRESS and serotonin syndrome, which can be a complication of therapy with serotonin-specific reuptake inhibitors (SSRIs), alone or in combination with other medication, notably the antibiotic linezolid.

ANTIBIOTIC COMPLICATIONS BY CLASS/AGENT
Fluoroquinolones

Quinolone antibiotics are associated with tendinopathy, in particular Achilles tendonitis and tendon rupture. Overall the rates of these complications are low, 3.2 cases per 1000 patient-years for tendonitis,[36] and even less frequent for tendon rupture, but there are likely some groups at higher risk for whom quinolones must be used with caution. It appears that the risk of tendonitis is higher in patients older than 60 years and those also on corticosteroids,[36] and there may also be an increased risk in patients with renal failure.

An additional rare adverse effect of quinolones is retinal detachment. Given the high rates of vision loss with this complication, this is a potential complication that providers should be aware of. It is estimated that the absolute increase in risk of retinal detachment in patients on fluoroquinolones is 4 per 10,000 person-years,[37] although it is difficult to be precise in the quantification of this risk given its rarity. Based on available evidence, it is unknown if any one fluoroquinolone is more likely to causes this side effect than others, and also unknown if there are specific patient groups at higher risk. This uncommon side effect should not preclude use of the antibiotic, but it is yet another reminder that antibiotics must always be used judiciously, assuring that the potential risks do not outweigh the benefits. In addition, should a patient on a fluoroquinolone develop symptoms that could be consistent with retinal detachment, such as new "floaters," they should be referred quickly to an ophthalmologist for evaluation.

Linezolid

Serotonin syndrome is a potentially life-threatening condition that results from toxic elevations of serotonin in the central nervous system. Symptoms include neuromuscular hyperactivity such as clonus and rigidity, autonomic hyperactivity such as tachycardia, hyperthermia, and hypertension, and changes in mental status such as agitated delirium. Development can result from use of an SSRI in combination with another medication that alters serotonin metabolism, such as the well-known drug interaction between antidepressant monoamine oxidase (MAO) inhibitors and SSRIs. Perhaps less widely known is that linezolid is a weak MAO inhibitor, and there have been many cases of serotonin syndrome in the setting of concomitant linezolid and SSRI therapy.[38] This combination is also therefore contraindicated, and it is not adequate to simply stop the SSRI on initiation of linezolid therapy; there needs to be an adequate washout period for the SSRI to be completely inactive in the patient's body, which may take several weeks. Should a patient develop serotonin syndrome, treatment involves discontinuation of all serotonergic medications, and use of benzodiazepines as needed for agitation. Cyproheptadine, an antihistamine with serotonin receptor–blocking activity, can be considered, although it should be noted that this is not an indication for use of this agent that is approved by the Food and Drug Administration.

IMPORTANT DRUG-DRUG INTERACTIONS

There are thousands of potential drug-drug interactions involving antibiotic agents. This section is not intended to be comprehensive, but rather highlights a few common and important interactions to be aware of.

Warfarin

Warfarin, an oral anticoagulant prescribed in the setting of atrial fibrillation, venous thromboembolism, and mechanical heart valve replacement, and by nature of the indications more commonly prescribed to older patients, has many known potential drug interactions. Some studies would indicate that prescription for any antibiotic increases the risk of bleeding in stable outpatients on warfarin,[39] but there are several classes of antibiotics that are particularly problematic. Azole antifungals and TMP/SMX have both been consistently shown to increase the International Normalized Ratio (INR) of patients on stable doses of warfarin and to lead to increased hospitalizations for bleeding complications. Studies estimate a 4.5-fold increased risk of hospitalization for bleeding complication in patients on warfarin recently prescribed an azole antifungal, and a 2.7-fold increase in risk for patients prescribed TMP/SMX.[39] Perhaps not as widely known is that there is also an interaction between warfarin and other antibiotics including macrolides, quinolones, and metronidazole. In a study assessing for changes in INR in patients on stable outpatient doses of warfarin, during and immediately after prescription of antibiotics 16% of patients on azithromycin and 19% of patients on levofloxacin had INR elevations to greater than 4, although again the TMP/SMX interaction was clearly more potent, with 44% of patients having an INR increase to greater than 4.[40] In a study assessing for risk of hospitalization for upper gastrointestinal bleeding in elderly patients on warfarin with a prescription for antibiotics to treat urinary tract infections in the 14 days before hospitalization, TMP/SMX and ciprofloxacin were associated with an approximately 4-fold and a 2-fold increase in risk, respectively. Amoxicillin, nitrofurantoin, and norfloxacin were not associated with an increased risk when compared with controls[41]; when appropriate, these may be safer agents to prescribe.

Trimethoprim/Sulfamethoxazole

In addition to interactions with warfarin, there a few additional important drug interactions one must be aware of when prescribing TMP/SMX. As reviewed earlier in this article, TMP/SMX can lead to hyperkalemia, especially in the setting of concomitant prescription of angiotensin receptor blockers and spironolactone. Use of TMP/SMX with methotrexate is associated with a higher risk of bone marrow suppression than with methotrexate alone, even at low methotrexate doses such as 5 mg weekly.[42] TMP/SMX also interacts with sulfonylureas and meglitinides, increasing their potential to cause hypoglycemia. Studies have indicated that the risk of hospitalization for hypoglycemia for patients on sulfonylureas increases 4- to 6-fold following prescription of TMP/SMX.[43] Finally, there is an interaction between TMP/SMX and the commonly prescribed antiepileptic phenytoin, the result of which is increased phenytoin levels and an increased potential for toxicity.

Clarithromycin

Many of the drug interactions seen with TMP/SMX are due to its effects on cytochrome P450 enzymes. Another drug with several important drug interactions owing to its potent inhibition of the cytochrome P450 3A4 isoenzyme is clarithromycin. In ambulatory medicine, clarithromycin is commonly used in *Helicobacter pylori* eradication therapy; other indications include treatment of bacterial respiratory infections and mycobacterial infections. Potentially dangerous and even fatal complications to be aware of include interactions with statins, especially simvastatin and lovastatin, resulting in increased statin levels and an increased risk of rhabdomyolysis. Decreased metabolism of calcium-channel blockers can result in bradycardia and hypotension, and decreased metabolism of digoxin can result in digoxin toxicity. These interactions are all clinically significant; for example, studies indicate that elderly patients hospitalized for digoxin toxicity were 12 times more likely than controls to have been prescribed clarithromycin in the week before their hospitalization.[44] Clarithromycin has an important and dangerous interaction with colchicine, especially in patients who have renal insufficiency. Multiple case reports of death from this interaction, caused by refractory agranulocytosis and rhabdomyolysis, have surfaced. Azithromycin has the same spectrum of activity as clarithromycin, and because it has far fewer and much less severe drug interactions, it should be used instead of clarithromycin in almost all clinical settings where a macrolide is needed.

Rifampin

Rifampin, frequently used for adjuvant treatment of staphylococcal osteomyelitis and orthopedic hardware infections, is another antibiotic fraught with interactions. Rifampin is an inducer of many cytochrome P450 enzymes, therefore it increases the metabolism of many medications, at times resulting in subtherapeutic drug levels. There are many clinical scenarios in which this becomes important, including patients on immunosuppressant medications such as cyclosporine and tacrolimus; in this case increased doses may be needed, and immunosuppressant levels should be followed to guide this. When coadministered with methadone for the management of heroin addiction, patients may need an increase in their daily methadone dose to avoid going into drug withdrawal. Patients on oral contraceptive agents should be advised to use a second form of birth control if placed on rifampin. Patients on warfarin need close monitoring of their INR and likely an increase in their warfarin dose. Given the large number of potential drug interactions, all patients started on rifampin need a thorough review of their medication lists for potential interactions. Baciewicz and colleagues[45] offer a comprehensive review of this topic.

Oral Contraceptives

Rifampin has a well-established interaction with combined oral contraceptive pills, resulting in a subtherapeutic contraceptive effect and a potential for unintended pregnancy, but it is less clear if other antibiotics have clinically significant interactions with contraceptive pills. It has proved difficult to study this potential interaction, and beyond the previously mentioned interaction with rifampin there is no convincing evidence that antibiotics result in decreased efficacy of contraceptive medications.[46,47] This is a difficult issue to study because the outcome is rare, and there is potential for significant recall bias in the retrospective studies that led to initial concerns regarding this potential interaction[48]; moreover, unfortunately oral contraceptive failure is not uncommon even outside the setting of concomitant antibiotic use. Overall it appears very unlikely that use of antibiotics, other than rifampin, result in decreased efficacy of oral contraceptives.

Metronidazole

Many providers were taught in medical school that there is an interaction between metronidazole and alcohol, a disulfiram-like reaction resulting in nausea and vomiting. As a result, patients are frequently warned to avoid alcohol while taking this medication. However, it is likely that this is a media myth, as there is little evidence that this interaction exists. There has even been a small experiment on human volunteers in which they were treated with metronidazole and then given alcohol, which showed no results of laboratory tests and physical examination, or symptoms, consistent with a disulfiram-like reaction.[49] It is likely that the symptoms that initially raised concern for this interaction simply represent common side effects of metronidazole treatment itself: nausea, headache, and a bitter/metallic taste.

SUMMARY

Antibiotics are powerful agents that have brought about great advances in medicine, but they are not without potential side effects. When given a prescription, patients should be informed not only of the benefits but also the potential risks of therapy. Judicious use is the best form of prevention overall, but there are some patient populations of whom one needs to be particularly mindful when prescribing. Patient groups at risk include the elderly, those with renal dysfunction, patients with significant cardiac disease, and those on multiple medications. Antibiotics particularly fraught with dangerous interactions include TMP/SMX and, less commonly, rifampin and clarithromycin. Patients on warfarin are also at high risk of dangerous alterations in anticoagulant effect, and deserve special attention.

REFERENCES

1. Garratty G. Immune hemolytic anemia associated with drug therapy. Blood Rev 2010;24(4–5):143–50.
2. Young NS. Acquired aplastic anemia. Ann Intern Med 2002;136(7):534–46.
3. Available at: http://www.ouhsc.edu/platelets/ditp.html. last accessed 11/1/2012.
4. van der Klauw MM, Goudsmit R, Halie MR, et al. A population-based case-cohort study of drug-associated agranulocytosis. Arch Intern Med 1999;159(4):369–74.
5. Andersohn F, Konzen C, Garbe E. Systematic review: agranulocytosis induced by nonchemotherapy drugs. Ann Intern Med 2007;146(9):657–65.
6. Cunha BA. Antibiotic side effects. Med Clin North Am 2001;85(1):149–85.
7. Ray WA, Murray KT, Hall K, et al. Azithromycin and the risk of cardiovascular death. N Engl J Med 2012;366:1881–90.
8. Bril F, Gonzalez CD, Di Girolamo G. Antimicrobial agents associated with QT interval prolongation. Curr Drug Saf 2010;5(1):85–92.
9. Lapi F, Wilchesky M, Kezouh A, et al. Fluoroquinolones and the risk of serious arrhythmia: a population-based study. Clin Infect Dis 2012;55(11):1457–65.
10. Vahid B, Wildemore BM. Nitrofurantoin pulmonary toxicity: a brief review. Internet J Pulm Med 2006;6(2).
11. Bartlett JG. Clinical practice. Antibiotic-associated diarrhea. N Engl J Med 2002; 346(5):334–9.
12. Hempel S, Newberry SJ, Maher AR, et al. Probiotics for the prevention and treatment of antibiotic-associated diarrhea: a systematic review and meta-analysis. JAMA 2012;307(18):1959–69.
13. Available at: http://webedition.sanfordguide.com.
14. Gröchenig HP, Tilg H, Vogetseder W. Clinical challenges and images in GI. Pill esophagitis. Gastroenterology 2006;131(4):996, 1365.
15. Leitner JM, Graninger W, Thalhammer F. Hepatotoxicity of antibacterials: pathomechanisms and clinical data. Infection 2010;38:3–11.
16. Carson JL, Strom BL, Duff A, et al. Acute liver disease associated with erythromycins, sulfonamides, and tetracyclines. Ann Intern Med 1993;119(7 Pt 1):576–83.
17. Wong-Beringer A, Joo J, Tse E, et al. Vancomycin-associated nephrotoxicity: a critical appraisal of risk with high-dose therapy. Int J Antimicrob Agents 2011; 37(2):95–101.
18. Perazella MA, Markowitz GS. Drug-Induced acute interstitial nephritis. Nat Rev Nephrol 2010;6:461–70.
19. Antoniou T, Gomes T, Juurlink DN, et al. Trimethoprim-sulfamethoxazole-induced hyperkalemia in patients receiving inhibitors of the renin-angiotensin system. Arch Intern Med 2010;170(10):1045–9.

20. Antoniou T, Gomes T, Mamdani MM, et al. Trimethoprim-sulfamethoxazole induced hyperkalemia in elderly patients receiving spironolactone: nested case-control study. BMJ 2011;343:d5228.
21. Zietse R, Zoutendijk R, Hoorn EJ. Fluid, electrolyte and acid-base disorders associated with antibiotic therapy. Nat Rev Nephrol 2009;5(4):193–202.
22. Mohr JA, Clark RM, Waack TC, et al. Nafcillin-associated hypokalemia. JAMA 1979;242(6):544.
23. Xu J, Schwartw K. Effect of antibiotics on vulvovaginal candidiasis: a MetroNet Study. J Am Board Fam Med 2008;21:261–8.
24. Pirotta MV, Garland SM. Genital candida species detected from women in Melbourne, Australia, before and after treatment with antibiotics. J Clin Microbiol 2006;44:3212–7.
25. Pirotta M, Gunn J, Chondros P, et al. Effect of lactobacillus in preventing post-antibiotic vulvovaginal candidiasis: a randomised controlled trial. BMJ 2004; 329(7465):548.
26. Falagas ME, Betsi GI, Athanasiou S. Probiotics for prevention of recurrent vulvovaginal candidiasis: a review. J Antimicrob Chemother 2006;58(2):266–72.
27. Borchers AT, Keen CL, Gershwin ME. Drug-induced lupus. Ann N Y Acad Sci 2007;1108:166–82.
28. Diaz L, Ciurea AM. Cutaneous and systemic adverse reactions to antibiotics. Dermatol Ther 2012;25(1):12–22.
29. Cacoub P, Musette P, Descamps V, et al. The DRESS syndrome: a literature review. Am J Med 2011;124(7):588–97.
30. Usatine RP, Sandy N. Dermatologic emergencies. Am Fam Physician 2010;82(7): 773–80.
31. Romano A, Guéant-Rodriguez RM, Viola M, et al. Cross-reactivity and tolerability of cephalosporins in patients with immediate hypersensitivity to penicillins. Ann Intern Med 2004;141(1):16–22.
32. Vassileva SG, Mateev G, Parish LC. Antimicrobial photosensitive reactions. Arch Intern Med 1998;158(18):1993–2000.
33. Agbaht K, Bitik B, Piskinpasa S, et al. Ciprofloxacin-associated seizures in a patient with underlying thyrotoxicosis: case report and literature review. Int J Clin Pharmacol Ther 2009;47(5):303–10.
34. Tomé AM, Filipe A. Quinolones: review of psychiatric and neurological adverse reactions. Drug Saf 2011;34(6):465–88.
35. Catic AG. Identification and management of in-hospital drug-induced delirium in older patients. Drugs Aging 2011;28(9):737–48.
36. Wise BL, Peloquin C, Choi H, et al. Impact of age, sex, obesity and steroid use on quinolone-associated tendon rupture. Am J Med 2012;125:1228.e23–8.
37. Etminan M, Forooghian F, Brophy JM, et al. Oral fluoroquinolones and the risk of retinal detachment. JAMA 2012;307(13):1414–9.
38. Clark DB, Andrus MR, Byrd DC. Drug Interactions between linezolid and selective serotonin reuptake inhibitors: case reports involving sertraline and review of the literature. Pharmacotherapy 2006;26(2):269–76.
39. Baillargeon J, Holmes HM. Concurrent use of warfarin and antibiotics and the risk of bleeding in older adults. Am J Med 2012;125:183–9.
40. Glasheen JJ, Fugit RV, Prochazka AV. The risk of overanticoagulation with antibiotic use in outpatients on stable warfarin regimens. J Gen Intern Med 2005;20:653–6.
41. Fischer HD, Juurlink DN, Mamdani MM, et al. Hemorrhage during warfarin therapy associated with cotrimoxazole and other urinary tract anti-infective agents. Arch Intern Med 2010;170(7):617–21.

42. Bourre-tessier J, Haraoui B. Methotrexate drug interactions in the treatment of rheumatoid arthritis: a systematic review. J Rheumatol 2010;37:1416–21.

43. Ho JM, Juurlink DN. Considerations when prescribing trimethoprim-sulfamethoxazole. CMAJ 2011;183(16):1851–8.

44. Juurlink DN, Mamdani M, Kopp A, et al. Drug-drug interactions among elderly patients hospitalized for drug toxicity. JAMA 2003;289:1652–8.

45. Baciewicz AM, Chrisman CR, Finch CK, et al. Update on rifampin, rifabutin, and rifapentine drug interactions. Curr Med Res Opin 2013;29:1–12.

46. Archer JS, Archer DF. Oral contraceptive efficacy and antibiotic interaction: a myth debunked. J Am Acad Dermatol 2002;46:917–23.

47. Toh S, Mitchell AA, Anderka M, et al. Antibiotics and oral contraceptive failure—a case-crossover study. Contraception 2011;83:418–25.

48. Dickinson BD, Altman RD, Nielsen NH, et al. Drug interactions between oral contraceptives and antibiotics. Obstet Gynecol 2001;98:853–60.

49. Visapaa JP, Tillonen JS, Kaihavaara PS, et al. Lack of disulfiram-like reaction with metronidazole and ethanol. Ann Pharmacother 2002;36:971–4.

Enterohemorrhagic *Escherichia coli* Infections and the Hemolytic-Uremic Syndrome

Andrea V. Page, MD, MSc[a],*, W. Conrad Liles, MD, PhD[a,b]

KEYWORDS

- *Escherichia coli* O157:H7 • *Escherichia coli* O104:H4 • Shiga toxin
- Enterohemorrhagic *Escherichia coli* • Hemolytic-uremic syndrome • Eculizumab

KEY POINTS

- Enterohemorrhagic *Escherichia coli* (EHEC) should be considered in all patients with bloody diarrhea, particularly if accompanied by severe abdominal pain. Fever, while often reported on history, is usually absent at presentation.
- Stool samples from all patients with bloody diarrhea should be tested for *E. coli* O157:H7 and for non-O157 serotypes of EHEC.
- HUS is the most severe complication of EHEC infection, and is characterized by nonimmune hemolytic anemia, thrombocytopenia, and acute kidney injury.
- Supportive care is the mainstay of therapy for EHEC infections; this includes intravenous fluid replacement and, in the case of HUS, antihypertensive medications, red blood cell transfusions, and renal replacement therapy (hemodialysis) as necessary.
- Strict adherence to proper food handling and hand hygiene measures is the best way to prevent both primary and secondary transmission of EHEC.

INTRODUCTION

Enterohemorrhagic *Escherichia coli* (EHEC; Shiga toxin/verotoxin-producing *E. coli*) is well known to the public as a potentially serious cause of infectious diarrhea based on several recent and well-publicized outbreaks associated with contaminated food sources. Whereas uncomplicated bloody diarrhea is the typical outcome of a Shiga toxin–producing *E. coli* infection, some patients progress to life-threatening

Financial Disclosures or Conflicts of Interest: None.
[a] Division of Infectious Diseases, Department of Medicine, Mount Sinai Hospital – University Health Network, University of Toronto, 200 Elizabeth Street, Toronto, Ontario, M5G 2C4, Canada; [b] Division of Allergy and Infectious Diseases, Department of Medicine, University of Washington School of Medicine, 1959 NE Pacific Street, Seattle, WA 98195-6420, USA
* Corresponding author. Mount Sinai Hospital, Suite 436, 600 University Avenue, Toronto, Ontario M5G 1X5, Canada.
E-mail address: APage@mtsinai.on.ca

Med Clin N Am 97 (2013) 681–695
http://dx.doi.org/10.1016/j.mcna.2013.04.001
medical.theclinics.com

hemolytic-uremic syndrome (HUS), defined by the triad of nonimmune hemolytic anemia, thrombocytopenia, and acute kidney injury. In the 2011 outbreak centered in Germany, 3842 people fell ill, many after consuming contaminated fenugreek sprouts, the suspected source. More than half of these individuals required hospitalization, and 855 developed HUS. Fifty-three patients died. The serotype responsible, *E. coli* O104:H4, was previously thought to be of limited pathogenic potential in humans; however, the outbreak strain was subsequently found to have acquired new virulence factors. Although *E. coli* O157:H7 remains the most common serotype isolated in North America, the outbreak in Germany illustrates both the emerging importance of non-O157 serotypes as agents of human disease and the potential for modern, large-scale methods of food production and distribution to result in widespread illness. This review addresses the pathogenesis, clinical presentation, diagnosis, and treatment of both EHEC infection and HUS, with a focus on the most commonly reported EHEC serotype (O157:H7), the serotype responsible for the most recent large outbreak (O104:H4), and the differences between the two.

EPIDEMIOLOGY

In the United States, the FoodNet (Foodborne Diseases Active Surveillance Network) system actively tracks laboratory-confirmed cases of foodborne bacterial and parasitic pathogens in multiple catchment areas encompassing 15% of the country's population.[1] Surveillance data from 2011 revealed 0.97 infections with *E. coli* O157:H7 for every 100,000 individuals. The combined incidence for non-O157 Shiga toxin–producing serotypes was only slightly higher at 1.10 per 100,000 population. Individual serotypes O157 (47%), O26 (14%), and O103 (11%) were most frequently isolated, and all occurred most often in children younger than 5 years. HUS was most common in the same age group. Although the incidence of *E. coli* O157:H7 infection has declined in recent years, that of non-O157 serotypes and postdiarrheal HUS has not. Furthermore, significant underdiagnosis of both O157:H7 and non-O157 serotypes is likely, as patients may not seek medical attention for less severe infections and even when they do, appropriate diagnostic testing may not always be performed.[2]

The reported incidence of EHEC infection in Europe before the 2011 outbreak was similar to that in the United States. In 2009, 3573 cases of Shiga toxin–producing *E. coli* were identified in the European Union, and the EHEC-related mortality rate had stabilized at 2 to 3 deaths per year.[3] The 2011 *E. coli* O104:H4 outbreak was unique, in size (3842 patients infected) and in that it preferentially affected adults (median age: 42 years) and women (68% of those infected). Although this may have been related to a particular virulence factor associated with this serotype, behavioral patterns (ie, increased likelihood of consumption of the suspected vector, fenugreek sprouts) may also have resulted in the peculiar distribution of illness.

Also atypical was the lack of a known animal reservoir for *E. coli* O104:H4. *E. coli* O157:H7 and common non-O157 EHEC serotypes reside in the gastrointestinal tracts of cattle and other ruminants (eg, deer, goats, and sheep), and can survive and proliferate in both the environment (including in the watershed of key growing regions) and foodstuffs.[4] EHEC infections in both cattle and humans follow a consistent seasonal pattern and occur much more commonly in the spring (June to September in the Northern hemisphere).[5] Because EHEC are extremely virulent, even a low infectious dose (100–1000 organisms) can result in clinically significant infection.[6,7] Recent outbreaks of EHEC have been linked to fresh produce, undercooked beef, and various types of processed, prepackaged, and even frozen foods (**Table 1**). **Table 1** also

Table 1
Selected outbreaks of enterohemorrhagic *E. coli* infections with known source

Source	Serotype	Location	Year	Number Affected	Hospital	HUS	Deaths
Frozen foods (chicken quesadillas suspected)[a],[61]	O121	15 US states	2013	24	7	1	0
Raw clover sprouts[62]	O26	Chain restaurant in 11 US states	2012	29	7	0	0
Spinach and packaged leafy greens[63,64]	O157:H7	Single producer, 5 US states	2012	33	13	2	0
	O157:H7	USA and Canada	2006	205	103	31	3
Ground beef or beef sausage[25,65,66]	O157:H7	Denmark	2012	13	NR	8	NR
	O26:H11	Denmark	2007	20	NR	0	0
	O157:H7	Western USA	1993	501	151	45	3
Romaine lettuce[67,68]	O157:H7	Single farm, 10 US states	2011	58	34	3	0
	O145	Five US states	2010	31	11	3	0
Fenugreek sprouts (suspected)[69–72]	O104:H4	Germany	2011	3842	64%	855	53
		France	2011	24	8	7	NR
Unpasteurized milk, cheese, or other dairy products[73]	O157	Connecticut	2008	7	5	3	0
Ready-to-bake prepackaged cookie dough[74]	O157:H7	Single producer, 30 US states	2009	77	35	10	0
Petting zoos and close contact with farm animals[75,76]	O157	England	2009	93	27	17	NR
	O157:H7	North Carolina	2004	108	NR	15	0
Municipal or recreational (lakes, pools, and parks) water[52,77]	O157:H7	British Columbia, Canada	2004	10	6	1	0
	O157:H7	Ontario, Canada	2000	≈2300	65	27	7
Unpasteurized juice or cider[78]	O157:H7	Western USA and Canada	1996	70	25	14	1
White radish sprouts[79]	O157:H7	Japan	1996	9492	758	121	3

Abbreviation: NR, not reported.
[a] Outbreak ongoing at the time of publication.

illustrates how modern systems of food processing and distribution can result in widespread disease after contamination at a single source (whether grower, producer, or processor), and emphasizes the importance of disease recognition and reporting to a national food safety organization that can collate reports and explore potential relationships among illnesses in multiple jurisdictions.

In addition to contaminated food and water, EHEC infections have been acquired through person-to-person (household) transmission. Up to 20% of infections during *E. coli* O157:H7 outbreaks are estimated to occur via secondary transmission rather than exposure to the original contaminated source.[8] In the absence of a single identifiable source of infection, poor food handling and hygiene practices have been implicated in outbreaks associated with restaurants and day-care centers.[9,10]

PATHOGENESIS

EHEC combine the virulence features of 2 other *E. coli* pathotypes that cause diarrheal disease in humans (**Box 1**). With Shiga toxin–producing *E. coli* (STEC), they share bacteriophage-encoded Shiga toxins; and with enteropathogenic *E. coli* (EPEC), they share a chromosomally located pathogenicity island (the locus of enterocyte effacement [LEE]). The LEE encodes proteins necessary to produce an "attaching and effacing effect," whereby the bacteria attach to intestinal epithelial cells and induce loss of the microvilli on the apical surface.[11] These proteins include intimin, which brings the bacteria into close contact with the epithelial cell, and a type III secretion system (T3SS), by which bacterial proteins can be injected through the intestinal epithelial cell membrane. The regulation of these proteins is particularly well adapted to cause human disease. EHEC are able to survive exposure to gastric acid during passage through the stomach and to use the stimulus of the low pH to induce expression of intimin and T3SS, facilitating adhesion to epithelial cells and resulting in diarrhea once the bacteria reach the lower gastrointestinal (GI) tract.[12]

Box 1
Nomenclature of *E. coli* pathotypes causing intestinal infection in humans

Enteroaggregative *E. coli* (EAEC): Named for the pattern of adherence to cultured cells, EAEC may cause acute (including traveler's) or chronic (particularly in patients with human immunodeficiency virus) diarrhea

Enteroinvasive *E. coli* (EIEC): Possessing a plasmid-encoded type III secretion system that allows them to inject proteins through host cell membranes and subsequently to invade, multiply, and spread within intestinal epithelial cells, EIEC cause severe diarrhea with systemic symptoms, indistinguishable from shigellosis/bacillary dysentery

Enterotoxigenic *E. coli* (ETEC): Contracted through the ingestion of contaminated food and water, ETEC produce either or both of a heat-labile and heat-stable enterotoxin, and are a common cause of acute, watery, secretory diarrhea in children and travelers to resource-limited countries

Enteropathogenic *E. coli* (EPEC): Characterized by a unique attaching and effacing effect on intestinal epithelial cells, EPEC are spread by person-to-person transmission and are a common cause of severe diarrhea in infants in resource-limited settings

Shiga toxin–producing *E. coli* (STEC): Acquired through contaminated food or water, STEC harbor bacteriophages that encode the virulence factors Shiga-like toxins 1 and 2

Enterohemorrhagic *E. coli* (EHEC): A potentially severe cause of bloody diarrhea that may be complicated by HUS, EHEC shares characteristics of EPEC (attaching and effacing effect) and STEC (Shiga-like toxin 1 and/or 2 production)

Severe disease can result from other combinations of virulence factors. The EHEC serotype responsible for the European outbreak in 2011, *E. coli* O104:H4, is unique in that it has an enteroaggregative *E. coli* (EAEC) background (see **Box 1**). It possesses an EAEC virulence plasmid that encodes aggregative adherence fimbriae, rather than intimin and the T3SS.[13] Only 2 sporadic cases of HUS had previously been associated with this serotype, so the increased pathogenicity of the outbreak strain likely arose after acquisition of additional virulence factors. Unlike typical EAEC, the outbreak *E. coli* O104:H4 possessed a bacteriophage-encoded Shiga toxin (Stx2) and its promoter region, both similar to that found in EHEC serotypes. In addition, the outbreak strain also possessed a CTX-M-15 class extended-spectrum β-lactamase (ESBL), as well as a unique combination of enzymes known as SPATEs (Serine Protease Autotransporters of Enterobacteriaceae) that contributed to greater intestinal adherence and colonization.[14,15]

Once adhered to intestinal epithelial cells, EHEC produce and release Shiga-like toxin 1 (Stx1) and/or Shiga-like toxin 2 (Stx2). Stx2 and certain of its subtypes are most commonly associated with EHEC infections and HUS in humans, but for the purposes of this review the two are considered together. After release, the Shiga toxin is translocated across the intestinal epithelium and delivered to its receptor, globotriaosylceramide (Gb3), by circulating neutrophils.[16] Density of the Gb3 receptor mediates the susceptibility of individual vascular beds to the action of the Shiga toxin, and is particularly high in the kidneys, as well as the colon and brain.[17–19] Shiga toxin–mediated injury to the colonic microvasculature is the proposed mechanism leading to bloody diarrhea in EHEC infections, whereas toxin-mediated injury to renal endothelial cells leads to the acute kidney injury of HUS. Once bound to the Gb3 receptor and internalized, high intracellular concentrations of Shiga toxin induce cell death by modifying the ribosome and inhibiting elongation of the peptide chain, whereas lower intracellular concentrations of Shiga toxin alter gene expression and endothelial cell phenotype.[20]

Both Shiga toxin–induced mechanisms of cellular damage are apparent in the characteristic pathologic lesion of HUS, thrombotic microangiopathy (TMA). TMA is characterized by endothelial cell swelling and detachment from the basement membrane, and thrombosis of the microvasculature of the GI tract and kidneys.[21] Shiga toxin upregulates the expression of adhesion molecules (including E-selectin, intercellular cell adhesion molecule 1, and vascular cell adhesion molecule 1) on the endothelial cell surface, and facilitates the adherence and subsequent degranulation of neutrophils.[22] Neutrophil degranulation releases elastase, which can disrupt the extracellular matrix and result in endothelial cell detachment. Shiga toxins also increase cell-surface expression of P-selectin, and both induce the release and prevent cleavage of ultralarge von Willebrand factor. In doing so, the toxins promote platelet adhesion to the endothelial cell surface and subsequent thrombosis.[23,24]

Therefore, whereas diarrhea in EHEC infection occurs as a result of a direct interaction between intestinal epithelial cells and bacteria, bloody diarrhea and HUS both occur as a consequence of the actions of the Shiga toxin on the microvascular endothelial cells of the kidney and GI tract.

CLINICAL PRESENTATION

For *E. coli* O157:H7 infection, the incubation period between ingestion of bacteria and onset of diarrhea is approximately 3 days, although this can vary between 2 and 12 days.[25] Although not all patients with *E. coli* O157:H7 in the stool are symptomatic, severe abdominal cramping (often worse with defecation) and nonbloody diarrhea typically occur during the first 1 to 3 days of illness, and may be accompanied by vomiting.[26] Fever may be present or reported in up to 50% of patients during this initial phase of illness, but has usually resolved by the time of presentation to medical care. In approximately 90% of patients, bloody diarrhea follows the initial phase of illness and prompts patients or their caregivers to seek medical attention.

Although no components of history or physical examination are sufficiently specific to replace microbiologic diagnosis, bloody diarrhea, severe abdominal pain, and absent fever are more consistent with EHEC infection than that caused by other enteric bacteria including *Salmonella*, non–Shiga toxin-producing *Shigella*, and *Campylobacter* species. If a source or suspected exposure can be documented, the incubation period tends to be slightly longer with EHEC than with other enteric bacteria, and was particularly prolonged in the *E. coli* O104:H4 outbreak. The clinical presentation, risk of complications, and outcome of infection with *E. coli* O157:H7, non-O157 EHEC serotypes, *E. coli* O104:H4, and other enteric bacteria are outlined in **Table 2**.

The most feared complication of EHEC infection is HUS, defined by the triad of nonimmune hemolytic anemia, thrombocytopenia, and acute renal injury. An elevated white blood cell count and vomiting before hospital admission have been associated with an increased likelihood of subsequent development of HUS.[27,28] HUS is distinguishable from other thrombotic microangiopathies by the presence of a diarrheal prodrome, and the absence of other precipitating factors or comorbidities (**Box 2**).

DIAGNOSTIC TESTING

Culture of loose stool specimens is the current gold-standard method for diagnosis of EHEC infections. Patients with EHEC infections are not typically bacteremic (even during HUS), so blood cultures, though potentially useful for ruling out other infectious causes in patients with fever, are rarely useful in diagnosing EHEC. In addition, even in EHEC infections complicated by HUS, Shiga toxin can be detected in blood only transiently, and hence is not a means of diagnosis.[29]

Current guidelines from the Centers for Disease Control and Prevention (CDC) in the United States recommend that all stool samples submitted with the diagnosis of acute, community-acquired diarrhea be tested for Shiga toxin–producing *E. coli*, a process that requires selective and differential culture media (Sorbitol MacConkey [SMAC] agar).[30] Unlike most of the *E. coli* strains found in the human GI tract, *E. coli* O157:H7 cannot ferment sorbitol, and therefore appears as colorless colonies on SMAC. Normal GI tract flora–associated *E. coli* and non-O157 serotypes of EHEC typically ferment both sorbitol and lactose, and therefore appear as pink colonies on the same media. Latex agglutination tests can then be used to confirm the O157 serotype of any colorless colonies.

With the increasing recognition of the clinical importance of non-O157 Shiga toxin–producing serotypes, the CDC recommends that all samples submitted for acute diarrhea be simultaneously tested for non-O157 serotypes. Non-O157 serotypes, including the *E. coli* O104:H4 outbreak strain, can be cultured on either MacConkey agar or SMAC and can be confirmed as Shiga toxin producers by enzyme immunoassay for the Shiga toxin, or by polymerase chain reaction for the Shiga toxin genes *stx1* and *stx2*. Agglutination with O-specific antisera for the most common serotypes may also be performed. Although initial nonculture detection methods are acceptable, the lack of a viable isolate for serotyping hinders clinical prognostication and epidemiologic follow-up. Testing for non-O157 serotypes is not done in all clinical laboratories, therefore isolates should be sent to the local Public Health (or reference) Laboratory for specialized testing.

Table 2
Clinical characteristics of infection for enterohemorrhagic *E. coli* versus other enteric bacteria

	E. coli O157:H7[1,55]	Non-O157 *E. coli* Serotypes[28,80,81]	*E. coli* O104:H4[47,70,71,82]	Other Enterics[a,1,83]
Median incubation (range)	3 d (2–12)	4 d	8 d (6–10)	Hours to days
History of recent travel (Central or South America, the Caribbean)	<5%	15%	Rare	8%–16%
Bloody diarrhea	>90%	60%	79% with HUS 56% with GI	Possible
Abdominal pain	Severe, common	Common	>90%	30%–50%
Vomiting		Common early in illness		
Documented fever at presentation	Rare	Rar	Rare	50%–70%
Stool leukocytes	50%	36%	Not reported	Common
Need for hospitalization	43%	18%	≈64%	15%–30%
HUS				
Incidence	10%–15%	<10%	22%	0%
Diarrheal prodrome	7 d (5–13)	6 d	5 d	0%
Neurologic complications[b]	Common	Common	48% of adults 26% of children	0%
Case fatality rate	<1% GI <5% HUS	<0.5% GI <5% HUS	0.6% GI 4.1% HUS	<0.5%

[a] Non–Shiga toxin–producing *Campylobacter*, *Salmonella*, or *Shigella* species.
[b] Neurologic complications include cognitive impairment, aphasia, or seizures.

> **Box 2**
> **Differential diagnosis of thrombotic microangiopathy**
>
> Hemolytic-uremic syndrome
>
> Thrombotic thrombocytopenic purpura (congenital or idiopathic)
>
> Antiphospholipid antibody syndrome
>
> Disseminated intravascular coagulation
>
> Malignant hypertension
>
> Scleroderma renal crisis
>
> Drug-induced (eg, calcineurin inhibitors)

At present, there is no diagnostic test to predict which patients, from among all those with EHEC infection, will develop HUS. However, evidence of early vascular injury can be detected even in the pre-HUS stage. Children with EHEC infection who will eventually develop HUS (but have yet to do so) have levels of prothrombotic factors and endothelial-active cytokines that are significantly higher than those in children with uncomplicated EHEC infection.[31,32] By contrast, serum levels of angiopoietin-1, a key mediator of endothelial cell quiescence, decline with progressive stages of complicated *E. coli* O157:H7 infection, and can partially discriminate between those children who will have an uncomplicated course of EHEC infection and those who will develop HUS.[33] Although none of these markers are sufficiently specific to be used as the sole predictors of progression to HUS, combinations of markers may ultimately aid clinicians in prognostication.

MANAGEMENT

For EHEC-associated gastroenteritis, supportive care and intravenous fluid replacement are the cornerstones of therapy. Judicious administration of intravenous fluid and sodium early in illness in children with bloody diarrhea appears to improve outcomes in the subgroup which eventually develops HUS.[34] Antimotility agents and, possibly, other drugs with antimotility effects (such as narcotics) should not be administered, as these have been associated with an increased risk of development of HUS in some, but not all, studies.[28,35] Nonsteroidal anti-inflammatory drugs should also be avoided because of a theoretical risk of worsening of gastrointestinal bleeding and/or acute kidney injury.

Perhaps the most contentious issue in the therapy for EHEC-associated gastroenteritis is the use of antibiotics. Many studies have reported a strong association between receipt of antibiotics and the eventual development of HUS, whereas other studies and a meta-analysis found no association.[36–39] When studied in vitro certain antibiotics, particularly the quinolones and trimethoprim, can stimulate the bacterial SOS response, which in turn induces the bacteriophage that encodes the Shiga toxin, resulting in increased toxin production, cell lysis, and toxin release.[40] Because the association between antibiotic use and HUS has been most consistent in children, expert opinion generally recommends that antibiotics be avoided in children with EHEC gastroenteritis.[26]

This issue was partially readdressed during the recent *E. coli* O104:H4 outbreak. In vitro studies using the outbreak strain were inconsistent, with conflicting reports that exposure to ciprofloxacin did, or did not, induce Shiga toxin production depending on the strain used and the study conditions.[15,41,42] Exposure to azithromycin was not found to induce Shiga toxin production in vitro, and use of azithromycin in patients who had already developed HUS was associated with a shorter duration of fecal shedding of bacteria.[43] Nonetheless, neither this nor any other study yet published has examined the impact of early antimicrobial therapy on the subsequent development of HUS in a randomized, controlled fashion. At present, therefore, routine use of antibiotics in early EHEC infection is not recommended.

As with EHEC gastroenteritis, the mainstay of therapy for HUS is supportive care. All patients with HUS should be hospitalized, with frequent monitoring of laboratory markers of disease and receipt of intravenous volume replacement, antihypertensive therapy, renal replacement therapy, and packed red blood cells when necessary. No clinical benefit has been found with therapeutic anticoagulation, administration of fresh frozen plasma or glucocorticosteroids, or the use of specific Shiga toxin binders.[44]

Although therapeutic plasma exchange (TPE; plasmapheresis) is a key treatment strategy for thrombotic thrombocytopenic purpura and atypical (diarrhea-negative, EHEC-negative) HUS, its use in EHEC-associated HUS is controversial and has not been proved effective in any randomized controlled trial.[45] Because Shiga toxin is detectable in the circulation only very early in illness, and because Shiga toxin–induced endothelial and vascular dysfunction are known to precede the development of HUS, the pathophysiologic rationale for TPE in EHEC-associated HUS is lacking. A nonrandomized retrospective registry analysis of adult patients with HUS during the E. coli O104:H4 outbreak found no difference in neurologic symptoms or need for dialysis at the study end point of death or hospital discharge in patients who received TPE versus best supportive care. Although mortality was higher in those receiving best supportive care, such patients were older and more often had advance directives limiting care options.[46] The vast majority of pediatric patients with E. coli O104:H4 were treated with best supportive care (including dialysis) only, and had favorable outcomes.[47] Consequently, most investigators are circumspect about the potential benefits of TPE in EHEC-associated HUS.[48]

Eculizumab, a humanized monoclonal antibody that binds to C5 of the complement system to prevent propagation of the complement cascade, is an established therapy for atypical (diarrhea-negative) HUS that was also used during the E. coli O104:H4 outbreak. The rationale for its use derived from recent evidence of complement activation in typical EHEC-induced HUS and a report of the successful use of eculizumab in 3 young children with severe EHEC-induced HUS.[49,50] In the European O104 outbreak, administration of eculizumab was at the physicians' discretion and did not affect the need for dialysis or mechanical ventilation nor the occurrence of seizures and death.[51] While data from randomized trials is awaited, current evidence does not support the use of eculizumab for the treatment of EHEC-induced HUS.

PROGNOSIS

For most patients who develop uncomplicated EHEC-associated gastroenteritis and are treated with best supportive care, the prognosis is excellent. However, recent evidence suggests that long-term sequelae are possible in the adult population. Among 1977 adult patients, 1067 of whom developed gastroenteritis after exposure to a municipal water source contaminated with E. coli O157:H7 and Campylobacter species, new-onset hypertension, a combination of microalbuminuria and impaired glomerular filtration rate (GFR), and a physician-diagnosed cardiovascular event were all more common in those who had experienced symptomatic gastrointestinal illness 8 years earlier.[52]

For children who develop EHEC-associated HUS, there appears to be a small but significant risk (<5%) of end-stage renal disease, and a higher risk of hypertension, proteinuria, or a reduced GFR (25% pooled risk). Consequently, some investigators recommend screening children at least once per year for occult renal disease after an episode of EHEC-associated HUS.[53] A recent prospective study of 226 children with HUS documented full recovery in 70% after 5 years, with proteinuria (18%), hypertension (9%), decreased GFR (7%) and/or neurologic symptoms (4%) in the remainder.[54] Of note, half of these patients demonstrated late sequelae with onset more than 1 year after the acute event, again emphasizing the need for long-term follow-up.

Death is rare in both complicated and uncomplicated EHEC infections, occurring in less than 1% of patients with EHEC-associated gastroenteritis and in less than 5% of patients with EHEC-associated HUS.[55] Mortality with either syndrome is highest in those aged 60 years and older.

PREVENTION

Primary prevention of EHEC infections involves avoidance of common sources of bacteria or elimination of the bacteria through cooking or hand washing. Unpasteurized foods should be avoided, and care should be taken during food preparation to prevent cross-contamination between uncooked meat and foods that are to be served raw.[56] Raw foods, particularly leafy greens, should be washed thoroughly before eating even if prepackaged and prewashed. Ground beef should be cooked to an internal temperature of 160°F/71°C, verified by a meat thermometer. Lake or pool water should not be swallowed while swimming, and strict hand-hygiene protocols should be followed in petting zoos and after contact with animals.

Hand hygiene for both the infected patient and close contacts is also the key element in the prevention of secondary transmission. For hospitalized patients, contact precautions that include the use of gowns, gloves, and a single-bedded room are recommended. Because stringent infection control procedures such as these are impossible in homes, some investigators have advocated admitting young children with confirmed or suspected E. coli O157:H7 infection to hospital to avoid secondary transmission, particularly when there is another young child in the household.[57,58]

In the European outbreak of E. coli O104:H4, the median duration of shedding of bacteria in the stool was estimated to be 10 to 18 days, although long-term asymptomatic shedding of 7 months' duration was also described.[59] Of note, children and patients without HUS shed for a longer median duration (>30 days), as did those who received no antibiotic therapy, indicating that prolonged vigilance and compliance with hygiene measures is likely required to prevent secondary transmission.[60] Patients with ongoing fecal shedding of EHEC should be temporarily excluded from settings with a high risk of transmission (commercial food preparation, day-care centers) in accordance with local public health guidelines.

SUMMARY

EHEC continue to cause foodborne infectious diarrhea worldwide, typically resulting from a breach of proper food handling, sanitation and water processing, or hand-hygiene procedures. Clinicians therefore need to remain vigilant and consider EHEC in the differential diagnosis of diarrhea, particularly if bloody. Appropriate laboratory testing and reporting for both O157 and non-O157 serotypes, as well as prompt initiation of infection control procedures for confirmed or suspected cases, will facilitate follow-up investigation to identify the source of infection and will help to prevent secondary transmission. Supportive care and close monitoring for complications such as HUS are also crucial. Despite the frequency and severity of EHEC outbreaks, there are as yet no proven means to predict which patients will develop HUS, and no specific therapies to either prevent progression or treat HUS once it develops. Research in these areas will be key to improving the care of patients with EHEC infection in the years to come.

REFERENCES

1. CDC. Foodborne Diseases Active Surveillance Network (FoodNet): FoodNet surveillance report for 2011 (final report). Atlanta (GA): U.S. Department of Health and Human Services, CDC; 2012.
2. Scallan E, Hoekstra RM, Angulo FJ, et al. Foodborne illness acquired in the United States—major pathogens. Emerg Infect Dis 2011;17:7–15.
3. Kielstein JT. The German 2011 epidemic of Shiga toxin-producing *E. coli*—the nephrological view. Nephrol Dial transplant 2011;29:2723–6.
4. Cooley M, Carychao D, Crawford-Miksza L. Incidence and tracking of *Escherichia coli* O157:H7 in a major produce production region in California. PLoS One 2007;2:e1159.
5. Stanford K, Croy D, Bach SJ, et al. Ecology of *Escherichia coli* O157:H7 in commercial dairies in Southern Alberta. J Dairy Sci 2005;88:4441–51.
6. Tuttle J, Gomez T, Doyle MP, et al. Lessons from a large outbreak of *Escherichia coli* O157:H7 infections: insights into the infectious dose and method of widespread contamination of hamburger patties. Epidemiol Infect 1999;122: 185–92.
7. Tilden J, Young W, McNamara AM, et al. A new route of transmission for *Escherichia coli*: infection from dry fermented salami. Am J Public Health 1996;86: 1142–5.
8. Snedeker KG, Shaw DJ, Locking MR, et al. Primary and secondary cases in *Escherichia coli* O157 outbreaks: a statistical analysis. BMC Infect Dis 2009; 9:144.
9. Bradley KK, Williams JM, Burnsed LJ, et al. Epidemiology of a large restaurant-associated outbreak of Shiga toxin-producing *Escherichia coli* O111:NM. Epidemiol Infect 2012;140:1644–54.
10. Brown JA, Hite DS, Gillim-Ross LA, et al. Outbreak of shiga toxin-producing *Escherichia coli* serotype O26: H11 infection at a child care center in Colorado. Pediatr Infect Dis J 2012;31:379–83.
11. Pennington H. *Escherichia coli* O157. Lancet 2010;376:1428–35.
12. House B, Kus JV, Prayitno N, et al. Acid-stress-induced changes in enterohaemorrhagic *Escherichia coli* O157: H7 virulence. Microbiology 2009;155: 2907–18.
13. Bielaszewska M, Mellmann A, Zhang W, et al. Characterisation of the *Escherichia coli* strain associated with an outbreak of haemolytic uraemic syndrome in Germany, 2011: a microbiologic study. Lancet Infect Dis 2011;11:671–6.
14. Rohde H, Quin J, Cui Y, et al. Open-source genomic analysis of Shiga-toxin-producing *E. coli* O104:H4. N Engl J Med 2011;365:718–24.
15. Rasko DA, Webster DR, Sahl JW, et al. Origins of the *E. coli* strain causing an outbreak of hemolytic-uremic syndrome in Germany. N Engl J Med 2011;365: 709–17.
16. Brigotti M, Tazzari PL, Ravanelli E, et al. Endothelial damage induced by Shiga toxins delivered by neutrophils during transmigration. J Leuk Biol 2010;88:201–10.

17. Obrig TG, Louise CB, Lingwood CA, et al. Endothelial heterogeneity in Shiga toxin receptors and responses. J Biol Chem 1993;268:15484–8.
18. Richardson SE, Rotman TA, Jay V, et al. Experimental verocytotoxemia in rabbits. Infect Immun 1992;60:4154–67.
19. Obata F, Tohyama K, Bonev AD, et al. Shiga toxin 2 affects the central nervous system through receptor globotriaosylceramide localized to neurons. J Infect Dis 2008;198:1398–406.
20. Bitzan MM, Wang Y, Lin J, et al. Verotoxin and ricin have novel effects on preproendothelin-1 expression but fail to modify nitric oxide Synthase (ecNOS) expression and NO production in vascular endothelium. J Clin Invest 1998;101: 372–82.
21. Richardson SE, Karmali MA, Becker LE, et al. The histopathology of the hemolytic uremic syndrome associated with verocytotoxin-producing *Escherichia coli* infections. Hum Pathol 1988;19:1102–8.
22. Morigi M, Micheletti G, Figliuzzi M, et al. Verotoxin-1 promotes leukocyte adhesion to cultured endothelial cells under physiologic flow conditions. Blood 1995; 86:4553–8.
23. Morigi M, Galbusera M, Binda E, et al. Verotoxin-1-induced up-regulation of adhesive molecules renders microvascular endothelial cells thrombogenic at high shear stress. Blood 2001;98:1828–35.
24. Nolasco LH, Turner NA, Bernardo A, et al. Hemolytic uremic syndrome-associated Shiga toxins promote endothelial-cell secretion and impair ADAMTS13 cleavage of unusually large von Willebrand factor multimers. Blood 2005;106:4199–209.
25. Bell BP, Goldoft M, Griffin PM, et al. A multistate outbreak of *Escherichia coli* O157:H7-associated bloody diarrhea and hemolytic uremic syndrome from hamburgers. The Washington experience. JAMA 1994;272:1349–53.
26. Tarr PI, Gordon CA, Chandler WL. Shiga-toxin-producing *Escherichia coli* and haemolytic uraemic syndrome. Lancet 2005;365:1073–86.
27. Buteau C, Proulx F, Chaibou M, et al. Leukocytosis in children with *Escherichia coli* O157:H7 enteritis developing the hemolytic-uremic syndrome. Pediatr Infect Dis J 2000;19:642–7.
28. Piercefield EW, Bradley KK, Coffman RL, et al. Hemolytic uremic syndrome after an *Escherichia coli* O111 outbreak. Arch Intern Med 2010;170:1656–63.
29. Lopez EL, Contrini MM, Glatstein E, et al. An epidemiologic surveillance of Shiga-like toxin-producing *Escherichia coli* infection in Argentinean children: risk factor and serum Shiga-like toxin 2 values. Pediatr Infect Dis J 2012;31: 20–4.
30. Gould LH, Bopp C, Strockbine N, et al. Recommendations for diagnosis of shiga toxin-producing *Escherichia coli* infections by clinical laboratories. MMWR Recomm Rep 2009;58:1–14.
31. Chandler WL, Jelacic S, Boster DR, et al. Prothrombotic coagulation abnormalities preceding the haemolytic-uremic syndrome. N Engl J Med 2002; 346:23–32.
32. Petruzziello-Pellegrini TN, Yuen DA, Page AV, et al. The CXCR4/CXCR7/SDF-1 pathway contributes to the pathogenesis of Shiga toxin-associated hemolytic uremic syndrome in humans and mice. J Clin Invest 2012;122: 759–76.
33. Page AV, Tarr PI, Watkins SL, et al. Dysregulation of angiopoietin-1 and -2 in *Escherichia coli* O157:H7 infection and the hemolytic-uremic syndrome. J Infect Dis, in press.

34. Ake JA, Jelacic S, Ciol MA, et al. Relative nephroprotection during *Escherichia coli* O157:H7 infections: association with intravenous volume expansion. Pediatrics 2005;115:e673–80.
35. Bell BP, Griffin PM, Lozano P, et al. Predictors of hemolytic uremic syndrome in children during a large outbreak of *Escherichia coli* O157:H7 infections. Pediatrics 1997;100:E12.
36. Wong CS, Jelacic S, Habeeb RL, et al. The risk of the hemolytic-uremic syndrome after antibiotic treatment of *Escherichia coli* O157:H7 infections. N Engl J Med 2000;342:1930–6.
37. Wong CS, Mooney JC, Brandt JR, et al. Risk factors for the hemolytic uremic syndrome in children infected with *Escherichia coli* O157:H7: a multivariable analysis. Clin Infect Dis 2012;55:33–41.
38. Smith KE, Wilker PR, Reiter PL, et al. Antibiotic treatment of *Escherichia coli* O157 infection and the risk of hemolytic uremic syndrome, Minnesota. Pediatr Infect Dis J 2012;31:37–41.
39. Safdar N, Said A, Gangnon RE, et al. Risk of hemolytic uremic syndrome after antibiotic treatment of *Escherichia coli* O157:H7 enteritis: a meta-analysis. JAMA 2002;288:996–1001.
40. Kimmitt PT, Harwood CR, Barer MR. Toxin gene expression by Shiga toxin-producing *Escherichia coli*: the role of antibiotics and the bacterial SOS response. Emerg Infect Dis 2000;6:458–65.
41. Bielaszewska M, Idelevich EA, Zhang W, et al. Effects of antibiotics on Shiga toxin 2 production and bacteriophage induction by epidemic *Escherichia coli* O104:H4 strain. Antimicrob Agents Chemother 2012;56:3277–82.
42. Corogeanu D, Willmes R, Wolke M, et al. Therapeutic concentrations of antibiotics inhibit Shiga toxin release from enterohemorrhagic *E. coli* O104:H4 from the 2011 German outbreak. BMC Microbiol 2012;12:160.
43. Nitschke M, Sayk F, Hartel C, et al. Association between azithromycin therapy and duration of bacterial shedding among patients with Shiga toxin-producing enteroaggregative *Escherichia coli* O104:H4. JAMA 2012;307:1046–52.
44. Bitzan M, Shaefer F, Reymond D. Treatment of typical (enteropathic) hemolytic uremic syndrome. Semin Thromb Hemost 2010;36:594–610.
45. Tarr PI, Sadler JE, Chandler WL, et al. Should all adult patients with diarrhoea-associated HUS receive plasma exchange? Lancet 2012;379:516.
46. Kielstein JT, Beutel G, Fleig S, et al. Best supportive care and therapeutic plasma exchange with or without eculizumab in Shiga-toxin-producing *E. coli* O104:H4 induced haemolytic-uraemic syndrome: an analysis of the German STEC-HUS registry. Nephrol Dial Transplant 2012;27:3807–15.
47. Loos S, Ahlenstiel T, Kranz B, et al. An outbreak of Shiga toxin-producing *Escherichia coli* O104:H4 hemolytic uremic syndrome in Germany: presentation and short-term outcome in children. Clin Infect Dis 2012;55:753–9.
48. Tarr PI, Karpman D. *Escherichia coli* O104:H4 and hemolytic uremic syndrome: the analysis begins. Clin Infect Dis 2012;55:760–3.
49. Stahl AL, Sartz L, Karpman D. Complement activation on platelet-leukocyte complexes and microparticles in enterohemorrhagic *Escherichia coli*-induced hemolytic uremic syndrome. Blood 2011;117:5503–13.
50. Lapeyraque AL, Malina M, Fremeaux-Bacchi V, et al. Eculizumab in severe Shiga-toxin-associated HUS. N Engl J Med 2011;364:2561–3.
51. Menne J, Nitschke M, Stingele R, et al. Validation of treatment strategies for enterohaemorrhagic *Escherichia coli* O104:H4 induced haemolytic uraemic syndrome: case-control study. BMJ 2012;345:e4565.

52. Clark WF, Sontrop JM, Macnab JJ, et al. Long term risk for hypertension, renal impairment, and cardiovascular disease after gastroenteritis from drinking water contaminated with *Escherichia coli* O157:H7: a prospective cohort study. BMJ 2010;341:c6020.

53. Garg AX, Suri RS, Barrowman N, et al. Long-term renal prognosis of diarrhea-associated hemolytic uremic syndrome. JAMA 2003;290:1360–70.

54. Rosales A, Hofer J, Zimmerhackl LB, et al. Need for long-term follow-up in enterohemorrhagic *Escherichia coli*-associated hemolytic uremic syndrome due to late-emerging sequelae. Clin Infect Dis 2012;54:1413–21.

55. Gould HL, Demma L, Jones TF, et al. Hemolytic uremic syndrome and death in persons with *Escherichia coli* O157:H7 infection, Foodborne Diseases Active Surveillance Network Sites, 2000-2006. Clin Infect Dis 2009;49:1480–5.

56. Centers for Disease Control (CDC). *E. coli* infection. Available at: http://www.cdc.gov/Features/EcoliInfection/. Accessed April 4, 2013.

57. Werber D, Mason BW, Evans MR, et al. Preventing household transmission of Shiga toxin-producing *Escherichia coli* O157 infection: promptly separating siblings might be the key. Clin Infect Dis 2008;46:1189–96.

58. Ahn CK, Klein E, Tarr PI. Isolation of patients acutely infected with *Escherichia coli* O157:H7: low-tech, highly effective prevention of hemolytic uremic syndrome. Clin Infect Dis 2008;46:1197–9.

59. Abu Sin M, Takla A, Flieger A, et al. Carrier prevalence, secondary household transmission, and long-term shedding in 2 districts during the *Escherichia coli* O104:H4 outbreak in Germany, 2011. J Infect Dis 2013;207:432–8.

60. Vonberg RP, Hohle M, Aepfelbacker M, et al. Duration of fecal shedding of Shiga toxin-producing *Escherichia coli* O104:H4 in patients infected during the 2011 outbreak in Germany: a multicenter study. Clin Infect Dis 2013;56:1132–40.

61. Centers for Disease Control (CDC). Multistate outbreak of shiga toxin-producing *Escherichia coli* O121 infections linked to farm rich brand frozen food products. Available at: http://www.cdc.gov/ecoli/2013/O121-03-13/index.html. Accessed April 4, 2013.

62. Centers for Disease Control (CDC). Multistate outbreak of Shiga toxin-producing *Escherichia coli* O26 infections linked to raw clover sprouts at Jimmy John's restaurants. 2012. Available at: http://www.cdc.gov/ecoli/2012/o26-02-12/index.html. Accessed April 4, 2013.

63. Centers for Disease Control (CDC). Multistate outbreak of Shiga toxin-producing *Escherichia coli* O157:H7 infections linked to organic spinach and spring mix blend. 2012. Available at: http://www.cdc.gov/ecoli/2012/O157H7-11-12/index.html. Accessed April 4, 2013.

64. Wendel AM, Johnson DH, Sharapov U, et al. Multistate outbreak of *Escherichia coli* O157:H7 infection associated with consumption of packaged spinach, August-September, 2006: the Wisconsin Investigation. Clin Infect Dis 2009;48:1079–86.

65. Soborg B, Lassen SG, Muller L, et al. A verocytotoxin-producing *E. coli* outbreak with a surprisingly high risk of haemolytic uraemic syndrome, Denmark, September-October, 2012. Euro Surveill 2013;18. pii:20350.

66. Ethelberg S, Smith B, Torpdahl M, et al. Outbreak of non-O157 Shiga toxin-producing *Escherichia coli* infection from consumption of beef sausage. Clin Infect Dis 2009;48:e78–81.

67. Slayton RB, Turabelidze G, Bennett SD, et al. Outbreak of Shiga toxin-producing *Escherichia coli* (STEC) O157:H7 associated with romaine lettuce consumption, 2011. PLoS One 2013;8:e55300.

68. Folster JP, Pecic G, Taylor E, et al. Characterization of isolates from an outbreak of multidrug-resistant, Shiga toxin-producing *Escherichia coli* O145 in the United States. Antimicrob Agents Chemother 2011;55:5955–6.

69. Karch H, Denamur E, Dobrindt U, et al. The enemy within us: lessons from the 2011 European *Escherichia coli* O104:H4 outbreak. EMBO Mol Med 2012;4: 841–8.

70. Frank C, Werber D, Cramer JP, et al. Epidemic profile of Shiga-toxin-producing *Escherichia coli* O104:H4 outbreak in Germany. N Engl J Med 2011;365:1771–80.

71. Robert Koch Institute. Report: final presentation and evaluation of epidemiological findings in the EHEC O104:H4 outbreak, Germany 2011. Berlin: Robert Koch Institute; 2011.

72. King LA, Nogareda F, Weill FX, et al. Outbreak of Shiga toxin-producing *Escherichia coli* O104:H4 associated with organic fenugreek sprouts, France, June, 2011. Clin Infect Dis 2012;54:1588–94.

73. Guh A, Phan Q, Nelson R, et al. Outbreak of *Escherichia coli* O157 associated with raw milk, Connecticut, 2008. Clin Infect Dis 2010;51:1411–7.

74. Neil KP, Biggerstaff G, MacDonald JK, et al. A novel vehicle for transmission of *Escherichia coli* O157:H7 to humans: multistate outbreak of *E. coli* O157:H7 infections associated with consumption of ready-to-bake commercial prepackaged cookie dough—United States, 2009. Clin Infect Dis 2012;54:511–8.

75. Ihekweazu C, Carroll K, Adak B, et al. Large outbreak of verocytotoxin-producing *Escherichia coli* O157 infection in visitors to a petting farm in South East England, 2009. Epidemiol Infect 2012;140:1400–13.

76. Goode B, O'Reilly C, Dunn J, et al. Outbreak of *Escherichia coli* O157: H7 infections after Petting Zoo visits, North Carolina State Fair, October-November, 2004. Arch Pediatr Adolesc Med 2009;163:42–8.

77. An outbreak of *Escherichia coli* O157:H7 associated with a children's water spray park and identified by two rounds of pulsed-field gel electrophoresis testing. Can Commun Dis Rep 2005;31:133–40 [in English, French].

78. Cody SH, Glynn MK, Farrar JA, et al. An outbreak of *Escherichia coli* O157:H7 infection from unpasteurized commercial apple juice. Ann Intern Med 1999;130: 202–9.

79. Yoshioka K, Yagi K, Moriguchi N. Clinical features and treatment of children with hemolytic uremic syndrome caused by enterohemorrhagic *Escherichia coli* O157:H7 infection: experience of an outbreak in Sakai City, 1996. Pediatr Int 1999;41:223–7.

80. Hadler JL, Clogher P, Hurd S, et al. Ten-year trends and risk factors for non-O157 Shiga toxin-producing *Escherichia coli* found through Shiga toxin testing, Connecticut, 2000-2009. Clin Infect Dis 2011;53:269–76.

81. Klein EJ, Stapp JR, Clausen CR, et al. Shiga toxin-producing *Escherichia coli* in children with diarrhea: a prospective point-of-care study. J Pediatr 2002;141: 172–7.

82. Magnus T, Rother J, Simova O, et al. The neurological syndrome in adults during the 2011 northern German *E. coli* serotype O104:H4 outbreak. Brain 2012;135: 1850–9.

83. Slutsker L, Ries AA, Greene KD, et al. *Escherichia coli* O157:H7 diarrhea in the United States: clinical and epidemiologic features. Ann Intern Med 1997;126: 505–13.

Infections in Travelers

Mayan Bomsztyk, MD*, Richard W. Arnold, MD

KEYWORDS

- Travel medicine • Traveler's diarrhea • Malaria • Dengue • Leishmaniasis
- Immunosuppressed traveler

KEY POINTS

- The pretravel clinic visit is an integral part of disease prevention for travel.
- Traveler's diarrhea is common and generally occurs between 4 and 14 days after arrival.
- Fever in a returning travel is malaria until proved otherwise and can present months after return from endemic area.
- Most rashes and upper respiratory symptoms in travelers are not specifically related to a travel-related cause.
- The US Centers for Disease Control and the World Health Organization maintain helpful Web sites for both patient and physician.

INTRODUCTION

Every year more than 50 million people from developed nations visit the developing world.[1] Many of these travelers experience some sort of health issue and seek medical attention. In a 2000 study of 784 American travelers,[2] 64% reported some form of illness, and 12% of these travelers sought medical attention. Travelers seek medical attention for many different reasons, but the causes of their concerns can be broadly categorized as trauma-related, routine, or travel-associated illness. This article primarily focuses on the prevention and treatment of travel-associated illnesses.

The pretravel clinic visit is critical in the prevention of travel-related illness. It has 4 aims: baseline health assessment, review of itinerary, administration of appropriate vaccines, and counseling.[2] Although it is impossible to completely eliminate all risks associated with travel, a pretravel clinic visit can help prepare the patient to minimize risk and self-manage many diseases that may develop.

Once home, the 4 most common complaints of the returning traveler are diarrhea, rash, fever, and upper respiratory infection (URI).

Department of Medicine, University of Washington, 4245 Roosevelt Way Northeast, Seattle, WA 98105, USA
* Corresponding author.
E-mail address: mayanb@uw.edu

Med Clin N Am 97 (2013) 697–720
http://dx.doi.org/10.1016/j.mcna.2013.03.004
0025-7125/13/$ – see front matter © 2013 Elsevier Inc. All rights reserved.

PRETRAVEL VISIT

A thorough preclinic visit should include the following elements: (1) review of the itinerary; (2) review of past medication history and chronic medications; (3) administration of appropriate immunizations; (4) advice on prevention and self-treatment of common travel-related infections and assembling a medical kit; (5) provision of prescriptions and medical records when relevant.

Itinerary review should include dates of travel, specific sites of travel (eg, cities and regions), including layovers. During the itinerary review, the lodging arrangements and the style of trip should also be assessed. For instance, there are different risk factors for travelers staying at large hotel franchises and spas, travelers staying in youth hostels, and trekkers who are camping. In addition, the risk for travelers who reside in areas for substantial periods is increased over short-stay travelers.

The health assessment should include a review of past medical history, focusing on conditions that might be affected by travel, for instance, pulmonary diseases and air travel or coagulopathies and long periods of sitting. Current prescriptions should be reviewed and refilled to ensure that the patient has an adequate supply of appropriate medications during travel. Patients on antiretroviral medications or immunosuppression for organ transplant should take a supply equal to twice the anticipated quantity of pills needed for the duration of their travel. Other specific considerations for immunosuppressed patients are covered in a separate section.

Insurance coverage for travel visits varies by insurance carrier, as does appropriate bill coding. Some insurance plans allow billing of new (99201-99205) and established (99241-99245) patient evaluation/management (E/M) service for travel medicine visits. If the patient has been referred by a primary care physician, some plans allow billing outpatient consultation E/M service codes (99241-99245). Patients need to contact their insurer before their visit to see what services are covered.

Immunizations

Immunizations are an integral part of the pretravel visit. Multiple factors should be taken into consideration, including travel destination and climate, travel duration, severity of potential disease versus the risk of adverse effect from vaccination, activities planned, whether the trip is urban, rural, or remote from medical care, time remaining before departure, vaccine availability, cost, and the number of doses needed, history of allergy to vaccines or their components, pregnancy, and immunosuppression (**Box 1**). Multiple inactive vaccines can be conveniently and effectively administered at a single clinic visit.[3] Administration of multiple live vaccines sequentially can impair the immune response; therefore, they should be given either simultaneously or separated by at least 4 weeks. Interruption in a vaccine series does not require restarting the series; generally the series can resume from the last

---

Box 1
Considerations for administering vaccines

History of allergy

Pregnancy or immunosuppression

Destination and travel duration

Severity of disease versus risk of adverse effect from vaccination

Urban, rural, or remote from medical care

Vaccine availability, cost, and number of doses needed

administered dose. For instance, if a patient is receiving the hepatitis B series and receives the first and second injection at the appropriate interval (0 and 1 month) but misses the 6-month shot, the patient can receive it as soon as convenient without restarting the series de novo.

The US Centers for Disease Control (CDC) divides immunizations into routine, required, and recommended. Routine vaccines are necessary for protection from diseases that are potential risks in many parts of the world, for instance influenza or tetanus. Some patients may need boosters, especially for tetanus, pertussis, and diphtheria.

The only required vaccination by International Health Regulations, an international legal entity subscribed to by all member states of the World Health Organization (WHO), is yellow fever for travel to specific countries in sub-Saharan Africa and tropical South America. The Saudi Arabian government requires meningococcal vaccine for annual travel during the Hajj,[4] a ritual pilgrimage to Mecca made by more than 3 million Muslims annually.

Recommended vaccines may protect travelers from disease present in other parts of the world and prevent importation of nonendemic infectious diseases when the traveler returns home. Recommendations change frequently and up-to-date information can be found on the CDC Web site (http://www.cdc.gov/vaccines/). Examples of recommended vaccines (depending on travel destination) include hepatitis A, typhoid fever, meningococcus, and Japanese encephalitis (**Table 1**).

COUNSELING
Traveler's Diarrhea

Because it is impossible to tell which foods and water are safe, travelers should be educated in prevention and self-treatment of traveler's diarrhea. There are passive and active precautions. Passive actions include avoiding tap water and ice, salads, unpasteurized dairy products, thin-skinned fruits, and raw seafood. Active measures include drinking only boiled water or carbonated beverages or using a portable water filter. Iodine and chlorine alone are inadequate, because they do not eliminate all enteric pathogens. Taking bismuth prophylactically has been shown to provide up to 65% protection from diarrhea, although 2 tabs must be used 4 times a day to achieve the anticipated efficacy. Less frequent and lower doses still provide some protection, but efficacy may be reduced to between 30% and 40%.[5] Studies on

Table 1
Vaccines and abbreviated recommendations

Vaccine	Notes
Hepatitis A	Travelers to Central or South America, parts of Asia and Africa
Japanese encephalitis	Travelers who plan to spend >1 mo in endemic areas (most of Asia and parts of Western Pacific) during Japanese encephalitis virus transmission season (varies depending on destination)
Meningococcal	Travelers visiting sub-Saharan Africa during dry season (December–June)
Typhoid	Travelers to Asia, Africa, the Caribbean, and Central or South America, especially those who will have prolonged exposure to potentially contaminated food or drink
Yellow fever	Travelers to endemic areas in South America and sub-Saharan Africa

Data from Centers for Disease Control and Prevention. CDC Health Information for International Travel 2012. New York: Oxford University Press; 2012; and Hill DR, Ericsson CD, Pearson RD, et al. The practice of travel medicine: guidelines by the Infectious Diseases Society of America. Clin Infect Dis 2006;43:1499–539.

probiotics for prophylaxis of traveler's diarrhea have been variable and inconclusive.[6] Antibiotic prophylaxis of traveler's diarrhea is generally inappropriate in a healthy host.

Counseling on how to self-manage traveler's diarrhea is invaluable. Mild cases, defined as 1 to 2 unformed stools in 24 hours, may require no treatment other than oral fluids to maintain hydration. More severe cases benefit from antibiotic treatment. Self-treatment with antibiotics generally improves symptoms within 36 hours. A 2000 Cochrane meta-analysis[7] found that antibiotics reduced both the duration and the severity of traveler's diarrhea. Choice of antibiotic and duration of treatment depend on location of travel.

For otherwise healthy travelers, it is reasonable to provide a 3-day course of ciprofloxacin 500 mg twice a day with instructions to take if unformed stool count exceeds more than 3 per day and is associated with other gastrointestinal symptoms or fever.[8] A shorter course of ciprofloxacin has also proved effective,[9] and patients should be counseled that symptoms need to be reassessed after the first 24 hours, and if resolved, the course can be shortened. Otherwise, completion of the 3-day course is advised. For patients traveling to Southeast Asian countries, where quinolone-resistant *Campylobacter* is prevalent (check the CDC Web site for up-to-date resistance patterns), azithromycin is the preferred antimicrobial agent.[10] For these patients, azithromycin 1000 mg by mouth once should be provided.[11] Rifaxamin is an alternative for otherwise uncomplicated traveler's diarrhea in a healthy host; however, it is not first-line therapy, because of concern for decreased efficacy in more severe cases.[8]

Insect-Borne Diseases

In areas where insect-borne diseases are a significant risk, travelers should wear protective clothing, use bed netting and N,N-diethylmetatoluamide (DEET). Other types of insect repellant have been found inferior. The length of effectiveness is directly related to concentration of DEET. For example, 23.8% DEET is effective for approximately 5 hours, whereas 4.75% is effective for only 88 minutes.[12] Permethrin-based insecticide should be sprayed on clothing and bed nets to decrease risk of mosquitos and tick bites.[11,13]

Malaria deserves special mention, because it infects approximately 30,000 European and North American travelers per year.[14] The Infectious Disease Society of America (IDSA) recommends the ABCD approach to malaria. A stands for risk-awareness. The risk of contracting malaria varies with the destination, season, climate, altitude, and number of mosquito bites; up-to-date information is available on the CDC Web site. B is for bite-avoidance (see earlier discussion on avoiding insect bites in general). C is for chemoprophylaxis compliance. Prophylaxis is recommended for all travelers to endemic areas. Prophylaxis medications suppress malaria by killing asexual blood stages of the parasite before they can cause disease. Therefore, protective levels must be present when parasites emerge from the liver. Effective prophylaxis must start before first possible exposure and continue for a period after the last potential mosquito bite. The timing of starting and stopping prophylaxis varies by regimen, with some regimens needing to be started several weeks before departure, whereas others must be continued after the traveler returns home.[11] There are many options for malaria prophylaxis, although in practice the decision is often made easier by the combination of timing of departure, willingness to take a daily medication, and tolerance of potential side effects. One recommended approach is depicted in **Table 2**.

Table 2
Malaria prophylaxis options by destination

Destination	Suspected Organism	Medication	Special Considerations
Central America (west of the Panama Canal), Mexico, Haiti, Dominican Republic, most of the Middle East, states of former Soviet Union, northern Africa, Argentina, Paraguay and parts of China	Chloroquine-sensitive *P falciparum*	Chloroquine	**Chloroquine** Needs to be taken 1–2 wk before departure and 4 wk after return Once weekly
South America, including Panama (east of Panama Canal) but excluding Argentina and Paraguay, Asia, Southeast Asia, sub-Saharan Africa and Oceania	Chloroquine-resistant *P falciparum*	Atovaquone-proguanil Doxycycline Mefloquine	**Atovaquone-proguanil** Needs to be taken daily More expensive **Doxycycline** Needs to be taken daily and for 4 wk after return Can cause sun sensitivity **Mefloquine:** Avoid in patients with seizures, psychiatric or cardiac conduction issues Needs to be started 2 wk before and continued 4 wk after
Rural, forested areas of the Thailand-Burma and Thailand-Cambodia borders, western provinces of Cambodia	Multidrug-resistant *P falciparum*	Atovaquone-proguanil Doxycycline	**Atovaquone-proguanil** Needs to be taken daily More expensive **Doxycycline** Needs to be taken daily and for 4 wk after return Can cause sun sensitivity

Data from Centers for Disease Control and Prevention. CDC Health Information for International Travel 2012. New York: Oxford University Press; 2012; and Hill DR, Ericsson CD, Pearson RD, et al. The practice of travel medicine: guidelines by the Infectious Diseases Society of America. Clin Infect Dis 2006;43:1499–539.

Sexual Activity

Studies suggest that travelers may engage in more high-risk sexual behavior than they would otherwise, including sex with new partners and unprotected sex. The percentage of travelers who are sexually active with a new partner abroad depends on the population surveyed. A UK study surveying travelers 18 to 35 years old who traveled without a partner found a sexual activity rate of 10%, and of these only 75% used condoms consistently.[15] A Norwegian study that surveyed clients of a sexually transmitted infection clinic found a sexual activity rate of 41%.[16] High-risk sexual activity increases the risk of human immunodeficiency virus (HIV), hepatitis B, and other sexually transmitted diseases. Travelers who may have sex with new partners abroad should bring latex condoms, because some studies have shown those manufactured abroad may be more prone to breakage.[11,17,18] Populations found to be more likely to engage in sexual activity with new partners abroad or to have unprotected sex include younger travelers (<25 years age), men who have sex with men,[19] expatriates,[19] military personnel,[20] and sex tourists[18] (defined as those who travel with explicit intention of engaging in sexual activity). In these populations, discussion about how to obtain pre-exposure or postexposure prophylaxis for sexually transmitted infections is appropriate. Symptoms and signs of sexually transmitted infections, such as dysuria, purulent drainage, pruritus, and genital lesions, should be discussed with all patients.

Animal Exposure

In many parts of the world, rabies is present in the dog population. Travelers from countries with universal rabies vaccination of dogs are rarely aware of rabies risk. Rabies transmission from dog bites is a major problem in Africa, parts of Asia, and Central and South America. Travelers should be advised to avoid dogs when traveling and assume that there are no friendly dogs. If travelers are bitten by dogs while traveling in a high-risk area, they need postexposure prophylaxis as soon as possible.

Reptile and amphibian exposure is more likely in travelers. Turtles, iguanas, geckos, snakes, frogs, and toads are all prevalent in many warm climates, and may be featured in petting zoos and for hire photographic opportunities. All these creatures frequently spread *Salmonella*. It is best to advise to avoid them to decrease *Salmonella* transmission. If there is any exposure, good hand washing and use of antibacterial hand gel is a must. Antibacterial hand gel is a crucial part of the travel medical kit.

SYMPTOMS IN THE RETURNING TRAVELER
Traveler's Diarrhea

Background
Traveler's diarrhea affects 20% to 60% of travelers to resource-poor destinations[21] and is defined by 3 or more loose stools in 24 hours with or without cramps, nausea, fever, or vomiting. The destinations with highest risk are South Asia, Africa, and Latin America. Travel to other developed countries carries some risk but is lower (<10%).[22] The median time of onset of symptoms is approximately 1 week after arrival to destination. The illness tends to be self-limited, lasting several days, although it can occasionally last more than 2 weeks in 5% to 10% of cases. Although rarely life threatening, traveler's diarrhea can significantly affect the planned activities of a traveler.

Epidemiology
Most cases of traveler's diarrhea do not have an identifiable cause. In a 1999 study of 322 travelers returning from Jamaica,[23] only 32% had an identifiable cause. Of those with an identifiable cause, the most common pathogens were bacterial, but viruses and parasites were also common. The most common bacterial cause was enterotoxic *Escherichia coli*, followed by *Salmonella* species, *Campylobacter jejuni,* and *Shigella* species. The most common viral causes were rotavirus and enteric adenovirus. Parasitic causes included *Giardia lamblia, Cryptosporidium, Cyclospora* and *Entamoeba histolytica*.

Diagnosis
For patients with mild to moderate traveler's diarrhea and no fever, hematochezia or tenesmus, the diagnosis of traveler's diarrhea may be made on clinical grounds. One recommended approach is outlined in **Fig. 1**. Routine stool culture should not be reflexively ordered because it cannot distinguish between pathogenic and nonpathogenic strains of *Escherichia coli*, and the results of the stool culture might not affect management. However, if the patient reports fever, bloody, stool or tenesmus, a culture is warranted. Any patient who has recently taken antibiotics should have stool sent for testing for *Clostridium difficile*. Because parasitic infections are less common, an examination of stool for ova and parasites is often not initially indicated. If diarrhea persists more than 1 week despite appropriate antibiotic

Clinical Diagnosis	Species , geographic distribution	Recommended Drug	Additional Comments
Uncomplicated Malaria	P. ovale, P. malariae, P knowlesi malaria OR P. Falciparum from Central America (West of the Panama Canal), Haiti, the Dominican Republic and most of the Middle East Or P. vivax from all regions except Papa New Guinea or Indonesia	Chloroquine	For P. vivax and P. ovale, add primaquine
	Chloroquine-resistant P. falciparum from all other malarious regions not specified elsewhere OR P. vivax from Papau New Guinea or Indonesia	Atovaquone-proguanil OR Artemether-lumefantrine OR Quinine+ doxycycline, tetracycline or clindamycin OR Mefloquine	For P. vivax, add primaquine
	Multidrug-resistant P. falciparum from Southeast Asia	Atovaquone-proguanil OR Artemether-lumefantrine OR Quinine+ doxycycline, tetracycline or clindamycin	
Complicated Malaria	P. falciparum	Quinidine gluconate+ doxycycline, tetracycline or clindamycin OR Artesunate	Considered exchange transfusion in patients with parasitemia >10%, altered mental status, pulmonary edema or renal complications

Fig. 1. Approach to workup of traveler's diarrhea by patient history.

treatment, then parasitic infections should be considered. In this setting, stool should be examined for ova and parasites to assess for *Cryptosporidium* and *Cyclospora*, antigen testing for *Entamoeba histolytica* and immunoassay for *Giardia*.

Treatment

Treatment has 3 main components: volume repletion, symptom management, and treatment of the underlying infection. The most common serious complication of traveler's diarrhea is volume depletion. In mild to moderate cases, broth, juice, or similar liquids suffice. In the case of severe diarrhea, oral rehydration solution should be used. Commercial products are available, or the solution can be made inexpensively by mixing one-half tablespoon of table salt, one-half tablespoon of baking soda, and 4 tablespoons of sugar into 1 L of water.

The second component of treatment is aimed at helping symptoms. Bismuth is helpful in controlling nausea, and loperamide can help with decreasing number of loose stools. Several studies have shown that combination of an antibiotic and loperamide is safe and provides more rapid symptom relief than either agent alone.[24]

The infection must be addressed. Antibiotic regimens do not vary from self-treatment recommendations.

SKIN LESIONS IN THE TRAVELER
Background

The differential for skin lesions in a returning traveler can be overwhelming; this section focuses on the most common and the most serious infections with cutaneous manifestations. Approximately 10% of returning travelers experience some form of a skin disorder,[2] and skin disorders account for 18% of posttravel clinic visits.[25] Despite travel to exotic locales, many travel-related skin lesions have pedestrian causes. Travelers frequently experience sexually transmitted infections, sunburns, allergic reactions, scabies, staphylococcal, and streptococcal infections. Chronic skin conditions like acne or allergic dermatitis can flare in tropical locations.

Epidemiology

The GeoSentinel network, a collaboration between the International Society for Tropical Medicine and the CDC, found the most common skin-related diagnoses in returning travelers were cutaneous larva migrans (CLM) and insect bite-related disease, including superinfected bites, skin abscess, and allergic reaction (**Table 3**).

Leishmaniasis and dengue accounted for approximately 3% of cases in the GeoSentinel study and should be included in the differential diagnosis, given their potential severity. The largest study before the GeoSentinel study was a 1995 French study[26] that found similar results, but myiasis (9%) and tungiasis (6%) were also common. In the French study, there was a disproportionate travel to Africa, which likely explains the higher frequency of these generally uncommon diseases. The distinctive characteristics of CLM, leishmaniasis, myiasis, and tungiasis are described in this section, but discussion of dengue infections is deferred to the section on fever and the returning traveler.

CLM

CLM is caused by animal hook worms that can be found worldwide, but infection is more frequent in Southeast Asia, Africa, South America, Caribbean, and the southeastern part of the United States.[27] Humans are infected with CLM after contact with ground contaminated with feces from infected animals, generally dogs and cats. The larvae penetrate human skin and migrate through the subcutaneous tissue. The migration causes the characteristic serpiginous pattern of CLM (**Fig. 2**). The rash

Table 3
Most frequent diagnosis in returning travelers with dermatologic diagnoses

Diagnosis (N)	% of all Dermatologic Diagnoses
All (4742)	100
CLM (465)[a]	9.8
Insect bite (388)	8.2
Skin abscess (366)	7.7
Superinfected skin bite (324)	6.8
Allergic rash (263)	5.5
Rash, unknown cause (262)	5.5
Dog bite (203)	4.3
Superficial fungal infection (190)	4
Dengue (159)[a]	3.4
Leishmaniasis (158)[a]	3.3
Myiasis (126)[a]	2.7
Spotted fever group rickettsiae (72)[a]	1.5
Scabies (71)	1.5
Cellulitis (70)	1.5

[a] Travel-related illness.

Data from Lederman ER, Weld LH, Elyazar IR, et al. Dermatologic conditions of the ill returned traveler: an analysis from the GeoSentinel Surveillance Network. Int J Infect Dis 2008;12:593.

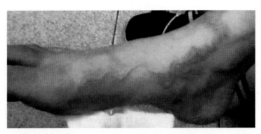

Fig. 2. A cutaneous serpentinelike track characteristic of CLM. (*From* Hamat RA, Rahman AA, Osman M, et al. Cutaneous larva migrans: a neglected disease and possible association with the use of long socks. Trans R Soc Trop Med Hyg 2010;104:171; with permission.)

is usually seen within days of exposure. Lesions may be papular or vesiculobullous and are prone to bacterial superinfection. Common locations are buttocks, thighs, and feet. Lesions may be associated with pruritus or pain. Diagnosis is made from clinical history and appearance. Eosinophilia is rarely present. Although cutaneous disease is self-limited, treatment shortens duration and reduces risk of superinfection. The preferred agent is ivermectin, although albendazole may be used as an alternative.[28] Hematogenous spread to the lungs is a rare complication, commonly presenting as respiratory symptoms approximately 1 week after the cutaneous eruption. No specific diagnostic test is available, and the treatment is the same as for the cutaneous infection.

Leishmaniasis

Leishmaniasis is present in more than 80 countries throughout Africa, Asia, southern Europe, and Latin America. Cutaneous leishmaniasis has 4 superficial manifestations: localized, recidivans, diffuse, and mucosal. The localized cutaneous form occurs on any exposed area of skin, starting as a red papule that enlarges to form a painless ulcer with heaped up margins and granulomatous tissue at the base (**Fig. 3**). These lesions are self-limited and the rate of resolution is determined by the particular infective species. A hypopigmented scar after ulcer resolution is common. Leishmaniasis recidivans is uncommon, and is caused by *Leishmania tropica* infections in the Middle East. After resolution of the primary lesion, a few remaining pathogens cause new papules to occur around the margins of the scar. These papules can appear, ulcerate, and heal repeatedly over decades. In patients with an impaired cell-mediated immune response, diffuse cutaneous leishmaniasis can occur. Instead of a primary lesion that ulcerates, the organism disseminates to macrophages in other areas of the skin. Diffuse cutaneous leishmaniasis characteristically has a relapsing or chronically progressive course that may cause significant deformity. Mucosal leishmaniasis occurs as a late-stage complication of less than 5% of cases of *L braziliensis* infection, which is endemic to Latin America. Months to years after primary lesion has resolved, recurrence at a distant mucosal site may occur.

Leishmaniasis traditionally has been diagnosed by microscopic visualization of the organism in a tissue sample. The burden of disease is determined by duration of infection (more chronic lesions have a lower burden[29]), and therefore lack of organism does not necessarily exclude diagnosis. Depending on the clinical facility, 4 processes are recommended: direct microscopy, culture, histology, and polymerase chain reaction (PCR).[30] PCR can be used for speciation when the location of travel has more than 1 endemic species. Speciation can be important because different species are associated with different clinical entities and prognosis. Tissue samples

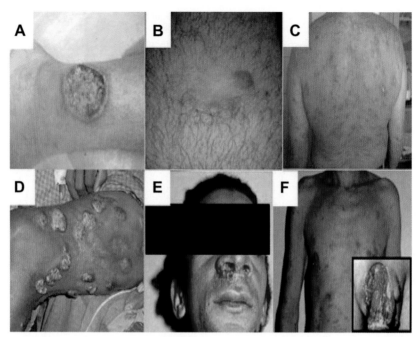

Fig. 3. Clinical forms of tegumentary leishmaniasis. (*A*) Localized cutaneous leishmaniasis presenting as a single ulcer on the leg. (*B*) Leishmaniasis recidiva cutis presenting as papules and vesicles around the healed lesion of cutaneous leishmaniasis on the leg. (*C*) Disseminated cutaneous leishmaniasis presenting as numerous small ulcers on the back. (*D*) Disseminated cutaneous leishmaniasis presenting as tumoral lesions and nodules associated with crusts and several scars from previous injuries on the left thigh. (*E*) Mucocutaneous leishmaniasis lesion in the nose and infiltration in the nasal mucosa. (*F*) Atypical cutaneous leishmaniasis in a patient infected with HIV presenting with multiple macules on the chest and abdomen. (*Insert* in *F*) Extensive ulcer on the penis of a patient with AIDS. (*Courtesy of* [*A*] Luiza K. Oyafuso, Instituto de Infectologia Emilio Ribas, São Paulo, Brazil; [*B*] Maria Edileuza Brito, Centro de Pesquisas Aggeu Magalhães, Fundação Oswaldo Cruz, Brazil; [*C*] Edgar M. Carvalho, Universidade Federal da Bahia, Brazil; and [*D*] Jackson M.L. Costa, Centro de Pesquisas Gonçalo Muniz, Fundação Oswaldo Cruz, Brazil.)

can be obtained by skin scraping, aspirate, or biopsy, which is preferred. If biopsy is possible, the lesion should be biopsied at the active edge, which is likely to have a higher parasite burden.

The treatment goals for leishmaniasis include resolution of active infection, reducing scarring, and decreasing recurrence. Choice and duration of therapy depend on its manifestation (cutaneous versus mucosal) and warrants involvement of a specialist. Traditionally, courses of intravenous (IV) pentavalent antimonials were used for 20 to 28 days. Single-dose IV liposomal amphotericin is becoming more commonly used.[30]

Myiasis

Myiasis is found in tropical and subtropical areas. The most common presentation of myiasis in a returning traveler is furuncular myiasis, caused by the botfly or the tumbu fly. In each instance, larvae penetrate skin and develop in subdermal tissue. There is typically 1 larva per lesion, although multiple lesions may be present. Patients may describe an enlarging insect bite of up to 3 cm in diameter and a crawling sensation or episodic pain near the lesion. There may be serosanguineous discharge from a central punctum or a small, white structure protruding from the lesion. Diagnosis is made by clinical history and physical examination. Removal of the intact larvae is curative. Different approaches for removal can be used. One option is to occlude with petroleum jelly the skin aperture through which the larva breathes and extract the larva when it moves closer to the surfaces to get air (**Fig. 4**). Larvae that die during occlusion are difficult to remove and often trigger an intense inflammatory reaction. Removal via manual expression and extraction through a small incision are preferable when possible.

Tungiasis

Like myiasis, tungiasis is found in subtropical and tropical destinations. Tungiasis is caused by the female sand flea, which can penetrate the human skin, usually on the feet or hands. Tungiasis causes skin inflammation, severe pain, itching, and a lesion at the site of infection that is characterized by a black dot at the center of a swollen red papule, surrounded by what looks like a white halo. The flea produces eggs that are expelled through the host's skin. Diagnosis is made by the clinical history and physical examination. Confirmation is made by identification of the organism after removal. Treatment is achieved by removal of the flea.

THE RETURNING TRAVELER AND FEVER
Background

Fever in a returning traveler can herald significant illness. In the GeoSentinel study, fever was the chief complaint for 28% of patients seeking posttravel care. In this study, 26% of patients with fever required hospitalization.[31] Globally, on return from the developing world, approximately 3% of travelers experience fever.[2] More than 17% of travelers with fever have a vaccine-preventable infection or *falciparum* malaria, which is preventable with chemoprophylaxis, underscoring the importance of the pre-travel visit.

Epidemiology of Fever in Returning Travelers

In the GeoSentinel study, the most common causes of fever in returning travelers were malaria, dengue, rickettsial infections, typhoid, or paratyphoid fever (otherwise known

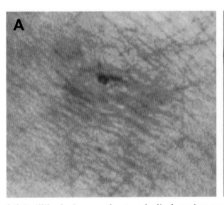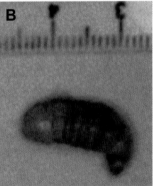

Fig. 4. (*A*) Boillike lesion on the trunk discharging serosanguineous fluid secondary to botfly myiasis infestation. (*B*) Botfly larva after removal from the boillike lesion. (*Data from* Morris-Jones R, Morris-Jones S. Travel-associated skin disease. Infect Dis Clin North Am 2012;26(3):680.)

as enteric fever).[31] Depending on travel destinations, leptospirosis, Chikungunya fever, and hepatitis A should also be considered as the cause of febrile systemic illness in returning travelers.

Diagnostic Algorithm of Fever in Returning Travelers

If a returning traveler presents with fever, the diagnosis of malaria must first be considered. If malaria is possible, based on timing and location of travel, obtain thin and thick smears. Repeat serial blood smears every 6 to 8 hours for 48 hours. If the malaria evaluation is negative or is unlikely based on other factors, evaluate based on localizing symptoms and signs as you would in any febrile patient. If there are no localizing symptoms or signs, consider dengue, rickettsiosis, enteric fever, and other causes of fever based on location of travel.

MALARIA
Background

Any patient who has visited a malaria endemic area in the last 4 years and reports fever should be evaluated for malaria, even if afebrile at presentation. In the GeoSentinel study, 20% of travelers who sought medical attention for fever eventually were diagnosed with malaria.[31] Thirty-three percent of patients with febrile illness who eventually died had malaria.

Malaria is caused by 1 of 5 protozoan species of the genus *Plasmodium: falciparum, vivax, ovale, malariae,* or *knowlesi. Anopheles* mosquito is the vector for malaria. After introduction of the organism through mosquito bite, the incubation period depends on the malaria species, but it is generally between 10 and 35 days, although *P vivax* and *ovale* can present up to 4 years after exposure, because of latent forms hiding in the liver. Fever is caused when the intracellular pathogen bursts from the erythrocyte.

Classification

Uncomplicated malaria is characterized by absence of end-organ dysfunction, although it can be associated with anemia and jaundice. Additional criteria for uncomplicated malaria include a parasite burden (defined as percent of infected erythrocytes) of less than 5% and the ability to take medications orally.[14] Complicated malaria is usually caused by *P falciparum*, although increasingly *P vivax* and *P knowlesi* are recognized to cause complicated malaria.

Cerebral malaria is defined by altered mental status, seizure, or coma. Risk factors include extremes of age, immunocompromised status (including HIV and asplenia), and pregnancy. Without treatment, cerebral malaria is uniformly fatal. Thus, prompt recognition and initiation of therapy are critical. Even with therapy, mortality remains 15% and 20%, and some patients may have permanent cognitive sequelae from infection.[32]

Clinical Presentation

Initially, patients with malaria may experience high fevers at irregular intervals throughout the day. As the infection progresses, rupture of infected red cells tends to synchronize, leading to characteristic day-to-day fever patterns. The pattern of fever depends on the particular species of malaria. *P falciparum, vivax* and *ovale* have a roughly 48-hour cycle, and *P malaria,* 72 hours.

There is no symptom or sign that is pathognomonic for malaria. Clinical features that may suggest malaria include fever without localizing symptoms, enlarged spleen, thrombocytopenia, and hyperbilirubinemia.[33]

The pathophysiology of malaria is related to the cytoadherence of red blood cells. This factor can lead to small infarcts, capillary leakage, and organ dysfunction. Clinical manifestations may include altered mental status, seizure, acute respiratory distress syndrome, metabolic acidosis, renal failure, hemoglobinuria (blackwater fever), hepatic failure, coagulopathy with or without disseminated intravascular coagulation, severe anemia or massive intravascular hemolysis, and hypoglycemia.

Diagnosis

The classic diagnostic test for malaria is examination of Giemsa-stained blood smears by light microscopy (**Fig. 5**). Two different smear preparations are ordered when there is concern for malaria. Thin smear allows for speciation and staging of the parasite in its life cycle. Thick smear allows more sensitivity, because more red blood cells are lysed and therefore more parasites released in the same area compared with the thin smear. The first test is positive in 95% of infected patients, but given the nature of cyclic parasitemia, exclusion of malaria requires smear evaluation every 6 to 12 hours for 48 hours.

Light microscopy has several disadvantages: it is labor intensive, requires considerable training, and is time consuming. Rapid diagnostic tests detect malaria antigen in a small amount of blood by immunochromatographic assay, with monoclonal antibodies directed against parasite antigen impregnated on a test strip. Commercial tests are manufactured with different combinations of target antigens to suit the local malaria epidemiology.[34] In 2007, the US Food and Drug Administration approved the first rapid detection test for use in the United States. Any positive rapid detection test result must be confirmed by microscopy; microscopy is also important for speciation and determination of parasite burden. PCR is available, but it is not used in the initial evaluation. PCR is used in some settings to determine the species of parasite after the diagnosis of malaria has been established.[14]

Treatment

Treatment of malaria is influenced by patient-specific factors (age, background of immunity, pregnancy, ability to take oral medications), species-specific factors, and local

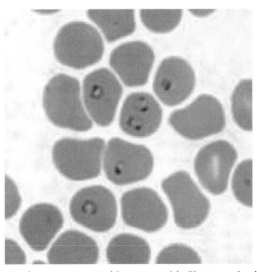

Fig. 5. P falciparum trophozyte seen on thin smear with Giemsa stain. (*Courtesy of* CDC.)

factors (drug resistance patterns, government treatment guidelines, tolerability, and drug availability) (**Table 4**). The same medication should not be used for treatment that the patient used for prophylaxis, in case a drug-resistant strain has been selected.

Non-*falciparum* malaria, (*vivax, malariae,* and *ovale*) should generally be treated with chloroquine, but chloroquine-resistant *vivax* has been reported recently in Papua New Guinea and Indonesia and chloroquine-resistant *malariae* has been reported in Sumatra.[35,36] In addition, primaquine is required in *P vivax* and *ovale* infections to eradicate the parasites that survive in the liver. Combination therapy generally prevents relapse in most *P vivax* and *ovale* infections, but primaquine-tolerant strains of *P vivax* have emerged in Oceania and East Africa, and longer and higher doses of primaquine are required in these areas for radical cure.

P falciparum treatment depends on sensitivity patterns in the particular area where the infection was acquired. *P falciparum* originating from Central America west of the Panama Canal, Haiti, the Dominican Republic, and much of the Middle East can be treated with chloroquine. However, there is developing resistance to this regimen. *P falciparum* acquired elsewhere should be treated with atovaquone-proguanil; artemether-lumefantrine; quinine plus doxycycline, tetracycline, or clindamycin; or mefloquine.[14,35] Mefloquine should not be used in patients who return from Cambodia and Thailand, because cases of mefloquine resistance have been reported.

Complicated disease, pregnancy, or severe nausea and vomiting necessitates admission to hospital and involvement of a specialist. Standard treatment of severe disease includes quinidine gluconate plus doxycycline, tetracycline, or clindamycin. Use of artesunate is becoming more common, and requires involvement of the CDC. Randomized controlled trials in endemic regions have shown a 30% reduction in mortality with artesunate-based regimens compared with quinine-based regimens.[37] Exchange transfusion should be considered in patients with parasite burden greater than 10%, altered mental status, pulmonary edema, or renal complications. The CDC Web site (http://www.cdc.gov/malaria/diagnosis_treatment/treatment.html) provides up-to-date information regarding the frequently changing epidemiology and resistance patterns and describes how to obtain artesunate in the United States. This Web site should be reviewed before initiation of malaria treatment.

DENGUE FEVER
Background

Dengue is endemic in Puerto Rico, Latin American, Africa, and Southeast Asia. There are periodic outbreaks in Samoa and Guam.[38] The dengue virus is a single-stranded RNA virus with 4 serotypes. Clinically, this description means that infection with 1 serotype provides immunity only for that particular serotype. The virus is carried by the *Aedes* mosquito, a silent daytime feeder with bites that frequently go unnoticed. The incubation period ranges from 2 to 14 days, and therefore it is effectively excluded as a cause of febrile illness in a traveler whose symptoms started more than 14 days after return.

Both viral and host characteristics influence the clinical presentation of dengue. There are several theories as to which combination of factors results in a more severe presentation.[39] Most evidence suggests that most severe dengue fever occurs in individuals who have been infected with dengue more than 1 time. Other theories include the hypothesis that different dengue viruses have inherently different levels of virulence, or that more severe clinical presentations involve abnormalities in T-cell response or autoimmune phenomena.

Table 4
Malaria treatment

Clinical Diagnosis	Species, Geographic Distribution	Recommended Drug	Additional Comments
Uncomplicated malaria	P ovale, P malariae, P knowlesi malaria or P falciparum from Central America (west of the Panama Canal), Haiti, the Dominican Republic and most of the Middle East or P vivax from all regions except Papa New Guinea or Indonesia	Chloroquine	For P vivax and P ovale, add primaquine
	Chloroquine-resistant P falciparum from all other malarious regions not specified elsewhere or P vivax from Papua New Guinea or Indonesia	Atovaquone-proguanil or artemether-lumefantrine or quinine + doxycycline, tetracycline or clindamycin or mefloquine	For P vivax, add primaquine
	Multidrug-resistant P falciparum from Southeast Asia		Atovaquone-proguanil or artemether-lumefantrine or quinine + doxycycline, tetracycline or clindamycin
Complicated malaria	P falciparum	Quinidine gluconate + doxycycline, tetracycline or clindamycin or artesunate	Considered exchange transfusion in patients with parasitemia >10%, altered mental status, pulmonary edema, or renal complications

Data from Centers for Disease Control and Prevention. Treatment of malaria (guidelines for clinicians). Available at: http://www.cdc.gov/malaria/diagnosis_treatment/treatment.html. Accessed April 10, 2013.

Classification and Clinical Presentation

Dengue disease occurs as a spectrum of disease severity. WHO guidelines categorize dengue disease as nonsevere and severe. Nonsevere dengue fever is an acute febrile illness with 2 more of the following manifestations: headache, retro-orbital pain, myalgia, arthralgia (which prompted the name breakbone fever), rash, leucopenia, and mild hemorrhagic symptoms. The triad of skin rash (**Fig. 6**), thrombocytopenia, and leukopenia in a febrile returning traveler is suggestive of dengue infection.[33]

The nonsevere group is further subdivided by the presence of warning signs.[40] Warning signs that usually arise between day 3 and 7 of fever may indicate the development of severe dengue fever. The warning signs include mucosal bleeding, emesis, hematemesis, severe abdominal pain, painful hepatomegaly, breathing discomfort, lethargy, and fatigue. These symptoms often occur as patients defervesce.

Severe dengue is defined by plasma leakage, fluid accumulation, respiratory distress, severe bleeding, and organ impairment. Patients with severe dengue manifest many or all of the warning signs. Severe dengue seems to occur less frequently among travelers than it does in native populations. Native populations might be more susceptible because they are more likely to be infected sequentially by 2 dengue serotypes (secondary infection hypothesis). An alternative explanation is that most exposed travelers are younger adults, who are less likely to develop severe disease compared with the very old or very young.[41]

Diagnosis

Diagnosis is often made based on clinical presentation, but serology and molecular tests are available. The choice of confirmatory diagnostic test depends on timing of the patient's presentation. If the patient presents with at least 3 days of acute febrile illness, measurement of antidengue IgM is recommended. If before 3 days or the antidengue IgM is negative and clinic suspicion remains high, PCR for dengue viral RNA can be performed, although viral RNA clears from the bloodstream early in the course of the infection.

Treatment

Supportive care is the only management available for treatment of dengue.

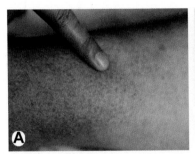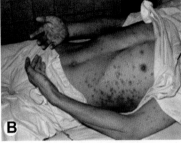

Fig. 6. Cutaneous manifestations of dengue. (*A*) Early maculopapular nonpruritic rash usually seen at the time of defervescence. (*B*) Late hemorrhagic and purpuric skin changes of a patient with severe dengue fever. (*Courtesy of* James H. Maguire, MD, Centers for Disease Control and Prevention, Atlanta, GA.)

RICKETTSIAL INFECTIONS
Background

Rickettsiosis is the term used for a spectrum of diseases caused by the intracellular bacteria *Rickettsia*, which invade endothelial cells and produce a vasculitis. There are multiple ectoparasite vectors for *Rickettsia*, including lice, ticks, fleas, and mites.

Classification

Rickettsiosis is divided into 3 main biogroups: typhus, spotted fever, and scrub typhus. The 4 most common rickettsioses seen in the traveler include murine typhus, Mediterranean spotted fever, African tick bite fever, and scrub typhus.[42] Each disease is caused by a different species, carried by different vector, has a different geographic distribution, and has different clinical presentation and sequelae.

Clinical Presentation

The combination of fever and cutaneous eruptions (**Fig. 7**) suggests rickettsiosis in a traveler returning from an endemic region.[33]

Diagnosis

As with Rocky Mountain spotted fever, rickettsial infections are primarily diagnosed clinically based on epidemiology and the history and physical examination findings. Rickettsiosis can be confirmed by 1 of 4 methods: isolation of the organism, serology, PCR, and immunologic detection in tissue samples.

Treatment

First-line treatment of all rickettsioses is doxycycline. Presumptive treatment is recommended whenever the diagnosis is suspected, because making the diagnosis during the acute phase can be difficult.

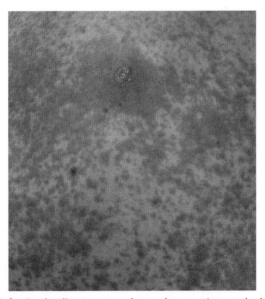

Fig. 7. Rickettsial infection leading to a maculopapular eruption on the back with a central necrotic area where the tick bite occurred. (*Data from* Morris-Jones R, Morris-Jones S. Travel-associated skin disease. Infect Dis Clin North Am 2012;26(3):688.)

ENTERIC FEVER
Background

Enteric fever encompasses both typhoid and paratyphoid fever and is common through most parts of the world except industrialized regions in North America, western Europe, Australia, and Japan.[43] *Salmonella enterica* serotypes *typhi* and *paratyphi* cause clinically indistinguishable entities; however, there are vaccines against serotype *typhi*, but not *paratyphi*. This gram-negative organism is ingested, survives gastric acidity, and invades gut epithelium. From there, it invades lymphatic tissue and can spread hematogenously and lymphatically.

Incubation period depends on amount of pathogen ingested, host age, and immune status, but generally is 7 to 14 days.[44]

Clinical Presentation

The classic clinical triad is abdominal pain, fevers, and chills. The patient may experience incremental increase in fever over the first week, increasing at a rate of 0.5°C to 1.0°C a day. A plateau of fevers ranging from 39 to 41 for 2 weeks follows. Generally, this plateau phase is not seen in the traveler, as opposed to the endemic population in a developing country, because travelers are more apt to seek care at earlier stages. On examination, relative bradycardia may be seen as well as hepatosplenomegaly, although neither of these findings is specific. Rose spots are lightly erythematous, nonblanching plaques 2 to 4 mm in diameter and are seen in 5% to 30% of patients with typhoid. Children and patients with HIV are more likely to present with diarrhea, whereas adults are more likely to complain of constipation. Complications occur in 10% to 15% of patients and are particularly likely in patients who have been ill for more than 2 weeks. Among the numerous complications are gastrointestinal bleeding, intestinal perforation, and typhoid encephalopathy.

Diagnosis

Enteric fever is diagnosed by blood or stool culture, but cultures may be negative if antibiotics have been given before obtaining the sample. Blood cultures have 60% to 80% sensitivity and are the standard diagnostic test. Stool culture has a sensitivity of 35%. If cultures remain negative and diagnosis remains uncertain, bone marrow biopsy is the most useful test, with a sensitivity of 90%. Serologic tests are not useful.[45]

Vaccination and Treatment

First-line treatment of enteric fever is 3 to 5 days quinolone (except for norfloxacin) antibiotic therapy.[46] The first-line agent for quinolone-resistant typhoid has not been determined; azithromycin, third-generation cephalosporins, and long, high-dose courses of quinolones have been proposed. The CDC recommends injectable third-generation cephalosporins.[41]

There are 2 modestly effective vaccines available for typhoid fever. The parental version takes advantage of IgG-mediated cell immunity; the oral form takes advantage of IgA secretory immunity. At best, parental vaccination is only 70% efficacious for preventing typhoid fever; oral vaccination is estimated to be less effective.[47]

RESPIRATORY INFECTION
Background

Respiratory infections occur in up to 20% of travelers.[2] The GeoSentinel study found that the most common diagnosis for URI was nonspecified URI, followed by pharyngitis and tonsillitis. The most common diagnoses for lower respiratory tract infections were bronchitis, pneumonia, and influenza. Thus, most travelers returning with respiratory complaints have diagnoses that are common in the developed world.[48]

Outbreaks are often linked to group settings, such as cruises or tour groups. Several pathogens have been associated with outbreaks including *influenza, Legionella, coronavirus,* and *histoplasma.* The risk for tuberculosis among immunocompetent travelers is low.

Diagnosis

Identification of the specific agent in the outpatient setting causing respiratory symptoms in an immunocompetent host is usually unnecessary.

Treatment

In some patients with influenza, treatment with oseltamivir might be appropriate. There is no effective specific therapy for noninfluenza respiratory viruses in immunocompetent adults. Treatment of bacterial pneumonia should be based on antibiotic sensitivity and local guidelines.

THE IMMUNOSUPPRESSED TRAVELER
Special Considerations in Patients with HIV

Fifty-nine countries have restrictions regarding travelers with HIV visiting their country, including deportation if HIV status is discovered. Four countries bar entry to any patient with HIV: Sudan, Yemen, United Arab Emirates, and Brunei.[49] Up-to-date information is available at http://www.unaids.org and should be reviewed before travel.

Killed or inactivated vaccines are safe in HIV-positive patients. For maximal effectiveness, vaccines should be administered when CD4 counts have peaked on effective antiretroviral therapy.[50]

There is increased incidence, prevalence, and severity of malaria in HIV-infected individuals.[51] Although there is no special precaution for patients with HIV that would not be indicated for immunocompetent patients (ie, nets, DEET, and strict prophylaxis compliance), the increased risk of infection and severe disease underscores their importance. The incidence of clinical episodes of malaria was found to be higher in individual with CD4 cell counts less then 200 cells/μL than in those with CD4 cell counts greater than 500 cells/μL.[52] Patients with CD4 less than 200 should be advised to postpone their travel until their counts rebound. The pharmacy should review any possible interactions between antiretroviral medications and malaria prophylaxis.

Routine antimicrobial prophylaxis for traveler's diarrhea for patients with HIV is not recommended. If severe immunosuppression is present and the trip cannot be postponed, a preventive regimen of daily-dose quinolone or rifaximin is appropriate.[28,53] As is the case in the immunocompetent patient, most HIV-infected travelers who develop traveler's diarrhea can be treated with ciprofloxacin. However, if diarrhea persists, in addition, a stool sample should be submitted for *Giardia* antigen, specific instructions for *Microsporidia* and *Cryptosporidium parvum* staining and ova and parasite (O&P) examination to look for *Cyclospora cayatenensis* and *Isospora belli.*

Special Considerations in Solid Organ Transplant Patients

The greatest risk for infection is during the 6 months after transplantation, when immunosuppression is highest[54,55]; travel should be postponed until this period has lapsed. Patients on antirejection drugs should avoid volume depletion, because many antirejection drugs are nephrotoxic and are more likely to cause acute kidney injury. Therefore, patients on antirejection drugs should be counseled to start volume repletion and should be given antibiotics and loperamide to start promptly for even mild traveler's diarrhea. Malaria prophylaxis may interact with antirejection drugs; thus, levels need to be monitored by a pharmacist before departure.

Special Considerations in Asplenic Patients

Splenectomy (whether functional or surgical) is not a contraindication to any vaccine. In addition, asplenic patients are particularly susceptible to encapsulated organisms and should have already been vaccinated against *Streptococcus pneumoniae* (within 5 years), *Neisseria meningitis* (within 3 years) and *Haemophilus influenza* (once). These vaccinations should be administered at travel visit if the traveler has not previously received them.[56] Although patients with asplenia are not at higher risk of influenza, it may predispose to invasive *Streptococcus pneumoniae*, and thus should also be immunized for flu at their pretravel visit if this has not already been done. Patients with asplenia should be promptly treated with antibiotics at the onset of any febrile illness or after any animal bite. Given that travelers may not have ready access to medical care, asplenic patients should be given a course of amoxicillin/clauvanate, which should be adequate initial treatment of both fever and animal bite prophylaxis. Taking antibiotics in this setting is an adjunct to seeking prompt medical care, not a replacement, and this distinction needs to be explicitly stated. Asplenic patients should also wear an alert bracelet. Asplenic patients with malaria may have delayed clearance of parasites from the bloodstream despite appropriate treatment.[57] They should receive a follow-up blood smear after treatment is complete.

Special Consideration in Patients on Corticosteroids or Tumor Necrosis Factor α

Patients taking greater than the equivalent 20 mg/d prednisone for more than 2 weeks should be considered immunosuppressed.[58] Live vaccines should not be administered, and immune response to inactivated vaccines may be insufficient. Physicians should wait more than 1 month after steroid discontinuation before administering vaccines. There is a paucity of data on administration of live vaccines to patients on tumor necrosis factor α (TNF-α) inhibitors, and they should be avoided in these patients.

The differential diagnosis in patients on corticosteroids and TNF-α inhibitors is necessarily broad, because they may present atypically. In addition, these patients have an increased risk for infections not otherwise commonly seen in other travelers, including tuberculosis and invasive fungal diseases.

Special Consideration in Patients on Oncologic Medications

The CDC considers patients on alkylating agents (cyclophosphamide), antimetabolites (azathioprine), and chemotherapeutic agents (including weekly methotrexate but excluding tamoxifen) to be severely immunosuppressed. Live vaccines should not be administered for at least 3 months after therapy has been discontinued.

SUMMARY

The pretravel clinic visit is an integral part of disease prevention for travel. The intended trip should be reviewed in depth with the patient to assess for risks particular to certain countries and conditions. Appropriate immunizations should be reviewed and administered; up-to-date recommendations are listed by location on the CDC Web site. Patients should be counseled on insect bite and traveler's diarrhea avoidance measures. Safe sex practices should be reinforced. Patients can be given antibiotics to take in case of moderate or severe traveler's diarrhea.

Traveler's diarrhea is common and generally occurs between 4 and 14 days after arrival.[10] Viral causes as well as most bacterial causes are usually self-limited, lasting several days. Mild diarrhea should be treated with volume repletion and symptoms management with loperamide and bismuth. If symptoms last longer than a week or bloody diarrhea is present, stool cultures should be obtained. If diarrhea has been present for more than a week despite antibacterial treatment, parasitic causes should be considered and stool O&P, and examinations for *Cryptosporidium*, *Cyclospora*, and so forth should be sent.

Skin lesions in a returning traveler are often secondary to conditions commonly seen in developed countries. CLM develops its pathognomonic serpiginous appearance 2 to 3 days after the larva has entered the human host. Diagnosis is clinical and can be treated with ivermectin or albendazole. Leishmaniasis has 4 different cutaneous manifestations. The interval from infection to clinical manifestation can range from weeks to years depending on the particular species and host immune status. Leishmaniasis is diagnosed by obtaining a tissue sample and performing microscopy, histology, PCR, or culture. Treatment is lengthy and should involve a specialist. Myiasis and tungiasis are diagnosed clinically and are treated by removal of the parasite.

Fever in a returning traveler is malaria until proved otherwise and can present months after return from endemic area. Evaluation involves thin and thick blood smears, the decision whether to admit, and treatment based on species and resistance patterns. The dengue incubation period is less than a week and can be excluded in any patient who presents with a fever more than 14 days after return. Dengue has a spectrum of severity and treatment is supportive. The incubation period and clinical presentation of rickettsiosis depend on the particular infective species; diagnosis is primarily clinical and treatment is doxycycline. Enteric fever presents as abdominal pain, fever, and chills. Incubation is generally from 1 to 2 weeks and is less likely in patients who present more than 3 weeks after return from endemic countries. Blood cultures are the diagnostic standard and infections are treated with a quinolone.

Patients with underlying immunosuppression need to receive tailored advice at their pretravel clinic visit. Immunosuppressed patients may have contraindications to live vaccines and impaired immune response to inactive vaccines. On return, the differential to a returning immunosuppressed patient must be broader because they may present atypically and are also susceptible to a wider range of pathogens.

Travel medicine continues to grow as international tourism and patient medical complexity increases. This article reflects the state of the discipline, but new recommendations on immunizations, resistance patterns, and treatment modalities constantly change. The CDC and WHO maintain helpful Web sites for both patient and physician. With thoughtful preparation and prevention, risks can be minimized and travel can continue as safely as possible.

REFERENCES

1. Spira A. Preparing the traveler. Lancet 2003;361:1368–81.
2. Hill DR. Health problems in a large cohort of Americans traveling to developing countries. J Travel Med 2000;7:259–66.
3. National Center for Immunization and Respiratory Diseases. General recommendations on immunization: recommendations of the Advisory Committee on Immunization Practices. MMWR Recomm Rep 2011;60(2):1–64.
4. Health information for travelers to Saudi Arabia. On: CDC Travelers Health Website. Available at: http://wwwnc.cdc.gov/travel/destinations/saudi-arabia.htm. Accessed December 12, 2012.

5. Steffen R, DuPont HL, Heusser R, et al. Prevention of traveler's diarrhea by the tablet form of bismuth subsalicylate. Antimicrob Agents Chemother 1986;29:625–7.

6. Ericsson CD. Nonantimicrobial agents in the prevention and treatment of traveler's diarrhea. Clin Infect Dis 2005;41:S557–63.

7. De Bruyn G, Hahn S, Borwick A. Antibiotic treatment for travellers' diarrhea. Cochrane Database Syst Rev 2000;(3):CD002242.

8. Castelli F, Saleri N, Tomasoni LR, et al. Prevention and treatment of traveler's diarrhea: focus on antimicrobial agents. Digestion 2006;73(Suppl 1):109–18.

9. Salam I, Katelaris P, Leigh-Smith S, et al. Randomized trial of single-dose ciprofloxacin for travellers' diarrhoea. Lancet 1994;344:1537–9.

10. Kuschner RA, Trofa AF, Thomas RJ, et al. Use of azithromycin for the treatment of *Campylobacter* enteritis in travelers to Thailand, an area where ciprofloxacin resistance is prevalent. Clin Infect Dis 1995;21:536–41.

11. Hill DR, Ericsson CD, Pearson RD, et al. The practice of travel medicine: guidelines by the Infectious Diseases Society of America. Clin Infect Dis 2006;43:1499–539.

12. Fradin MS, Day JF. Comparative efficacy of insect repellents against mosquito bites. N Engl J Med 2002;347:13–8.

13. Nevill CG, Some ES, Mung'ala VO, et al. Insecticide-treated bednets reduce mortality and severe morbidity from malaria among children on the Kenyan coast. Trop Med Int Health 1996;1:139–46.

14. Malaria. In: World Health Organization Website. Available at: http://www.who.int/topics/malaria/en/. Accessed December 14, 2012.

15. Bloor M, Thomas M, Hood K, et al. Differences in sexual risk behaviour between young men and women travelling abroad from the UK. Lancet 1998;352:1664–8.

16. Tveit KS, Nilsen A, Nyfors A. Casual sexual experience abroad in patients attending an STD clinic and at high risk for HIV infection. Genitourin Med 1994;70:12–4.

17. Marrazzo JM. Sexual tourism: implications for travelers and the destination culture. Infect Dis Clin North Am 2005;19:103–20.

18. Hamlyn E, Peer A, Easterbrook P. Sexual health and HIV in travellers and expatriates. Occup Med 2007;57:313–21.

19. Hill DR. Occurrence and self-treatment of diarrhea in a large cohort of Americans traveling to developing countries. Am J Trop Med Hyg 2000;62:585–9.

20. Malone JD, Hyams KC, Hawkins RE, et al. Risk factors for sexually transmitted diseases among deployed U.S. military personnel. Sex Transm Dis 1993;20:294–8.

21. Hill DR, Beeching NJ. Traveler's diarrhea. Curr Opin Infect Dis 2010;23:481–7.

22. Steffen R. Epidemiologic studies of the travelers' diarrhea, severe gastrointestinal infections and cholera. Rev Infect Dis 1986;8(Suppl 2):S122–30.

23. Steffen R, Collard F, Tornieporth N, et al. Epidemiology, etiology, and impact of traveler's diarrhea in Jamaica. JAMA 1999;281:811–7.

24. Riddle MS, Arnold S, Tribble DR. Effect of adjunctive loperamide in combination with antibiotics on treatment outcomes in traveler's diarrhea: a systematic review and meta-analysis. Clin Infect Dis 2008;47:1007–14.

25. Lederman ER, Weld LH, Elyazar IR, et al. Dermatologic conditions of the ill returned traveler: an analysis from the GeoSentinel Surveillance Network. Int J Infect Dis 2008;12:593–602.

26. Caumes E, Carrière J, Guermonprez G, et al. Dermatoses associated with travel to tropical countries: a prospective study of the diagnosis and management of 269 patients presenting to a tropical disease unit. Clin Infect Dis 1995;20:542–8.

27. Hochedez P, Caumes E. Hookworm related cutaneous larva migrans. J Travel Med 2007;14:326–33.

28. Caumes E, Carriere J, Datry A, et al. A randomized trial of ivermectin versus albendazole for the treatment of cutaneous larva migrans. Am J Trop Med Hyg 1993;49:641–4.

29. Andrade-Narvaez FJ, Medina-Peralta S, Vargas-Gonzalez A, et al. The histopathology of cutaneous leishmaniasis due to *Leishmania (Leishmania) mexicana* in the Yucatan peninsula, Mexico. Rev Inst Med Trop Sao Paulo 2005;47:191–4.

30. Ameen M. Cutaneous leishmaniasis: advances in disease pathogenesis, diagnostics and therapeutics. Clin Exp Dermatol 2010;35:699–705.

31. Wilson ME, Weld LH, Boggild A, et al. Fever in returned travelers: results from the GeoSentinel Surveillance Network. Clin Infect Dis 2007;44:1560–8.

32. Kihara M, Carter JA, Newton CR. The effect of *Plasmodium falciparum* on cognition: a systematic review. Trop Med Int Health 2006;11:386–97.

33. Bottieau E, Clerinx J, Van den Enden E, et al. Fever after a stay in the tropics: diagnostic predictors of the leading tropical conditions. Medicine 2007;86:18–25.

34. Wongsrichanalai C, Barcus MJ, Muth S, et al. A review of malaria diagnostic tools. Am J Trop Med Hyg 2007;77:119–27.

35. White NJ. The treatment of malaria. N Engl J Med 1996;335:800–6.

36. Maguire JD, Sumawinata IW, Masbar S, et al. Chloroquine-resistant *Plasmodium malariae* in south Sumatra, Indonesia. Lancet 2002;360:58–60.

37. Dondorp A, Nosten F, Stepniewska K, et al. Artesunate versus quinine for treatment of severe *falciparum* malaria: a randomised trial. Lancet 2005;366:717–25.

38. Tomashek KM. Dengue fever and dengue hemorrhagic fever. In: 2012 Yellow Book-Traveler's Health. Available at: http://wwwnc.cdc.gov/travel/yellowbook/2012/chapter-3-infectious-diseases-related-to-travel/dengue-fever-and-dengue-hemorrhagic-fever.htm. Accessed January 3, 2013.

39. Halstead SB. Controversies in dengue pathogenesis. Paediatr Int Child Health 2012;32:5–9.

40. Nathan MB, Dayal-Drager R, Guzman M. Dengue: guidelines for diagnosis, treatment, prevention and control. 2009. Available at: http://whqlibdoc.who.int/publications/2009/9789241547871_eng.pdf. Accessed January 3, 2013.

41. Wilder-Smith A. Dengue infections in travelers. Paediatr Int Child Health 2012;32:28–32.

42. Jensenius M, Fournier PE, Raoult D. Rickettsioses and the international traveler. Clin Infect Dis 2004;39:1493–9.

43. Bhattarai A, Mintz E. Typhoid and paratyphoid fever. In: 2012 Yellow Book-Traveler's Health. Available at: http://wwwnc.cdc.gov/travel/yellowbook/2012/chapter-3-infectious-diseases-related-to-travel/typhoid-and-paratyphoid-fever.htm. Accessed January 3, 2013.

44. Parry CM, Hien TT, Dougan G, et al. Typhoid fever. N Engl J Med 2002;347:1770–82.

45. Edelman R, Levine MM. Summary of an international workshop on typhoid fever. Rev Infect Dis 1986;8:329–49.

46. White NJ, Parry CM. The treatment of typhoid fever. Curr Opin Infect Dis 1996;9:298–302.

47. Typhoid immunization: recommendations of the Advisory Committee on Immunization Practices (ACIP). MMWR Morb Mortal Wkly Rep 1994;43:1–7.

48. Leder K, Sundararajan V, Wald L, et al. Respiratory tract infections in travelers: a review of the GeoSentinel surveillance network. Clin Infect Dis 2003;36:399–406.

49. Mapping of restrictions on the entry, stay and residence of people living with HIV 2009. Available at: http://www.unaids.org/en/media/unaids/contentassets/dataimport/pub/report/2009/jc1727_mapping_en.pdf. Accessed January 3, 2013.

50. McCarthy AE, Mileno MD. Prevention and treatment of travel-related infections in compromised hosts. Curr Opin Infect Dis 2006;19:450–5.

51. Kublin JG, Steketee RW. HIV infection and malaria–understanding the interactions. J Infect Dis 2006;193:1–3.

52. Laufer MK, van Oosterhout JJ, Thesing PC, et al. HIV-associated immunosuppression on malaria infection and disease in Malawi. J Infect Dis 2006;193:872–8.

53. Franco-Paredes C, Hidron A, Tellez I, et al. HIV infection and travel: pretravel recommendations and health-related risks. Top HIV Med 2009;17:2–11.

54. Kofidis T, Pethig K, Ruther G, et al. Traveling after heart transplantation. Clin Transplant 2002;16:280–4.

55. Boggild AK, Sano M, Humar A, et al. Travel patterns and risk behavior in solid organ transplant recipients. J Travel Med 2004;11:37–43.

56. Watson DA. Pretravel health advice for asplenic individuals. J Travel Med 2003;10:117–21.

57. Chotivanich K, Udomsangpetch R, McGready R, et al. Central role of the spleen in malaria parasite clearance. J Infect Dis 2002;185:1538–41.

58. Jong EC, Freedman DO. Immunocompromised Traveler. In: 2012 Yellow Book-Traveler's Health. Available at: http://wwwnc.cdc.gov/travel/yellowbook/2012/chapter-8-advising-travelers-with-specific-needs/immunocompromised-travelers.htm. Accessed January 3, 2013.

Serious Group A Streptococcal Infections

Christopher J. Wong, MD[a],*, Dennis L. Stevens, PhD, MD[b,c]

KEYWORDS

- Group A *Streptococcus* • Necrotizing fasciitis • Cellulitis • Toxic shock syndrome
- Pneumonia • Penicillin • Clindamycin • Soft tissue infection

KEY POINTS

- Increasingly virulent group A streptococcal infections associated with high morbidity and mortality have been observed since the late 1980s and continue to be prevalent in North America and worldwide.
- The M protein of the cell wall, encoded by the *emm* gene, likely plays a critical role in the virulence of group A *Streptococcus*.
- Early clinical suspicion is key to early diagnosis of necrotizing fasciitis. Patients may have swelling (often beginning in the limbs), fever, and severe pain out of proportion to physical examination findings. Typical laboratory findings are hyponatremia, acute kidney injury, leukocytosis, and an increased creatine kinase level.
- If group A streptococcal toxic shock syndrome is suspected, antibiotic therapy should include both intravenous penicillin and clindamycin.

INTRODUCTION

Group A *Streptococcus* (GAS) has been prevalent throughout the centuries and causes a wide range of infections and nonsuppurative complications. Milder infections include acute pharyngitis, impetigo, cellulitis, and erysipelas. However, GAS also causes severe, invasive infections such as puerperal sepsis, bacteremia, pneumonia, necrotizing fasciitis, and toxic shock syndrome (TSS). Nonsuppurative complications include acute rheumatic fever, poststreptococcal glomerulonephritis, scarlet fever, and the PANDAS syndrome (pediatric autoimmune neuropsychiatric disorder associated with GAS).

Funding Sources: C.J. Wong: None. D.L. Stevens: Department of Veterans Affairs, National Institutes of Health.
Conflicts of Interest: None.
[a] Division of General Internal Medicine, Department of Medicine, University of Washington, 4245 Roosevelt Way Northeast, Box 354760, Seattle, WA 98105, USA; [b] Infectious Diseases Section, Veterans Administration Medical Center, 500 West Fort Street (Building 45), Boise, ID 83702, USA; [c] University of Washington School of Medicine, Seattle, WA, USA
* Corresponding author.
E-mail address: cjwong@uw.edu

Med Clin N Am 97 (2013) 721–736
http://dx.doi.org/10.1016/j.mcna.2013.03.003
medical.theclinics.com

The incidence of and mortality from severe infections caused by GAS declined from the late 1800s to the mid-twentieth century. GAS became more commonly known for its continuing role in the common syndromes of acute pharyngitis and erysipelas. The nonsuppurative complication of acute rheumatic fever continues to be prevalent worldwide, but is uncommon now in developed nations. Invasive infections were rare for many years.

Then, in the 1980s, emergent cases of virulent GAS were reported in the United States and Europe.[1–5] These cases were notable because they often occurred in otherwise healthy patients, with a frequent association of necrotizing fasciitis and multiorgan failure, and with a markedly fulminant course: deaths were common and occurred within a few days of presentation. Since that time, invasive GAS has continued its prevalence in North America and worldwide as a significant cause of morbidity and mortality.

PATHOPHYSIOLOGY AND MICROBIOLOGY

Streptococcus pyogenes is an aerobic, gram-positive coccus that grows in chains and causes a clear zone of hemolysis on blood agar plates (β-hemolysis). Humans are the only known host. Group A is distinguished from other streptococcal species by its carbohydrate cell wall antigens. In addition, subtypes of *S pyogenes* can be distinguished by M protein antigens also in the cell wall. More than 150 different M types have been described. β-hemolytic streptococcal disease is discussed in this article, although other nonhemolytic have been implicated in human disease.[6] Most commonly, clinicians encounter GAS as episodes of acute pharyngitis and skin and soft tissue infections such as erysipelas.

The question remains why such a prevalent organism, which generally causes common, milder skin and oropharyngeal infections, should infrequently cause severe invasive disease, and why the severe phenotype has continued to remain prevalent since its emergence in the late 1980s. The M protein and the pyrogenic exotoxins are perhaps the best studied of the virulence factors.

The M protein of the cell wall, encoded by the *emm* gene, likely plays a critical role in the virulence of GAS. The M protein is believed to increase virulence by inhibiting opsonization and phagocytosis in the absence of type-specific anti-M protein antibody. There is a multitude of different M protein types which comprise most cases of invasive GAS infections. More than 50% of cases were caused by M1, M3, M4, M12, and M28 in 2 series in Canada[7,8] and M1, M3, M28, M12, and M89 in the United States.[9] Outside North America, M1, M89, and M28 accounted for 59% of isolates in France in 2007[10]; in the Netherlands, most isolates from 1992 to 1996 comprised M1, M3, M28, M6, M12, and M89.[11] M1, M28, M3, M89, and M87 accounted for more than 50% of isolates in a 2003 to 2004 study across Europe, with notable variation by country, with M1 being the most prevalent in most countries.[12] In that study, M28 was the most prevalent M type in Finland and Sweden, but updated data from 2004 to 2007 showed an increase in M1 in Finland,[13] and a case cluster from Sweden in 2006 to 2007 also showed M1 predominance.[14] Thus the M1 protein seems to be consistently highly prevalent in studies of invasive GAS infections, frequently in many but not most cases. There is some evidence that specific M types increase virulence: in the United States the emm1, emm3, and emm12 genotypes have been associated with increased risk of mortality,[9,15] and the emm1 genotype was more common in invasive disease (31.9%) compared with noninvasive disease (9.5%) in a study in Spain.[16]

The streptococcal pyrogenic exotoxins (A, B, and C) function as superantigens and have been implicated in streptococcal TSS. These toxins function as superantigens by binding simultaneously to specific V-β regions of T lymphocytes and to the major histocompatibility complex II portion of antigen-presenting cells such as macrophages. The speA gene, encoding pyrogenic exotoxin A, has been associated with specific serotypes of S pyogenes such as M1.[2,7] SpeB encodes pyrogenic exotoxin B, a cysteine protease that is implicated in degradation of host extracellular matrix proteins, antibacterial peptides, and immunoglobulins, and is of importance in localizing the site of infection to the soft tissues in necrotizing fasciitis.[17] Other candidate virulence factors include immunoglobulin-binding M-like proteins,[18] a putative vimentin-binding protein,[19] complement-binding proteins,[20] NADase,[21] hyaluronidase, and cell envelope proteinase.

The presence of virulence factors alone does not explain the pathogenesis of highly destructive infections such as necrotizing fasciitis. Increased rate of toxin production and toxin-induced local ischemia may both play a role.[22] Despite the multiple virulence factors that have been identified, the absence of large epidemics suggests that host defenses nevertheless are a major determinant of the development of invasive disease.[1]

EPIDEMIOLOGY

The yearly incidence of invasive GAS disease in developed countries is estimated at 2.45 cases per 100,000 persons.[23] Because of limited data, the worldwide incidence is not well known, but is believed to be significantly higher in developing nations.[23] In the United States, surveillance by the Centers for Disease Control (CDC) in 2000 to 2004 estimated an incidence of 3.5 cases per 100,000 persons, with a high case fatality rate of 13.7%.[9] This incidence rate was believed to be stable between 1996 and 2004. However, smaller, more regional data suggest that the incidence of invasive GAS infections may be increasing. A survey in Utah using a laboratory surveillance system estimated an increase in annual incidence from 3.5 to 9.8 cases per 100,000 persons, with an increased incidence in Pacific Islanders. Acute rheumatic fever notably declined during this time. The most common sites of infection were skin/soft tissue, pneumonia, and primary bacteremia.[24]

Seasonal variation remains uncertain. An increase in GAS pneumonia has been reported in the winter months in Canada,[25] possibly as a result of increased influenza infection, and data from the United States suggest that most pharyngeal infections and invasive disease occur in the winter and early spring.[9]

CLINICAL PRESENTATION

There is a wide range of presentation of invasive GAS (**Tables 1** and **2**). Specific syndromes are discussed later.

Necrotizing Soft Tissue Infections

Necrotizing fasciitis is a dreaded, often lethal, form of deep soft tissue bacterial infection. Necrotizing soft tissue infections may be classified as type 1, of polymicrobial cause, and type 2, caused by a single organism, classically GAS. Roughly 30% to 55% of cases of necrotizing fasciitis are caused by polymicrobial infections[26–28] whereas GAS causes 10% to 40% (**Table 3**).[26–28] In 1 series, patients with GAS necrotizing fasciitis were younger and had fewer comorbidities, without a difference in clinical outcome compared with necrotizing fasciitis with other causes.[26] In another series, cases caused by GAS were not associated with increased mortality[27] unless shock and organ failure (TSS) were also present.

Table 1
Clinical features of invasive GAS infections (see text for details)

Syndrome	Clinical Features
Necrotizing fasciitis	Severe pain, often in extremities Predisposing trauma or infection, but may have no obvious risk factor High rate of TSS and organ failure Extremely rapid course of illness Treatment: surgical debridement necessary for both diagnosis and treatment; penicillin, clindamycin, ± IVIG High mortality
GAS TSS	Hypotension and multiorgan failure (see **Box 1**) Symptoms localized to site of primary infection. Rapid progression High mortality Treatment: IV fluid resuscitation, penicillin, clindamycin, IVIG
Pneumonia	Acute dyspnea, fever cough May have preceding viral syndrome or influenza Pleural effusions, empyema common, early in course Respiratory failure common
Septic arthritis	Usually monoarticular, often with fever, leukocytosis Treatment: penicillin, joint debridement
Puerperal sepsis	Peripartum, frequently complicated by shock, multiorgan failure, DIC May require surgical exploration
Meningitis	Uncommon, often with predisposing upper respiratory tract infection or neurosurgical procedure
Endocarditis	Uncommon, may be associated with varicella infection and injection drug use
Osteomyelitis	More common in children, may be associated with varicella infection. Septic arthritis may be present
Intra-abdominal infections	Uncommon; some cases of peritonitis reported
Pyomyositis	May be associated with septic arthritis or necrotizing fasciitis
Bacteremia without a focal source	Presents with fever, may develop TSS

On presentation, patients may have swelling (often beginning in the limbs), fever, and severe pain out of proportion to physical examination findings. The illness may be mistaken initially as cellulitis, deep venous thrombosis, or muscle strain. Late in the course, cutaneous bullae containing clear to violaceous fluid, ecchymosis, and marked swelling develop, followed quickly by hypotension and organ failure. Clinical suspicion remains essential; as few as 1 in 6 patients who develop necrotizing fasciitis are suspected of having it on admission.[27] There may be a predisposing history of penetrating injuries, trauma, cuts or burns, and in some cases, varicella infection.[26,27,29,30] However, in 49% to 54% of cases, there is no identified source (see **Table 3**)[26,27]; in such cases, blunt trauma or muscle strain may be the predisposing factor, and infection begins deep in the tissue at the site of muscle injury.[19]

The first step to diagnosis is clinical suspicion. Surgical consultation should be immediately obtained when there is suspicion of necrotizing fasciitis, and should not be delayed awaiting laboratory testing or imaging studies, because necrosis may spread rapidly during this time. Laboratory studies may show hyponatremia, acute kidney injury, leukocytosis, and an increased creatine kinase level.

Table 2
Invasive GAS manifestations reported in case series/epidemiology studies[a]

	Date Range	n	Cellulitis (%)	Bacteremia Without Source (%)	Toxic Shock (%)	Pneumonia (%)	Arthritis (%)	Necrotizing Fasciitis (%)	Other (%)
United States (Utah)[24]	2002–2010	1514	70.3	9.2	3.5	10.2	5.1	4.0	17.8 (abdominal peritoneal 9.1; puerperal, osteomyelitis, endocarditis, meningitis)
Spain[16]	1998–2009	247	41.3	19.0	12.6	7.7[b]	8.9	2.4	5.7 (puerperal sepsis, endocarditis, unknown)
United States (CDC)[9]	2000–2004	5400	36.4	29.4	5.7	14.7	7.7	7.2	17.6 (abscess, abdominal/ peritoneal infection, osteomyelitis, pregnancy-related, endocarditis, meningitis, epiglottitis or otitis media, other)

[a] Adults and children, unless otherwise noted. Cases may be represented in multiple categories.
[b] 10.1% if include empyema and lung abscess.

Table 3
Necrotizing fasciitis case series: microbiology and mortality

Study	N	Type	Years	% Polymicrobial	% Single Organism	No Organism	% Caused by Any Streptococcus	% Caused by GAS	Mortality	% Source (Portal of Entry) Identified
							Microbiology			
Singapore[27]	89	Case series	1997–2002	54	28	18	34.8	9	21	49
South Auckland, Australia[28]	82	Case series	2000–2006	32		10		40	30	[a]
Cook County, IL[26]	80	Case series	1999–2002	39	25		44	15	15[b]	54

[a] 41% had a surgical procedure, but other causes not reported.
[b] None of GAS patients died.

Treatment of necrotizing fasciitis consists of immediate intravenous (IV) antibiotic therapy and surgical debridement of infected tissue. Characteristic findings during surgery confirm the diagnosis of soft tissue necrosis, and in this way, diagnostic confirmation and treatment may take place concurrently. Surgical debridement is necessary to reduce mortality, and serial debridements are frequently required; in severe cases, amputation may be necessary. Necrotizing infections of the head, neck, thorax, and abdomen have been associated with higher mortality, probably because of the difficulty of debridement in these areas. Antibiotic therapy should be initiated immediately at suspicion of necrotizing fasciitis. Often the microbiologic cause from intraoperative or blood cultures is unknown at the time of initial presentation of necrotizing fasciitis; in that situation, broad-spectrum antibiotics should be immediately initiated. If GAS is suspected to be the causative organism, antibiotic therapy should include both IV penicillin and clindamycin. Penicillin should be administered at a dose of 4 million units IV every 4 hours. Dosing adjustments frequently have to be made because of acute kidney injury. Clindamycin, a protein synthesis inhibitor, may improve efficacy by several possible mechanisms: being less dependent on bacterial replication for its antibacterial effect and having a longer postantibiotic effect; suppressing synthesis of bacterial toxin, penicillin-binding protein synthesis, and M protein; and suppressing tumor necrosis factor production by macrophages.[31] A retrospective pediatric analysis showed less treatment failure when clindamycin was used in addition to a penicillin-based antibiotic regimen.[32]

Supportive care is crucial, because patients with necrotizing fasciitis, particularly those with streptococcal TSS, frequently have shock, require ventilator support, dialysis and impressive IV fluid requirements. Because approximately 20% of cases progress rapidly to hypotension,[26,27] patients commonly require early care in the intensive care unit (ICU) for hemodynamic support.

IV immunoglobulin (IVIG) may be considered; there is some evidence that IVIG may improve outcomes in patients with streptococcal TSS (see later discussion), a common complication of patients with necrotizing fasciitis.

Despite these treatments, necrotizing fasciitis remains a highly morbid disease. Mortality ranges from 15% to 45%.[7,26–28,33] Risk factors for mortality caused by necrotizing fasciitis vary depending on the study. Patient risk factors include age,[26,28] 2 or more comorbid conditions,[26] or comorbidities such as ischemic heart disease, congestive heart failure, gout, and chronic kidney disease (CKD),[28] and the use of corticosteroids.[26] Risk factors based on patient presentation include the examination finding of purple/violaceous skin discoloration, hypotension on admission, and positive blood cultures.[26] Treatment factors associated with increased mortality include a delay from the time of admission to surgical debridement, highlighting the need for clinical suspicion and prompt surgical consultation.[27,28] In most cases, these risk factors were not assessed for cases caused by GAS specifically. Morbidity is frequent and may be severe, including limb amputation (9% to 23%),[26–28] extended hospitalization, acute kidney injury, and streptococcal TSS.

Streptococcal TSS

GAS TSS is defined as invasive GAS (isolation of GAS from a normally sterile site), hypotension, and evidence of involvement of 2 or more organs: renal impairment, coagulopathy, acute liver injury, acute respiratory distress syndrome (ARDS), rash, or soft tissue necrosis.[34] **Box 1** outlines the diagnosis of GAS TSS.

The initial clinical presentation of streptococcal TSS is often localized to the primary infection site. This presentation may include pain in a limb or other location caused by necrotizing fasciitis, or pelvic pain associated with a uterine infection.[1] There may be a

---

Box 1
Diagnosis of GAS TSS

- Isolation of GAS from a normally sterile site
  - Blood, cerebrospinal fluid, pleural fluid, peritoneal fluid, wound/biopsy

and

- Hypotension
  - Systolic blood pressure (SBP) 90 mm Hg or less (adults) or SBP less than fifth percentile (children)

and

- 2 or more of the following:
  - Acute kidney injury
    - Creatinine 2 mg/dL or greater or 2 times or greater than baseline if CKD
  - Coagulopathy
    - For example, disseminated intravascular coagulation (DIC), thrombocytopenia
  - Liver injury
    - Transaminases greater than or equal to the upper limit of normal or 2 times baseline or greater if chronically increased at baseline
  - ARDS
  - Rash
    - Erythematous, macular, may be desquamating
  - Soft tissue necrosis
    - Necrotizing fasciitis, myositis, gangrene

Probable GAS TSS: GAS isolated from nonsterile site, but meets other criteria.

Data from Breiman RF, Davis JP, Facklam RR, et al. Defining the group A streptococcal toxic shock syndrome. Rationale and consensus definition. JAMA 1993;269:390–1.

---

preceding history of trauma (even minor), surgical procedures, or viral infections such as varicella or influenza.[2,35] However, in up to 55% of cases, the portal of entry is not identified.[2] Systemic symptoms including fever, chills, and myalgia may mimic a viral prodrome.[1] Patients frequently have altered mental status, and those who are initially normotensive may develop profound hypotension within 4 hours of presentation.[1] Laboratory studies typically show normal to increased white blood cell count, with left shift. Acute kidney injury is common, and often precedes hypotension.

Treatment must be provided with recognition of the rapid, dynamic course of the illness, especially in the first 24 hours. Patients should be evaluated immediately for possible sites of infection, including workup for soft tissue infection that may require early surgical debridement. Necrotizing fasciitis is the most common site of streptococcal infection in GAS TSS, present in 26% to 55% of cases,[2,7,11] followed by pneumonia and bacteremia without a focus.[7] IV fluid resuscitation should begin immediately and often requires massive volumes of crystalloid to maintain blood pressure support. Because a diffuse capillary leak syndrome develops, serum albumin levels commonly decrease to less than 1.5 g/dL, and thus albumin replacement may be necessary. Because GAS possesses 2 potent hemolysins, intravascular hemolysis, particularly in those with bacteremia, may be impressive. Thus, careful monitoring of the volume of packed red blood cells (hematocrit) is necessary and transfusion is frequently required. Vasopressors may be required in addition to adequate volume resuscitation to maintain blood pressure. Patients may develop respiratory failure from volume overload and ARDS and require ventilator support. Antibiotic therapy should be given IV with a β-lactam antibiotic concurrently with clindamycin, as discussed earlier. Often the initial microbiology is not identified on admission, and broad-spectrum antibiotics for sepsis should be administered; if there is the possibility of GAS, broad coverage should include a β-lactam and clindamycin.

There have been multiple case reports of the use of IVIG in streptococcal TSS. A nonrandomized case control study of patients with streptococcal TSS administered IVIG compared with usual care showed a higher 30-day survival rate.[36] A randomized trial of IVIG versus placebo in individuals with streptococcal TSS, most of whom had deep tissue infection, showed a trend toward decreased mortality in the IVIG group, but was limited by small sample size.[37]

Despite aggressive treatment, morbidity and mortality remain high for GAS TSS. Mortality has been reported between 20% and 80% (**Table 4**).[7,11,14,16,24,38] In 1 series of cases of invasive GAS in Utah, GAS TSS had an odds ratio of 12.7 (95% confidence interval, 7.5–21.3) for mortality.[9]

Pneumonia

Although GAS is an uncommon cause of pneumonia, the incidence of GAS pneumonia may be increasing. Studies from Utah suggest a disproportionate increase among children between 2002 and 2009,[24] with a parallel increase in GAS pneumonia associated with H1N1 influenza.[39] In Canada, different studies showed an increase in incidence between 1995 and 2001[8] and from 1992 to 1999.[25] There may be seasonal variation; some studies suggest that GAS pneumonia is more common in the winter months than in the summer.[25,40]

There is some evidence that the M1 genotype of M protein is more frequent in *S pyogenes* pneumonia.[16,40] Serotypes 1, 3, 6, and 12 were the predominant M types in 1 series.[25] Case series have implicated outbreaks of *S pyogenes* pneumonia in military settings,[41,42] in injection drug users,[43] and in nursing home residents.[25,44,45] Rarely, it may complicate varicella infection.[25]

Patients may present with acute onset of dyspnea, fever, and cough. There may be an antecedent viral illness (47% of cases in 1 series).[40] *S pyogenes* has been seen as a coinfection with influenza specifically, implicated in fatal cases during the 2009 H1N1 pandemic influenza season.[46,47] Laboratory studies typically but not universally show leukocytosis, and may show lymphopenia.[40] Bacteremia may portend a more serious clinical course. Pleuritic chest pain and pleural effusions may present early

Table 4			
Mortality associated with GAS TSS in published case series			
Study	**N**	**Years**	**Mortality (%)**
Ontario, ICU[38]	62	1992–2002	68
Utah[24]	1514	2002–2010	19
Uppsala, Sweden[14]	30	2006–2007	25
Netherlands[11]	880	1992–1996	59
Spain[16]	247	1998–2009	48
Ontario[7]	323	1992–1993	81[a]

[a] 65% for those who met consensus definition.

in the course of illness compared with other causes of bacterial pneumonia. Patients with GAS pneumonia may have concurrent sites of infection elsewhere; in 1 study in Canada, 10% also had a soft tissue infection.[25] However, preceding streptococcal pharyngitis is uncommon.

Recognition of GAS as the cause of pneumonia is of distinct clinical importance. Although most empiric treatments for community-acquired pneumonia typically have activity against GAS, including ceftriaxone/azithromycin, and fluoroquinolones, there are reports of fluoroquinolone-resistant GAS in regions with high fluoroquinolone use.[48] β-Lactams remain the treatment of choice for GAS pneumonia.

Clinical outcomes are severe. ICU admission is common (in about 50% of cases),[25] with respiratory failure being common, and a rate of ARDS of approximately 10%. Necrotizing pneumonitis has been reported.[49] Empyema occurs in approximately 20% of patients, and TSS occurs in one-third of cases.[25] The case fatality rate may be as high as 38%, and is often fulminant, causing death within a few days.[25] Mortality is associated with TSS, age, and other underlying illnesses.[25]

Arthritis

Although *Staphylococcus aureus* remains the most common cause of septic arthritis, streptococcal species are the second most common organism.[50] Isolation of GAS in cases of septic arthritis varies by location and time period; in 1 pediatric randomized trial of short versus long duration of antibiotic therapy, *S pyogenes* represented approximately 12% of cases,[51] and *S pyogenes* is the causative organism in 2% to 12% of cases in other series.[52–54]

Of patients with invasive GAS infections, approximately 5% to 9% present with septic arthritis (see **Table 2**).[9,16,24] Patients may have underlying risk factors such as rheumatologic disease or diabetes, very young or advanced age,[50] and may rarely present after varicella infection.[55] However, patients may present without known risk factors.

GAS tends to cause an acute monoarticular arthritis, with an erythematous, swollen joint that is painful with any motion. Systemic signs of fever and leukocytosis are common. Multifocal arthritis without endocarditis or other bacteremic source is uncommon, but has been reported.[56,57]

Prompt treatment is critical to reduce the risk of joint destruction and other complications. Empirical IV antibiotics should be initiated pending culture results. For GAS septic arthritis, 2 weeks of IV therapy is generally indicated. A portal of entry should be sought, but is not always found. Joint drainage, washout, or debridement is often required, necessitating early orthopedic consultation.

Other Manifestations of Invasive GAS

Approximately 80% of invasive GAS disease is represented by pneumonia, soft tissue infections, necrotizing fasciitis, septic arthritis, TSS, and bacteremia without a source (see **Table 2**). The remaining 20% include obstetric, intra-abdominal infections, meningitis, endocarditis, osteomyelitis, pyomyositis, and upper respiratory deep tissue infections (range 6%–18%, see **Table 2**).

Puerperal sepsis caused by hemolytic streptococci deserves discussion, because it was an entity that was historically a cause of childbed fever, a leading cause of maternal morbidity and death in the 1850s in Europe and the United States. That entity largely disappeared by the 1930s, with the exception of sporadic cases.[58] Then, in the late 1980s, coinciding with the virulent strains of GAS reported in North America,[2] reports emerged of GAS causing severe infections during pregnancy and the postpartum period, with complications of shock, multiorgan failure, and DIC.[59–61]

Meningitis is distinctly uncommon, representing approximately 1% of cases of invasive GAS.[9] GAS is an uncommon cause of meningitis in general. In the largest case series, most patients had an upper respiratory tract infection such as otitis media, sinusitis, or another predisposing factor contributing to direct spread of infection such as a previous neurosurgical procedure.[62] Patients may present with typical findings of meningitis, such as headache, fever, and neck stiffness; approximately one-third of cases in 1 series had focal neurologic deficits or seizures.[62] The mortality may be as high as 27%,[9,62] although some smaller case series[63] reported more favorable outcomes.

Endocarditis is uncommonly caused by GAS and accounts for approximately 1% of cases. Among patients with invasive GAS, endocarditis or pericarditis is present in 1% to 2%. Cases have been reported after varicella infection in children, and in injection drug users in adults. Osteomyelitis caused by GAS is more common in children than adults,[9] and has been associated with varicella infection.[64] Septic arthritis may be present concurrently. Intra-abdominal infections are uncommon. There are case reports of primary peritonitis caused by GAS, without an identified source. Pyomyositis has been reported and may be in association with septic arthritis or necrotizing fasciitis. Deep space infections of the upper respiratory tract have also been reported.

Other Clinical Syndromes Associated With GAS Infections

Rheumatologic and other immune-mediated manifestations such as rheumatic fever and poststreptococcal glomerulonephritis are not discussed here.

TREATMENT

The mainstay of treatment of invasive GAS remains a β-lactam such as penicillin. It should be treated with IV antibiotics (eg, penicillin 4 million units IV every 4 hours), with adjustment for renal impairment.

Clindamycin, 900 mg IV every 8 hours, should be administered concurrently with penicillin for severe disease. As discussed earlier, there are retrospective data in the pediatric population suggesting improved clinical outcomes with the use of clindamycin.[32] Animal models of myositis showed improved survival if given clindamycin, and it is postulated that the efficacy of clindamycin is less affected by the bacterial stage of growth compared with penicillin.[65,66] In addition, clindamycin has direct toxin inhibitory effects.[67–69]

As discussed earlier, the initial microbiological cause may be unknown; for cases of necrotizing fasciitis that are not known to be monomicrobial in origin, broad-spectrum antibiotics should cover gram-positive, gram-negative, and anaerobic bacteria, with consideration of the use of clindamycin. Similarly, patients presenting with pneumonia should be treated with antibiotics directed against either community-acquired or nosocomial pneumonia, depending on the clinical setting, and if there is suspicion for GAS, a β-lactam should be one of the initial choices of antibiotic therapy.

There is some evidence that IVIG may improve outcomes in patients with streptococcal TSS. The mechanism of IVIG may include decreasing the activity of virulence factors, including the pyrogenic exotoxins, by means of neutralizing antibodies,[70] and by decreasing the activity of tumor necrosis factor. Treatment protocols for IVIG, used in addition to appropriate antibiotic therapy with penicillin and clindamycin, vary in the published literature: 1 study used 1 g/kg body weight for the first day, then 0.5 g/kg for the following 2 days[37]; another used 2 g/kg as a single dose, with a repeat dose at 48 hours if the patient remained unstable.[36] There is practice variation regarding its use in patients with necrotizing fasciitis or systemic infections with hypotension that do not meet criteria for GAS TSS.[71] IVIG is contraindicated in patients with a history of anaphylactic reaction to IVIG, and in patients with IgA deficiency.

PREVENTION

A suitable vaccine directed against GAS has been sought for many years. Early concerns regarding vaccine development included the risk of developing autoantibodies as a result of cross-reactivity; studies from the 1960s[72] reported cases of acute rheumatic fever in vaccinated patients, but causality remains uncertain. Over the last 10 years, there have been increased efforts at vaccine development. In 2004, phase 1 trial results of a hexavalent vaccine based on the M protein were published,[73] and in 2005, a 26-valent vaccine based on the M protein was shown to induce immunogenicity in volunteers without cross-reactivity to human tissue samples.[74] The 26-valent vaccine uses the N terminus of the M protein, and includes M proteins implicated in rheumatic fever in addition to those causing invasive disease. At estimated 84% efficacy, this vaccine is projected to prevent 48% to 61% of deaths in children younger than 5 years, and 42% to 49% of deaths in adults age 65 years and older.[9] The large number of M types poses a challenge to vaccine development; vaccines targeted against the conserved regions of the M protein, or using other carriers to improve mucosal delivery, have not yet completed safety trials, and others using different epitopes are still in preclinical development.[72] For now, the mainstay of prevention of invasive GAS disease remains containing outbreaks with isolation and appropriate infection control.

SUMMARY

GAS remains an important pathogen, notable for its recent history of a resurgence in severe, invasive disease, starting in the late 1980s. Its persistence remains concerning, and it remains to be seen whether its incidence will increase, decrease, or stay at the same level over the next decades. Early recognition of invasive GAS infections is critical to initiate timely treatment. Mainstays of treatment are penicillin and clindamycin; the organism remains sensitive to penicillin, but should this situation change, a new epidemic may emerge. Vaccine development is a promising avenue for reducing the burden of GAS disease, both infectious and noninfectious, but is still under development.

REFERENCES

1. Stevens DL. Streptococcal toxic shock syndrome associated with necrotizing fasciitis. Annu Rev Med 2000;51:271–88.
2. Stevens DL, Tanner MH, Winship J, et al. Severe group A streptococcal infections associated with a toxic shock-like syndrome and scarlet fever toxin A. N Engl J Med 1989;321:1–7.
3. Bartter T, Dascal A, Carroll K, et al. "Toxic strep syndrome": a manifestation of group A streptococcal infection. Arch Intern Med 1988;148:1421–4.
4. Cone LA, Woodard DR, Schlievert PM, et al. Clinical and bacteriologic observations of a toxic shock-like syndrome due to *Streptococcus pyogenes*. N Engl J Med 1987;317:146–9.
5. Martin PR, Holby EA. Streptococcal serogroup A epidemic in Norway 1987-1988. Scand J Infect Dis 1990;22:421–9.

6. Taylor MB, Barkham T. Fatal case of pneumonia caused by a nonhemolytic strain of *Streptococcus pyogenes*. J Clin Microbiol 2002;40:2311–2.
7. Davies HD, McGeer A, Schwartz B, et al. Invasive group A streptococcal infections in Ontario, Canada. N Engl J Med 1996;335:547–54.
8. Hollm-Delgado MG, Allard R, Pilon PA. Invasive group A streptococcal infections, clinical manifestations and their predictors, Montreal, 1995–2001. Emerg Infect Dis 2005;11(1):77–82.
9. O'Loughlin RE, Roberson A, Cieslak PR, et al. The epidemiology of invasive group A streptococcal infection and potential vaccine implications: United States, 2000-2004. Clin Infect Dis 2007;45(7):853–62.
10. Lepoutre A, Doloy A, Bidet P, et al. Epidemiology of invasive *Streptococcus pyogenes* infections in France in 2007. J Clin Microbiol 2011;49:4094–100.
11. Vlaminckx B, van Pelt W, Schouls L, et al. Epidemiological features of invasive and noninvasive group A streptococcal disease in the Netherlands, 1992–1996. Eur J Clin Microbiol Infect Dis 2004;23:434–44.
12. Luca-Harari B, Darenberg J, Neal S, et al. Clinical and microbiological characteristics of severe *Streptococcus pyogenes* disease in Europe. J Clin Microbiol 2009;47:1155–65.
13. Siljander T, Lyytikainen O, Vahakuopus S, et al. Epidemiology, outcome and emm types of invasive group A streptococcal infections in Finland. Eur J Clin Microbiol Infect Dis 2010;29:1229–35.
14. Vikerfors A, Haggar A, Darenberg J, et al. Severe group A streptococcal infections in Uppsala County, Sweden: clinical and molecular characterization of a case cluster from 2006 to 2007. Scand J Infect Dis 2009;41:823–30.
15. O'Brien KL, Beall B, Barrett NL. Epidemiology of invasive group A streptococcus disease in the United States, 1995–1999. Clin Infect Dis 2002;35:268–76.
16. Montes M, Ardanuy C, Tamayo E, et al. Epidemiological and molecular analysis of *Streptococcus pyogenes* isolates causing invasive disease in Spain (1998-2009): comparison with non-invasive isolates. Eur J Clin Microbiol Infect Dis 2011;30(10):1295–302.
17. Johannson L, Thulin P, Low DE, et al. Getting under the skin: the immunopathogenesis of *Streptococcus pyogenes* deep tissue infections. Clin Infect Dis 2010; 51:58–65.
18. Stenberg L, O'Toole P, Lindahl G. Many group A streptococcal strains express two different immunoglobulin-binding proteins, encoded by closely linked genes: characterization of the proteins expressed by four strains of different M-type. Mol Microbiol 1992;6:1185–94.
19. Bryant AE, Bayer CR, Huntington JD, et al. Group A streptococcal myonecrosis: increased vimentin expression after skeletal-muscle injury mediates the binding of *Streptococcus pyogenes*. J Infect Dis 2006;193:1685–92.
20. Akesson P, Sjoholm AG, Bjorck L. Protein SIC, a novel extracellular protein of *Streptococcus pyogenes* interfering with complement function. J Biol Chem 1996;271:1081–8.
21. Stevens DL, Salmi DB, McIndoo ER, et al. Molecular epidemiology of NGA and NAD glycohydrolase/ADP-ribosyltransferase activity among *Streptococcus pyogenes* causing streptococcal toxic shock syndrome. J Infect Dis 2000;182:1117–28.
22. Bryant AE, Bayer CR, Chen RY, et al. Vascular dysfunction and ischemic destruction of tissue in *Streptococcus pyogenes* infection: the role of streptolysin O–induced platelet/neutrophil complexes. J Infect Dis 2005;192:1014–22.
23. Carapetis JR, Steer AC, Mulholland EK, et al. The global burden of group A streptococcal disease. Lancet Infect Dis 2005;5:685–94.

24. Stockmann C, Ampofo K, Hersh AL, et al. Evolving epidemiologic characteristics of invasive group A streptococcal disease in Utah, 2002-2010. Clin Infect Dis 2012;55(4):479–87.
25. Muller MP, Low DE, Green KA, et al. Clinical and epidemiologic features of group A streptococcal pneumonia in Ontario, Canada. Arch Intern Med 2003; 163(4):467–72.
26. Dworkin MS, Westercamp MD, Park L, et al. The epidemiology of necrotizing fasciitis including factors associated with death and amputation. Epidemiol Infect 2009;137(11):1609–14.
27. Wong CH, Chang HC, Pasupathy S, et al. Necrotizing fasciitis: clinical presentation, microbiology, and determinants of mortality. J Bone Joint Surg 2003; 85(8):1454–60.
28. Nisbet M, Lang S, Taylor S, et al. Necrotizing fasciitis: review of 82 cases in South Auckland. Intern Med J 2011;41(7):543–8.
29. Nuwayhid ZB, Aronoff DM, Mulla ZD. Blunt trauma as a risk factor for group A streptococcal necrotizing fasciitis. Ann Epidemiol 2007;17:878–81.
30. Imöhl M, van der Lindern M, Reinert RR, et al. Invasive group A streptococcal disease and association with varicella in Germany, 1996-2009. FEMS Immunol Med Microbiol 2011;62:101–19.
31. Stevens DL. Streptococcal toxic-shock syndrome: spectrum of disease, pathogenesis, and new concepts in treatment. Emerg Infect Dis 1995;1:69–78.
32. Zimbelman J, Palmer A, Todd J. Improved outcome of clindamycin compared with beta-lactam antibiotic treatment for invasive *Streptococcus pyogenes* infection. Pediatr Infect Dis J 1999;18:1096–100.
33. Kaul R, McGeer A, Low DE, et al. Population-based surveillance for group A streptococcal necrotizing fasciitis: clinical features, prognostic indicators, and microbiologic analysis of seventy-seven cases. Am J Med 1997;103:18–24.
34. Breiman RF, Davis JP, Facklam RR, et al. Defining the group A streptococcal toxic shock syndrome. Rationale and consensus definition. JAMA 1993;269: 390–1.
35. Laupland KB, Davies HD, Low DE, et al. Invasive group A streptococcal disease in children and association with varicella-zoster virus infection. Pediatrics 2000; 105:e60.
36. Kaul R, McGeer A, Norrby-Teglund A, et al. Intravenous immunoglobulin therapy for streptococcal toxic shock syndrome–a comparative observational study. The Canadian Streptococcal Study Group. Clin Infect Dis 1999;28:800–7.
37. Darenberg J, Ihendyane N, Sjolin J, et al. Intravenous immunoglobulin G therapy in streptococcal toxic shock syndrome: a European randomized, double-blind, placebo-controlled trial. Clin Infect Dis 2003;37:333–40.
38. Mehta S, McGeer A, Low DE, et al. Morbidity and mortality of patients with invasive group A streptococcal infections admitted to the ICU. Chest 2006;130: 1679–86.
39. Ampofo K, Herbener A, Blaschke AJ, et al. Association of 2009 pandemic influenza A (H1N1) infection and increased hospitalization with parapneumonic empyema in children in Utah. Pediatr Infect Dis J 2010;29:905–9.
40. Barnham M, Weightman N, Anderson A, et al. Review of 17 cases of pneumonia caused by *Streptococcus pyogenes*. Eur J Clin Microbiol Infect Dis 1999;18: 506–9.
41. Wasserzug O, Valinsky L, Klement E, et al. A cluster of ecthyma outbreaks caused by a single clone of invasive and highly infective *Streptococcus pyogenes*. Clin Infect Dis 2009;48:1213–9.

42. Crum NF, Russell KL, Kaplan EL, et al. Pneumonia outbreak associated with group a *Streptococcus* species at a military training facility. Clin Infect Dis 2005;40(4):511–8.

43. Lamagni TL, Neal S, Keshishian C, et al. Epidemic of severe *Streptococcus pyogenes* infections in injecting drug users in the UK, 2003-2004. Clin Microbiol Infect 2008;14(11):1002–9.

44. MMWR Weekly. Epidemiologic notes and reports nursing home outbreaks of invasive group A streptococcal infections – Illinois, Kansas, North Carolina, and Texas. MMWR Morb Mortal Wkly Rep 1990;39:577–9.

45. Thigpen MC, Thomas DM, Gloss D, et al. Nursing home outbreak of invasive group a streptococcal infections caused by 2 distinct strains. Infect Control Hosp Epidemiol 2007;28(1):68–74.

46. Jean C, Louie JK, Glaser CA, et al. Invasive group A streptococcal infection concurrent with 2009 H1N1 influenza. Clin Infect Dis 2010;50:e59–62.

47. MMWR. Bacterial coinfections in lung tissue specimens from fatal cases of 2009 pandemic influenza A (H1N1)–United States, May–August 2009. MMWR Morb Mortal Wkly Rep 2009;58:1071–4.

48. Van Heirstraeten L, Leten G, Lammens C, et al. Increase in fluoroquinolone non-susceptibility among clinical *Streptococcus pyogenes* in Belgium during 2007-10. J Antimicrob Chemother 2012;67(11):2602–5.

49. Kalima P, Riordan T, Berrisford RG, et al. Necrotizing pneumonia associated with group A streptococcal bacteraemia. Eur J Clin Microbiol Infect Dis 1998;17(4):296–8.

50. Garcia-Arias M, Balsa A, Mola EM. Septic arthritis. Best Pract Res Clin Rheumatol 2011;25:407–21.

51. Peltola H, Paakkonen M, Kallio P, et al. Prospective, randomized trial of 10 days versus 30 days of antimicrobial treatment, including a short- term course of parenteral therapy, for childhood septic arthritis. Clin Infect Dis 2009;48:1201–10.

52. Kaandorp CJ, Dinant HJ, van de Laar MA, et al. Incidence and sources of native and prosthetic joint infection: a community based prospective survey. Ann Rheum Dis 1997;56:470–5.

53. Dubost JJ, Soubrier M, De Champs C, et al. No changes in the distribution of organisms responsible for septic arthritis over a 20 year period. Ann Rheum Dis 2002;61:267–9.

54. Weston VC, Jones AC, Bradbury N, et al. Clinical features and outcome of septic arthritis in a single UK Health District 1982–1991. Ann Rheum Dis 1999;58:214–9.

55. Bradley TM, Dormans JP. *Streptococcus pyogenes* septic arthritis of the elbow complicating the chicken pox. Pediatr Emerg Care 1997;13:380–1.

56. Diaz-Borjon A, Lim S, Franco-Paredes C. Multifocal septic arthritis: an unusual complication of invasive *Streptococcus pyogenes* infection. Am J Med 2005;118:924–5.

57. Marti J, Anton E. Polyarticular septic arthritis caused by *Streptococcus pyogenes* in an immunocompetent woman. Eur J Intern Med 2007;18:80.

58. Nathan L, Leveno KJ. Group A streptococcal puerperal sepsis: historical review and 1990s resurgence. Infect Dis Obstet Gynecol 1994;1:252–5.

59. Swingler GR, Bigrigg MA, Hewitt BG, et al. Disseminated intravascular coagulation associated with group A streptococcal infection in pregnancy. Lancet 1988;1:1456–7.

60. Kavi J, Wise R. Group A beta-haemolytic *Streptococcus* causing disseminated intravascular coagulation and maternal death. Lancet 1988;1:993–4.

61. Acharya U, Lamont CA, Cooper K. Group A beta-haemolytic streptococcus causing disseminated intravascular coagulation and maternal death. Lancet 1988;1:595.

62. Van de Beek D, de Gans J, Spanjaard L, et al. Group A streptococcal meningitis in adults: report of 41 cases and a review of the literature. Clin Infect Dis 2002; 34:e32–6.

63. Sommer R, Rohner P, Garbino J, et al. Group A beta-hemolytic streptococcus meningitis: clinical and microbiological features of nine cases. Clin Infect Dis 1999;29:929–31.

64. Ibia EO, Imoisili M, Pikis A. Group A beta-hemolytic streptococcal osteomyelitis in children. Pediatrics 2003;112:e22–6.

65. Stevens DL, Bryant AE, Yan S. Invasive group A streptococcal infection: new concepts in antibiotic treatment. Int J Antimicrob Agents 1994;4:297–301.

66. Stevens DL, Yan S, Bryant AE. Penicillin-binding protein expression at different growth stages determines penicillin efficacy in vitro and in vivo: an explanation for the inoculum effect. J Infect Dis 1993;167:1401–5.

67. Coyle EA, Cha R, Rybak MJ. Influences of linezolid, penicillin, and clindamycin, alone and in combination, on streptococcal pyrogenic exotoxin a release. Antimicrobial Agents Chemother 2003;47:1752–5.

68. Mascini EM, Jansze M, Schouls LM, et al. Penicillin and clindamycin differentially inhibit the production of pyrogenic exotoxins A and B by group A streptococci. Int J Antimicrob Agents 2001;18:395–8.

69. Goscinski G, Tano E, Thulin P, et al. Penicillin and clindamycin differentially inhibit the production of pyrogenic exotoxins A and B by group A streptococci. Scand J Infect Dis 2006;38:983–7.

70. Norrby-Teglund A, Kaul R, Low DE, et al. Plasma from patients with severe invasive group A streptococcal infections treated with normal polyspecific IgG inhibits streptococcal superantigen-induced T cell proliferation and cytokine production. J Immunol 1996;156:3057–64.

71. Valiquette L, Low DE, Chow R. A survey of physician's attitudes regarding management of severe group A streptococcal infections. Scand J Infect Dis 2006; 38:977–82.

72. Carapetis JR, Steer AC, Mulholland EK. Group A streptococcal vaccine development: current status and issues of relevance to less developed countries. Geneva: World Health Organization; 2005. WHO/FCH/CAH/0.5.09.

73. Kotloff KL, Corretti M, Palmer K, et al. Safety and immunogenicity of a recombinant multivalent group A streptococcal vaccine in healthy adults. Phase 1 trial. JAMA 2004;292:709–15.

74. McNeil SA, Halperin SA, Langley JM, et al. Safety and immunogenicity of 26-valent group A streptococcus vaccine in healthy adult volunteers. Clin Infect Dis 2005; 41:1114–22.

Management of Urinary Tract Infections in the Era of Increasing Antimicrobial Resistance

Amanda Kay Shepherd, MD[a],*, Paul S. Pottinger, MD[b]

KEYWORDS

- Urinary tract infection • Acute cystitis • Resistance • Fosfomycin
- Trimethoprim-sulfamethoxazole • Nitrofurantoin • Recurrent UTI

KEY POINTS

- Antimicrobial resistance in common urinary pathogens is increasing at an alarming rate, as a result of overuse and misuse of antibiotics. Resistance patterns vary by geographic location, but are rising nationwide and globally.
- In the properly selected woman with suspected uncomplicated cystitis, evaluation by a symptom-based approach is both cost-effective and may improve patient satisfaction.
- Acute, uncomplicated urinary tract infections (UTIs) should be treated with fosfomycin, nitrofurantoin, or trimethoprim-sulfamethoxazole. Fluoroquinolones are no longer recommended as first-line therapy for uncomplicated UTI.
- Recurrent UTIs are common. Risk factors include recent intercourse, new sexual partner, and contraceptive type.
- Prevention of recurrent UTIs should begin with a history-based approach to identify associated factors. Antimicrobial prophylaxis should be reserved for use when all other considerations have failed.

INTRODUCTION

A previously healthy 32-year-old woman presents to primary care with dysuria and urinary frequency of 2 days' duration. She denies fevers, chills, or flank pain. You have seen her for this reason 3 times in the last 2 years.

This scenario is frustratingly common in modern medicine. The problem is becoming more complex. Despite the availability of oral antibiotics (in fact, because of that

---

[a] Department of Medicine, University of Washington, 1959 Northeast Pacific Street, Box #356421, Seattle, WA 98195, USA; [b] Division of Allergy and Infectious Diseases, University of Washington, 1959 Northeast Pacific Street, Box #356130, Seattle, WA 98195, USA
* Corresponding author.
E-mail address: Amanda24@uw.edu

Med Clin N Am 97 (2013) 737–757
http://dx.doi.org/10.1016/j.mcna.2013.03.006
0025-7125/13/$ – see front matter © 2013 Elsevier Inc. All rights reserved.

medical.theclinics.com

availability), antimicrobial-resistant gram-negative rods are becoming increasingly important for patients and physicians alike. This article provides an update and practical strategies for the prevention, diagnosis, and treatment of urinary tract infections (UTI) in the contemporary era.

INCIDENCE AND IMPACT

Acute uncomplicated bacterial cystitis is a frequent problem in the American outpatient setting, with an estimated 8.6 million cases annually,[1] accounting for 1.6 billion dollars in health care expenditures.[2] Acute cystitis is associated with an average of 6.1 days of symptoms and 1.2 productive days lost because of illness.[3] Of patients with acute cystitis, an estimated 59% present to primary care and 23% to emergency departments.[1]

MICROBIOLOGY, RESISTANCE MECHANISMS, AND RISK FACTORS

Staphylococcus saprophyticus and any member of the *Enterobacteriaceae* family (including *Escherichia coli, Klebsiella pneumonia* and *Proteus mirabilis)* and can cause cystitis. However, *E coli* remains the most common cause, responsible for an estimated 65% to 95% of cases. Because of the predominance of this bacteria, *E coli* resistance is often a focus of epidemiologic resistance studies.[4–6]

The most recent Infectious Disease Society of America (IDSA) guidelines for treatment of uncomplicated cystitis and pyelonephritis focused on the resistance of organisms responsible for uncomplicated cystitis.[7] The guidelines describe the association between antimicrobial prescribing and resistance development as collateral damage. For example, areas with high rates of fluoroquinolone prescribing for all reasons, in particular sinopulmonary infections, show higher *E coli* fluoroquinolone resistance compared with areas with lower prescription rates.[8] Despite clinical practice guidelines for a wide variety of common infections, studies continue to document improper antibiotic prescribing patterns, both in the hospital and in the ambulatory setting.[9,10]

Microbes have developed multiple antimicrobial resistance mechanisms, including alterations of the drug target, enhanced drug efflux, and limitation of drug influx.[11] Many resistance elements are chromosomal point mutations that provide a survival advantage in the setting of selective drug pressure.[12] In contrast, plasmid-mediated genes provide a highly mobile alternative mode of resistance of increasing prevalence. Microbes can exchange plasmids between members of the same or different species. Examples of plasmid-mediated resistance include carbapenem resistance of *Klebsiella pneumoniae* and fluoroquinolone resistance of *Enterobacteriaceae*. Resistant bacteria have increased survivorship under antibiotic selection, leading to increased prevalence.[11,12] Furthermore, plasmids often contain genes encoding for resistance against multiple drugs, and thus bacteria resistant to 1 antimicrobial agent are more likely to also be resistant to others.[5,6]

Resistance caused by extended spectrum β-lactamases (ESBL) deserve special mention. ESBLs are a family of plasmid-borne hydrolytic enzymes that inactivate penicillins and cephalosporins. Original descriptions of ESBL involved *E coli* and *K pneumoniae*, but the plasmids have been detected in a variety of gram-negative rods since then. The current frequency of ESBL expression probably varies substantially from region to region, although national and international numbers are difficult to come by. It is clear that these plasmids are seen routinely in areas where they were previously not found; for example, resistance increased from undetectable to detectable in 8 years' surveillance in Europe, although the overall frequency was low as of

2012.[6] Although penicillins and cephalosporins are rendered inactive by ESBLs, carbapenems are still generally active against them.

However, carbapenem-resistant *Enterobacteriaceae* are also on the increase, thanks to the expression of carbapenemases. Like ESBLs, these are β-lactamases, but they have activity against carbapenems in addition to penicillins and cephalosporins. Two of the most clinically important carbapenemases are the *Klebsiella pneumoniae* carbapenemase (KPC) and the New Delhi metallo-β-lactamase-1 (NDM-1).

KPC expression has been detected in many *Enterobacteriaceae* including *E coli* and *Proteus*, as well as non-*Enterobacteriaceae* such as *Pseudomonas aeruginosa*. It was first identified in North Carolina in 2001, and since then, has become endemic in many hospitals in the North Eastern United States.[13] In addition to β-lactams, cephalosporins, and carbapenems, these bacteria typically show resistance to quinolones and aminoglycosides.[14] KPC resistance was believed to be isolated to the United States until it was identified in France in 2005 (in a patient recently hospitalized in the United States).[15] This enzyme is encoded by a transposon capable of insertion into diverse plasmids, thereby providing rapid and interspecies transmission.[13] Another worrisome realization is that resistance detection by standard methods is not reliable. Sensitivity testing to meropenem and imipenem is inadequate to evaluate for in vitro carbapenem resistance,[13] because some carrier organisms remain in the susceptible range by in vitro testing. Ertapenem testing has shown better sensitivity than the other carbapenems. Those with increased minimum inhibitory concentrations (MICs) to carbapenems should be tested using the modified Hodge test for further resistance characterization.[14] However, this specialized technique is challenging to perform, and it is possible that many laboratories do not detect KPC expression.

NDM-1 was first recognized in a patient hospitalized in New Delhi, India in 2007.[16] Most cases since that time have been linked in some way to the Indian subcontinent, where prevalence estimates range from 5% to 18%. By August 2010, the resistance was found worldwide, with the exception of Central and South America.[17] By June 2012, a total of 13 cases had been reported in the United States.[16] Organisms with NDM-1 expression are usually sensitive to colistin and may be sensitive to tigecycline and fosfomycin.[17] The NDM-1 gene is transmitted on a variety of plasmids, some highly mobile, even between distantly related gram-negative organisms.[17] Bacterium with NDM resistance can colonize hosts and contaminate water and environmental surfaces.[18]

Regardless of the mechanisms involved, resistance patterns continue to change, in patterns that are geographically distinct and dynamic.[5] For example, overall *E coli* drug resistance is higher in Portugal and Spain when compared with Northern European nations and Canada.[4] There is a pressing need for a unified national American drug resistance surveillance system. One effort, the National Antimicrobial Resistance Monitoring System (available at http://www.NARMS.com), a coalition between the US Centers for Disease Control, Food and Drug Administration (FDA), and Department of Agriculture, monitors the resistance patterns of enteric bacteria cultured from humans and animals. However, this group is largely focused on food-borne illness, and is underfunded to investigate patterns of gram-negative resistance as they pertain to UTI.

Defining one's local resistance patterns is even more difficult. Many hospitals monitor resistance of organisms cultured in their microbiology laboratory. These data may reflect drug-exposed, hospital-acquired organisms more than community-acquired, outpatient-based illnesses. Thus, hospital antibiograms likely overestimate community resistance patterns.[19,20] However, the IDSA recommends avoiding antimicrobial agents when local resistance exceeds 20%,[7] implying that primary care providers should be familiar with local outpatient resistance patterns. We hope that local health departments will collaborate with outpatient providers and their laboratories to create local ambulatory antibiograms.

EVALUATION

Your patient is calling on Friday afternoon with her usual UTI symptoms. She does not have fevers, back pain, nausea or vomiting. Can empirical treatment be started? Should you obtain a urinalysis or culture before treatment?

Urine culture remains the gold standard to confirm suspected UTI, but bacterial colony count and resistance patterns require more than 24 hours of analysis, and therefore a probable diagnosis must be made by history, examination, and point-of-care diagnostics. Symptoms of dysuria, frequency, hematuria, nocturia, and urgency all increase the probability of UTI, with likelihood ratios between 1.10 and 1.72, whereas vaginal discharge decreases the likelihood of UTI (**Table 1**).[21]

Dipstick analysis is a quick and cheap diagnostic tool. But is it reliable? The positive predictive value is substantial in the setting of both positive leukocyte esterase (LE) and nitrite, but these tests are limited by low sensitivity, and therefore a low negative predictive value as well (**Table 2**).[22] For example, not all uropathogens can convert nitrate into nitrite. With limited negative predictive values, UTI may be difficult to rule out even when all features are negative.[22,23] Dipstick-positive hematuria has been shown to increase the likelihood for UTI and is additive with a positive nitrite.[21] Symptom-based evaluation provides only modest positive predictive value, whereas urine dipstick analysis is unable to effectively rule out UTI when there is moderate clinical suspicion.

Definitive diagnosis of cystitis can be made only with clinical symptoms and bacteriuria. IDSA guidelines recommend a colony-forming unit level of 10^5 or greater as diagnostic of UTI.[7] However, colony counts of 10^2 have shown improved sensitivity and retained specificity among symptomatic women.[24]

In some settings, empirical treatment has been found to be cost-effective and to reduce overall symptom duration when compared with dipstick and culture evaluations.[25] Guidelines have been proposed to help providers reduce expense and inconvenience to patients. **Fig. 1** represents 1 such guideline modified to reflect concerns regarding resistance. These guidelines have reduced the use of urinalysis, cultures,

Table 1
The accuracy of symptoms for diagnosis of UTI

Symptom	Sensitivity	Specificity	Positive Likelihood Ratio	Negative Likelihood Ratio
Dysuria	0.78	0.36	1.22 (1.11–1.34)	0.61 (0.50–0.74)
Frequency	0.90	0.17	1.09 (1.02–1.16)	0.58 (0.32–0.79)
Urgency	0.75	0.36	1.17 (1.04–1.31)	0.70 (0.57–0.86)
Fever	0.10	0.89	0.90 (0.45–1.80)	1.01 (0.93–1.10)
Vaginal discharge[a]			0.65 (0.51–0.83)	1.10 (1.01–1.20)
Hematuria[b]			1.68 (1.06–2.66)	0.89 (0.82–0.98)

[a] Based on $\geq 10^2$ CFU/mL.
[b] Based on $\geq 10^3$ CFU/mL.
Adapted from Giesen LG, Cousins G, Dimitrov BD, et al. Predicting acute uncomplicated urinary tract infection in women: a systematic review of the diagnostic accuracy of symptoms and signs. BMC Fam Pract 2010;11:78.

Table 2
The accuracy of dipstick for diagnosis of UTI

Dipstick	Sensitivity	Specificity	Positive Likelihood Ratio	Negative Likelihood Ratio
Positive LE[a]	0.62	0.70	2.01	0.54
Positive nitrite[b]	0.50	0.82	2.78	0.61
Positive LE or nitrate[b]	0.75	0.70	2.50	0.36
Both LE and nitrate positive[b]	0.45	0.99	45	0.56

Likelihood ratios calculated from published data.
  [a] Nonurologic population.
  [b] General population.
  Data from Deville WL, Yzermans JC, Van Duijn NP, et al. The urine dipstick test useful to rule out infections. A meta-analysis of the accuracy. BMC Urol 2004;4:4.

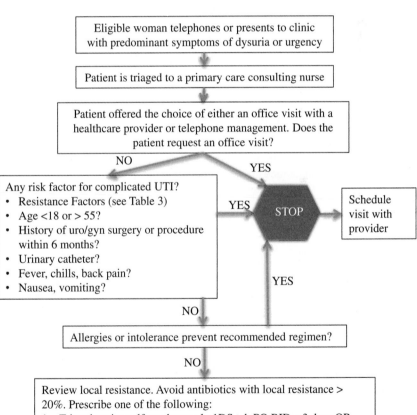

Fig. 1. Evaluation and management of acute, uncomplicated UTI. (*Adapted and modified from* Sanjay S, Scholes D, Fihn SD, et al. The effectiveness of a clinical practice guideline for the management of presumed uncomplicated urinary tract infection in women. Am J Med 1999;106(6):638.)

and office visits and have increased use of recommended antibiotics.[26,27] Cystitis is one of the few, if not the only, infectious diseases in which telephone triage antibiotic prescribing has been shown to be an acceptable option. In indeterminate cases, dipstick or culture should be used to assist with making the diagnosis and reducing antibiotic use for inappropriate cases. Culture is recommended if pyelonephritis is suspected or if the individual patient is at higher risk for resistance.

In cases in which the diagnosis remains unclear, it may be appropriate to delay initiation of antibiotics. In this scenario, the patient submits a urine culture, which is monitored for 48 hours. If positive, a prescription is provided. In a randomized, controlled trial evaluating this approach, patients in the delayed antibiotics arm received antibiotics less often, although those who ruled in for UTI had symptoms for 37% longer than those in the immediate arm. The severity of symptoms was not of significant increased severity in either arm, and there was no increased progression to pyelonephritis among those in the delayed arm.[28]

Because geographic resistance is difficult to estimate, many studies have examined individual factors believed to be predictive for development of resistant UTI. These factors include age older than 60 years,[29,30] recent international travel,[31] previous history of a UTI,[6] chronic medical conditions,[5,6] recent hospitalization,[8] and any recent antibiotic course[6,8,32] (with more recent treatment portraying a higher risk of resistance).[6] Risk factors should be considered when using empirical treatment guidelines (**Box 1**) and when they are present, urine culture should be considered before antibiotic start.

TREATMENT: RECOMMENDED DRUG AND COURSE

In choosing the best antimicrobial agent for uncomplicated cystitis, prescribers must take into account a patient's treatment history, allergies or intolerances, pregnancy or breastfeeding status, insurance coverage, and drug interactions. Because side effects vary by agent, these should be taken into account as applicable. Please see **Table 3**.

Nitrofurantoin

Nitrofurantoin is an inactive antiseptic that is largely activated in the urine by microbes. It is produced in 3 formulations that vary by crystal preparation. The smaller crystalline form of nitrofurantoin (Furadatin), is rapidly absorbed, leading to gastrointestinal (GI) upset, and thus it is rarely used.[33] Macrocrystalline nitrofurantoin (Macrodantin), a larger molecule, is more slowly absorbed. The third formulation, monohydrate macrocrystals, also known as modified-release nitrofurantoin (Macrobid), is composed of

---

Box 1
Risk factors for UTI caused by a resistant organism

Risk Factors for Antimicrobial Resistance

- Age older than 60 years
- Previous history of UTI
- Chronic medical conditions
- Recent hospitalization
- Any recent antibiotic treatment
- Recent travel abroad

Table 3
Commonly used antimicrobial agents and regimens

Drug	Dosing	Side Effects	Other Considerations	Pregnancy Class	Breastfeeding American Academy of Pediatrics[47]/LactMed[39]	Price
Nitrofurantoin	100 mg by mouth twice a day × 5 d	Nausea, vomiting, diarrhea, hypersensitivity reactions including hepatitis	Rare cases of pulmonary fibrosis in long term use	B[a,b]	Hemolysis with glucose-6-phosphate dehydrogenase (G-6PD)-deficient infant/avoid <1 mo old or G-6PD-deficient	100-mg tablets, 20, $70
Trimethoprim-sulfamethoxazole	1 double strength tablet by mouth twice a day × 3 d	Nausea, vomiting, rash including Stevens-Johnson-syndrome in rare cases	Increased bleeding risk with warfarin. Risk of hyperkalemia with low glomerular filtration rate or when combined with angiotensin-converting enzyme inhibitor, angiotensin receptor blockers, aldosterone antagonist. Multiple drug interactions	C[b]	None reported/avoid in ill or premature infants	800-mg to 160-mg tablets, 20, $4
Fosfomycin	3 g by mouth × 1	Nausea, diarrhea, vaginitis	After treatment improvement in symptoms over a few days should be expected	B	Not applicable/limited data, avoid <2 mo old	3-g tablet, 1, $80
Ciprofloxacin	250 mg by mouth twice a day × 3 d	Nausea, vomiting, headache	Risk of Clostridium difficile colitis and tendon rupture in those using corticosteroids	C	None reported/little risk	500-mg tablets, 100, $4 1000-mg XL tablets, 50, $465[c]

[a] Contraindicated at term.
[b] American College of Obstetricians and Gynecologists recommends using during first trimester only if no other options.[36]
[c] Prices estimated at http://www.target.com, http://www.walmart.com, and http://www.drugstore.com.

approximately 75% nitrofurantoin monohydrate and 25% macrocrystal, which produce a slow-release preparation by forming a gel matrix in the stomach.[34] The bioavailability is increased when taken with food.[34]

As a result of brisk renal excretion, blood levels rarely reach a therapeutic level, thus reducing effectiveness and making this drug not suitable in pyelonephritis, perinephric abscess, or prostatitis. The rate of clearance is proportional to the creatinine clearance, and dose adjustments are necessary with renal impairment.[35] The urinary excretion of modified-release nitrofurantoin is similar to that of macrocrystalline nitrufurantoin.[34]

The most common adverse effects of using nitrofurantoin are GI in origin, including nausea, vomiting, and diarrhea[35]; the macrocrystalline preparations are better tolerated.[33,35] Nitrofurantoin may color the urine brown. Less common side effects include several hypersensitivity reactions characterized by chills, fever, blood cell dyscrasias, and hepatitis, all of which are treated by discontinuation of the drug. Nerve effects have been reported, with neuropathies being most common in patients with chronic kidney disease. Acute pneumonitis is reported as a rare effect also treated by drug removal.[35]

Chronic nitrofurantoin pulmonary toxicity rates are difficult to estimate but are believed to be rare. For example, chronic lung reactions related to nitrofurantoin were 2.0%, 5.3%, and 3.4% of all adverse reactions reported in the United Kingdom, Sweden, and Holland, respectively, over approximately 3 decades.[36] In a Mayo Clinic retrospective review of cases believed to be secondary to nitrofurantoin, most subjects were women (94%), older (median age of 72 years), and patients who had received a prolonged preventative dosing exposure (median interval of 23 months).[37]

Nitrofurantoin has been associated with a variety of fetal malformations when used in the first trimester. The American College of Obstetricians and Gynecologists recommends using a different agent during this time if an alternative is available.[38] It is also recommended to avoid nitrofurantoin use between 38 weeks' gestation and delivery because of the possibility of hemolytic anemia.[34] Data are limited, but use seems safe for breastfeeding infants older than 1 month and without glucose-6-phosphate dehydrogenase deficiency.[39]

Nitrofurantoin has few drug interactions, probably because of reliance on microbial activation. However, an alternative therapy should be considered when fluconazole is used, because of reports of hepatic and pulmonary toxicity.[40] Antacids containing magnesium may also reduce absorption and subsequent urinary secretion.[34]

Microbes rarely produce new resistance to nitrofurantoin, making this an excellent choice when considering emerging resistance. However, the less common *Proteus*, *Pseudomonas*, *Enterobacter*, and *Klebsiella* species are usually inherently resistant.[35]

The efficacy of nitrofurantoin compared with other antimicrobials has been studied. When compared with 3 days of low-dose ciprofloxacin, ciprofloxacin showed higher bladder eradication rates but similar rates of clinical resolution.[41] No difference in outcomes was found when a 5-day course of nitrofurantoin was compared with a 7-day course of trimethoprim-sulfamethoxazole.[42]

Trimethoprim-Sulfamethoxazole

Trimethoprim-sulfamethoxazole (cotrimoxazole, Bactrim, Septra) was first introduced as a combination drug in the 1970s. It inhibits bacterial production of folate at 2 separate steps, causing a bacteriostatic effect. Trimethoprim-sulfamethoxazole is readily absorbed from the GI tract, has a half-life of approximately 10 hours, and is renally excreted between 25% and 60% in the first 24 hours.[35]

Adverse effects of trimethoprim-sulfamethoxazole are variable, but most commonly include GI upset and rash, which vary from transient eruptions to fixed drug reactions to catastrophic exfoliative syndromes (Stevens-Johnson syndrome and toxic epidermal necrolysis). Trimethoprim-sulfamethoxazole can cause a variety of anemias, some related to folate deficiency, as well as thrombocytopenia and rarely methemoglobinemia.[35]

Hyperkalemia may be a concern when prescribing trimethoprim-sulfamethoxazole. It is caused by a reduction in potassium elimination from the distal nephron and is potentiated by reduction in glomerular filtration rate, concomitant use of angiotensin-converting-enzyme inhibitors, angiotensin receptor blockers, or aldosterone blockers.[43] Elderly individuals are at greatest risk for hyperkalemia caused by trimethoprim-sulfamethoxazole. Severe hyperkalemia (>5.5 mmol/L) was found in 21% of treated hospitalized patients,[44] but less often in a prospective controlled trial of outpatients, among whom only 6% developed severe hyperkalemia after a 5-day course.[45]

Trimethoprim-sulfamethoxazole deserves special mention with regards to drug interactions. Both components inhibit separate P450 enzymes, leading to multiple interactions. The drug inhibits warfarin metabolism and is associated with a 3-fold higher risk of GI bleeding when used in combination with warfarin compared with use of other antibiotics.[46] Other interactions include sulfonylureas (hypoglycemia),[35,43] methotrexate (pancytopenia), and anticonvulsants (toxicity).[35]

When used in the first trimester of pregnancy, trimethoprim-sulfamethoxazole has been shown to be associated with rare cases of neural tube, cardiovascular, and possibly oral cleft palate and urinary system defects. After 32 weeks' gestation, a theoretic risk of fetal kernicterus exists and so the drug should be avoided if possible.[43] It seems to be safe during breastfeeding.[43,47]

Resistance mechanisms can occur by chromosomal mutation and selection but are largely based on plasmids, likely leading to the known distinct regional resistance patterns.[35] For example, in the ECO-SENS study evaluating European *E coli* resistance, trimethoprim-sulfamethoxazole resistance was found in 26.7% of uncomplicated UTIs in Portugal but only in 9.5% in Austria.[4]

Trials comparing trimethoprim-sulfamethoxazole with other antimicrobials for UTI treatment have shown similar efficacy to nitrofurantoin,[41] ciprofloxacin,[41] and fosfomycin.[48]

Fosfomycin

Fosfomycin is an inhibitor of cell wall synthesis, structurally unrelated to any other antibiotic,[49] and is active against most urinary tract pathogens.[21] It is approximately 40% bioavailable with a 4-hour half-life. The active drug is renally excreted, with excellent urinary concentrations, exceeding most MICs for pathogens.[49,50]

Fosfomycin is approved for a single 3-g dose in uncomplicated UTI.[49,51] With such dosing, no dose adjustment is needed for patients with renal or hepatic dysfunction.[52] Side effects of single 3-g dosing are typically mild and resolve within 1 to 2 days, and include diarrhea, nausea, abdominal pain, headache, dizziness, and vaginitis.[51] In a review of more than 800 patients,[53] side effects occurred in only 6.1% of patients and none was considered severe. Patients should be counseled that urinary symptoms slowly improve over 2 to 3 days, even after a single dose, and that this is not necessarily a sign of failure.[54]

Drug interactions are few, but include balsalazide and metoclopramide, the latter of which when used with fosfomycin may decrease fosfomycin serum and urinary concentrations.[52]

Fosfomycin is safe in pregnancy.[49] The drug is likely excreted in low levels in breast milk, but limited data suggest safety with breastfeeding.[39]

Resistance to fosfomycin is rare,[54] but when present, it is caused by decreased drug transport into the bacterium[50] and enzymatic modification of the drug.[52] Furthermore, many species resistant to other antibiotics, including ESBL-producing *E coli*, are susceptible to fosfomycin.[55]

Single-dose fosfomycin has been compared with a 7-day course of nitrofurantoin and a 5-day course of trimethoprim-sulfamethoxazole. Clinical efficacy was similar between trimethoprim-sulfamethoxazole and single-dose fosfomycin.[48] When fosfomycin was compared with nitrofurantoin, rates of clinical cure (resolution of symptoms) were similar for both treatments. Despite similar early clinical response rates, the microbiological cure rates (resolution of bacteriuria) at the first follow-up visit were lower for fosfomycin (78%) than nitrofurantoin (86%).[56] The drug costs about $80 for treatment course, which is more expensive than the other first-line agents (trimethoprim-sulfamethoxazole and nitrofurantoin). It is also not so easily available, because many pharmacy chains do not carry it.

Fluoroquinolones

Ciprofloxacin and levofloxacin, both fluorinated quinolones, are commonly (and often inappropriately) used for empirical UTI treatment.[10] The bactericidal effects of the drugs come from targeting DNA gyrase and topoisomerase IV.[35] Fluoroquinolones are well absorbed orally, have a half-life of about 4 hours, and are time-dependent and concentration-dependent agents.[35] Given this pharmacokinetic picture, once-daily extended release formations of ciprofloxacin have been found to be equally efficacious to twice-daily[57] dosing, but at a increased price. Ciprofloxacin is largely renally excreted and can lead to increased urinary concentrations.[35]

Side effects are most commonly GI in origin, with up to 17% of patients having nausea or other form of discomfort. Of the fluoroquinolones, ciprofloxacin is the most likely to cause *Clostridium difficile* colitis. Other common side effects include those of the central nervous system (mild headache to rarely seizure, usually when used with theophylline or nonsteroidal antiinflammatory drugs) and rash. Corrected QT interval (QTc) prolongation is usually associated with other drugs in the same class,[35] but should probably be avoided in patients using other prolonging agents or with a history of QTc disorder.

Fluoroquinolones have long been known to cause tendon rupture. However, this effect is rare. In a case control study,[58] it occurred in approximately 3.2 cases per 1000 and only in patients older than 60 years. Use of corticosteroids was found to be a risk factor for rupture. It is advisable to counsel all patients regarding this risk and to ask them to discontinue treatment and contact their physician with any unexpected tendon or joint pain, especially at the Achilles tendon. Ciprofloxacin is contraindicated in pregnancy because of the risk of fetal arthropathy.[35,59] A review performed by the American Academy of Pediatrics found no evidence for adverse outcome with breastfeeding.[47]

The main drug interaction to recall is that ciprofloxacin can lead to an increase in theophylline levels and subsequent toxicity.[35] It can also lead to increases in international normalized ratio in patients on warfarin.

Resistance to fluoroquinolones occurs secondary to changes in the drug target or to increased drug efflux.[35] Resistance may be mediated by acquisition of genes via plasmids.[59] The increase in fluoroquinolone resistance in *E coli* has occurred at an alarming rate in relation to increased prescribing practices. For example, in the Denver Health System, when the preferred antibiotic for UTI was changed from trimethoprim-sulfamethoxazole to levofloxacin because of baseline trimethoprim-sulfamethoxazole resistance, the rate of levofloxacin-resistant isolates increased from 1% to 9% in 6 years.[8]

OTHER ANTIBIOTICS

Cefpodoxime has been used for treatment of UTI, given its tolerability and twice-daily dosing. However, cefpodoxime has been found to be inferior to ciprofloxacin[60] and equivalent to trimethoprim-sulfamethoxazole in a study with limited power,[61] questioning overall efficacy. Amoxicillin-clavulanate was compared with ciprofloxacin and found to be inferior, even in cases in which strains were sensitive to amoxicillin-clavulanate. As recommended by the IDSA guidelines, β-lactams should be avoided if possible to avoid resistance and reduce collateral damage.[7]

ORAL CONTRACEPTIVES AND ANTIBIOTICS

Patients with UTI are often women of childbearing age, many of whom rely on oral contraceptive pills (OCPs) for birth control, and so the question of antibiotic interactions with OCPs should be addressed openly. Although more than 200 articles have been published on this question, it is difficult to establish a firm interaction in most cases. Although certain antibiotics that heavily inhibit cytochrome 3A4 (in particular, rifampin) may be expected to increase OCP metabolism, these drugs are virtually never used for UTI. However, based on the serious nature of the consequences, and in light of some continued uncertainty, it is customary to counsel patients to consider using an alternative method of birth control in addition to continuing OCPs until 1 menstrual cycle has completed after antibiotic treatment.[62,63]

PREVENTION AND OTHER CONSIDERATIONS

Another patient recalls that she has had 3 UTIs in the last 12 months and asks about preventative methods, including continuous antibiotics, cranberry juice, and probiotics.

Recurrent UTIs

An estimated 26.6% of women with initial UTI have a recurrence within 6 months.[64] Women with a history of recurrent UTI have an average of 2.6 episodes per patient-year (varying from 0.3–7.6 episodes).[65] Recurrent episodes seem to cluster in time, with the highest risk of recurrence immediately after a previous event.[65]

At first diagnosis, hematuria and urgency may be strong predictors of recurrent UTI.[64] These investigators propose that this finding may indicate that the initial causal bacterium was particularly virulent. Compared with other organisms, when *E coli* caused a first UTI, recurrence was more likely.[66]

Risks for recurrent UTI are similar to those of first UTI. These risks include recent sexual intercourse,[66–68] new sexual partner,[67] and use of diaphragm, cervical cap, or spermicide.[66,69] Other risk factors include age younger than 15 years at the time of first UTI,[67] mother or family with history of UTI,[67,70] and history of previous UTI.[68,71]

Anatomic factors have been implicated. Women with a shorter urethra-anus distance have more frequent UTIs compared with those with longer measurements.[72] Studies have also looked at individual genetic variables, including Lewis blood group[73] and toll-like receptor polymorphisms[74] for further understanding of recurrent UTI susceptibility. These factors remain unproved and are not modifiable.

Behavior and Habits

Evidence of the relationship between habits and recurrent UTI is limited. Habits not associated with a change in recurrence rates include voiding after sexual intercourse,[64,67] delayed voiding,[67,68] wiping patterns, douching, use of hot tubs, or pantyhose.[67] Caution should be exercised when interpreting these data, because in such small trials, a small effect may not be realized until larger studies are performed.

Mode of Contraception

Contraception method is related to acquisition of UTI. Recent condom use, both lubricated and nonlubricated, with or without spermicidal cream or gel, was found to strongly increase the risk of a first and recurrent UTI.[75,76] Diaphragm use is also highly associated with both first and recurrent UTI.[3,66,68]

Spermicide

Spermicide use is associated with increased frequency of first and recurrent UTI.[67,75] Nonoxynol-9, the most commonly used spermicide, is toxic to lactobacilli, and in particular hydrogen peroxide (H_2O_2)-producing lactobacilli including *Lactobacillus crispatus*.[77] The toxic effect to lactobacilli is greater than its toxic effect to *E coli*[77] and may enhance *E coli* attachment to urogenital epithelial cells,[78] with spermicide users more likely to be colonized with *E coli* than nonusers.[79] Unless there are no other options, spermicides should be avoided.

Probiotics

The use of probiotics has become popular in the age of increasing antimicrobial use and resistance; however, no probiotic agent has been approved for therapeutic use by the FDA.[80] *Lactobacillus* has been shown to be safe in studies of generally immunocompetent hosts.[81] Evidence for the use of probiotics is diverse and inconsistent, but the proposed mechanisms for prevention of urogenital infection by probiotics include modulating host immunity, preventing adherence of pathogenic organisms to the urogenital epithelium,[82] and modulating growth/colonization of these pathogens.[81] When comparing patients with recurrent UTI with those without UTIs, patients with recurrent UTIs were less likely to be colonized with H_2O_2-producing strains of lactobacilli and more likely to have *E coli* introital colonization, even when controlling for use of spermicide.[83] However, in a 2008 review that evaluated 4 studies looking at the efficacy of *Lactobacillus* for prevention of UTI, only 1 study reported a positive effect (reduction in rate of recurrent UTI), but many were underpowered and used a variety of *Lactobacillus* strains, including those not shown to produce H_2O_2.[84] Most recently, Lactin-V, a product containing an H_2O_2-producing strain of *Lactobacillus crispatus*, was evaluated in a phase 2 clinical study.[85] When used vaginally once per week after antibiotic treatment of UTI, a relative risk reduction of 50% (95% confidence interval, 0.2–1.2) was shown, but the study included only 100 participants, and was likely underpowered to see a statistically significant benefit. In a randomized trial comparing low-H_2O_2-producing *Lactobacillus* and trimethoprim-sulfamethoxazole prophylaxis, the *Lactobacillus* was shown to be inferior to trimethoprim-sulfamethoxazole.[86] Until further evidence is available in larger, randomized trials, using *L crispatus*, probiotics cannot be conclusively recommended. However, they are unlikely to be harmful and may provide benefit to individual patients.

Cranberries

Cranberries are often used for UTI treatment and prevention. Cranberry extract has been shown both ex vivo and in vivo to interfere with *E coli* adherence to the uroepithelium.[87] Many trials have studied the use of cranberry in various forms and concentrations, but with mixed results. A 2012 Cochrane review, limited because of article diversity, calculated a risk reduction of 0.62, with women, children, and consumers of cranberry juice having the most observed benefit.[88] Most recently, a randomized controlled trial comparing cranberry juice and placebo found no difference in time to UTI; however, this study did note reduction of infections with P-fimbriated *E coli* strains in the cranberry group.[89] Cranberry has been shown to be inferior when compared with trimethoprim-sulfamethoxazole for prophylaxis.[90] Results are discouraging, although patients may safely choose to try cranberry; those who cannot tolerate the sugar and acidity of juice might try extract capsules instead, although again the supporting evidence has been underwhelming.

Urinary Additives

Methenamine salts are proposed to prevent UTI by producing formaldehyde from hexamine, leading to urinary acidification, and thus making the bladder more hostile to microbial invasion. Few large trials have evaluated the efficacy of these additives. The salts come in 2 forms: methenamine hippurate and methanamine mandelate; the latter is not widely available. Typically well tolerated, methenamine salts were examined by a Cochrane review in 2012. With great study heterogeneity, subgroup analysis showed a relative risk (RR) of 0.24 when used by patients without renal tract abnormalities, a finding not shown in patients with such abnormalities. Furthermore, treatment duration of 1 week showed an RR of recurrent UTI of 0.14.[91] These medications are generally well tolerated, although some women discontinued use because of a sensation of urethral burning caused by chemical irritation.

Estrogen for Postmenopausal Women

After menopause, women are believed to lose the UTI-protective benefits of estrogen, with resultant increases in vaginal pH[92] and decrease in introital *Lactobacillus* colonization,[93] among other effects. Investigations of estrogens to prevent recurrent UTI have varied by dose, route (oral vs vaginal), and control group (placebo vs antimicrobial). In a 2008 Cochrane review, oral estrogen replacement was not found to reduce recurrent UTI, whereas vaginal estrogens showed a reduced risk (RR of 0.25 and 0.64 in 2 trials). Studies comparing estrogen replacement with prophylactic antibiotics were again heterogeneous in design and showed conflicting results.[94] Topical estrogen treatment could be considered in motivated, postmenopausal women with recurrent UTIs, especially when the risk of prophylactic antibiotic use is high.

Evaluation of Recurrent UTIs

The purpose of recurrent UTI workup is to evaluate and eliminate any cause that might predispose the patient to morbidity related to recurrent UTIs. The workup should start with a thorough history, including possible predisposing factors, such as temporal relationship to intercourse and method of contraception. Symptoms such as vaginal discharge or odor may point toward an alternative diagnosis. The physical examination should focus on vaginal and urethral disease, and in particular uterine or rectal prolapse.[95] Residual urinary volume should be measured with either bladder ultrasonography or catheterization to rule out retention (**Fig. 2**).[96]

After these tests are completed, imaging may be considered, although in many cases, it yields no information to change management. Cystoscopic or radiologic evaluation should be considered in patients with complicated, persistent, or febrile infections.[95] Patients without fever, flank pain, or hematuria can usually be managed without imaging.[96] In a prospective study of 100 patients referred for urologic work

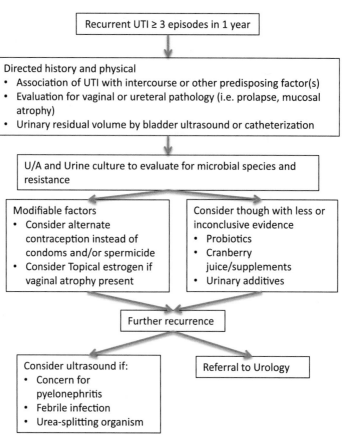

Fig. 2. Recommended management of women with recurrent cystitis.

up in the setting of UTI, the usefulness of imaging and subsequent findings was evaluated. Abdominal radiographs were performed in all 100 patients without an abnormal finding in any case. Renal ultrasonography was performed in 90 cases, with 5 abnormalities found, and in 16 intravenous urograms, 2 were abnormal. In total, 6 abnormalities were found, but only 1 was considered related to recurrent UTIs.[97] Those with pyelonephritis caused by urea-splitting organisms such as *Proteus vulgaris* should be considered for ultrasonography or plain radiography to rule out nephrolithiasis, because of the association between these bacteria and struvite calculi.[96]

Cystoscopy has been used in the evaluation of recurrent UTI to evaluate for structural abnormalities not found with imaging, such as urethral stricture, bladder calculus, or colovesicual fistula. In a study of 118 patients with recurrent UTI undergoing cystoscopy, all of whom had some form of previous imaging, only 8% of the women had a significant abnormality detected radiographically. Most of these abnormalities were in women older than 50 years. Furthermore, negative imaging before cystoscopy carried a negative predictive value of 99% for finding an abnormality.[98] Given these findings, in women without risk factors for structural abnormalities and with negative imaging, cystoscopy can usually be deferred. Furthermore, given the association of abnormal findings with age, it is likely not necessary to evaluate women younger than 40 years with cystoscopy.[97,98]

Antibiotic Prevention

When conservative, nonantimicrobial measures fail to prevent recurrent UTI, antibiotics are relied on. In a recent Cochrane review,[99] the effectiveness, safety and administration schemes of antibiotic prophylaxis were reviewed. This database defined recurrent UTI as 3 or more episodes within 1 year or 2 or more episodes within 6 months. Antibiotic prophylaxis prevented recurrence after treated UTIs with an RR of 0.21 and a number needed to treat to prevent 1 recurrence of 1.85. As expected, the rate of side effects was higher in the treatment group (RR 1.58 for severe side effects), with high dropout overall (exceeding 20% in some studies). Dropout was highest amongst the nitrofurantoin groups. After prophylaxis was discontinued, the protective effect was no longer evident. However, the investigators were unable to pose a best antibiotic, duration, or other mode because of the heterogeneity of the studies.

Prophylactic regimens are used in many schedules, including daily, weekly, monthly, and postcoital. With the pressure of antibiotic resistance, regimens with limited duration offer the benefit of less exposure. Postcoital administration of trimethoprim-sulfamethoxazole was more effective than placebo at preventing UTI (0.3 events per patient-year compared with 3.6 events per patient-year), although this was a small study,[100] and postcoital ciprofloxacin showed similar efficacy compared with daily administration in another study.[101]

Patient-initiated regimens have also been studied. In a randomized trial in 2011,[102] patients were randomized to continuous prophylaxis or patient-initiated treatment. The patient-initiated arm was instructed to take a single dose after an event known to be associated with recurrence in the individual's circumstance (eg, intercourse, delayed micturition, diarrhea). Groups had similar efficacy but fewer side effects in the patient-initiated arm (9.1%) compared with the continuous group (30%). Limitations of this study included inclusion of only postmenopausal women and a rotation of the continuous antibiotic every 2 to 4 weeks. Because recurrence is known to cluster near the time of initial UTI,[64,65] duration of prophylaxis might continue for 6 to 12 months, regardless of the method chosen.[99]

SUMMARY

In the era of increasing microbial resistance, caution should be taken when prescribing both for the individual patient's risk of resistant infection and for reducing community antimicrobial resistance. Practice guidelines have been shown to reduce cost and increase the rate of appropriate antibiotic use. Antibiotics with less potential for promoting resistance (nitrofurantoin, fosfomycin) should be used preferentially. Trimethoprim-sulfamethoxazole remains an important first-line agent in most settings. Fluoroquinolones and broad-spectrum antibiotics should be reserved as second-line agents. Some host factors may be modified to reduce risk of recurrence. Prophylactic antibiotics should be minimized and (if needed) used in a patient-initiated scheme.

REFERENCES

1. Schappert SM, Rechtsteiner EA. Ambulatory medical care utilization estimates for 2007. Vital Health Stat 13 2011;169:1–38.
2. Foxman B, Barlow R, D'Arcy H, et al. Urinary tract infection: self-reported incidence and associated costs. Ann Epidemiol 2000;10(8):509–15.

3. Foxman B, Frerichs RR. Epidemiology of urinary tract infection: I. Diaphragm use and sexual intercourse. Am J Public Health 1985;75(11):1308–13.

4. Kahlmeter G. An international survey of the antimicrobial susceptibility of pathogens from uncomplicated urinary tract infections: the ECO.SENS Project. J Antimicrob Chemother 2003;51(1):69–76.

5. Khawcharoenporn T, Vasoo S, Ward E, et al. High rates of quinolone resistance among urinary tract infections in the ED. Am J Emerg Med 2012;30(1):68–74.

6. Kahlmeter G, Poulsen HO. Antimicrobial susceptibility of Escherichia coli from community-acquired urinary tract infections in Europe: the ECO·SENS study revisited. Int J Antimicrob Agents 2012;39(1):45–51.

7. Gupta K, Hooton TM, Naber KG, et al. International clinical practice guidelines for the treatment of acute uncomplicated cystitis and pyelonephritis in women: a 2010 update by the Infectious Diseases Society of America and the European Society for Microbiology and Infectious Diseases. Clin Infect Dis 2011;52(5): e103–20.

8. Johnson L, Sabel A, Burman WJ, et al. Emergence of fluoroquinolone resistance in outpatient urinary Escherichia coli isolates. Am J Med 2008;121(10):876–84.

9. Grover ML, Bracamonte JD, Kanodia AK, et al. Assessing adherence to evidence-based guidelines for the diagnosis and management of uncomplicated urinary tract infection. Mayo Clin Proc 2007;82(2):181–5.

10. Kallen AJ, Welch HG, Sirovich BE. Current antibiotic therapy for isolated urinary tract infections in women. Arch Intern Med 2006;166(6):635–9.

11. Tenover FC. Mechanisms of antimicrobial resistance in bacteria. Am J Med 2006;119(6 Suppl 1):S3–10 [discussion: S62–70].

12. Opal S, Pop-Vicas A. Molecular mechanisms of antibiotic resistance in bacteria. In: Mandell, Douglas, and Bennet's principles and practice of infectious disease, vol. 1, 7th edition. Philadelphia: Churchill Livingstone Elsevier; 2010.

13. Arnold RS, Thom KA, Sharma S, et al. Emergence of Klebsiella pneumoniae carbapenemase-producing bacteria. Southampt Med J 2011;104(1):40–5.

14. Gupta N, Limbago BM, Patel JB, et al. Carbapenem-resistant Enterobacteriaceae: epidemiology and prevention. Clin Infect Dis 2011;53(1):60–7.

15. Naas T, Nordmann P, Vedel G, et al. Plasmid-mediated carbapenem-hydrolyzing -lactamase KPC in a Klebsiella pneumoniae isolate from France. Antimicrobial Agents Chemother 2005;49(10):4423–4.

16. Carbapenem-resistant Enterobacteriaceae containing New Delhi metallo-beta-lactamase in two patients–Rhode Island, March 2012. Available at: http://www.cdc.gov/mmwr/preview/mmwrhtml/mm6124a3.htm. Accessed December 27, 2012.

17. Nordmann P, Poirel L, Walsh TR, et al. The emerging NDM carbapenemases. Trends Microbiol 2011;19(12):588–95.

18. Wilson ME, Chen LH. NDM-1 and the role of travel in its dissemination. Curr Infect Dis Rep 2012;14(3):213–26.

19. Miller LG, Tang AW. Treatment of uncomplicated urinary tract infections in an era of increasing antimicrobial resistance. Mayo Clin Proc 2004;79(8):1048–53 [quiz: 1053–4].

20. Richards DA, Toop LJ, Chambers ST, et al. Antibiotic resistance in uncomplicated urinary tract infection: problems with interpreting cumulative resistance rates from local community laboratories. N Z Med J 2002;115(1146):12–4.

21. Giesen LG, Cousins G, Dimitrov BD, et al. Predicting acute uncomplicated urinary tract infection in women: a systematic review of the diagnostic accuracy of symptoms and signs. BMC Fam Pract 2010;11:78.

22. Devillé WL, Yzermans JC, Van Duijn NP, et al. The urine dipstick test useful to rule out infections. A meta-analysis of the accuracy. BMC Urol 2004;4:4.

23. Little P, Turner S, Rumsby K, et al. Validating the prediction of lower urinary tract infection in primary care: sensitivity and specificity of urinary dipsticks and clinical scores in women. Br J Gen Pract 2010;60(576):495–500.

24. Kunin CM, White LV, Hua TH. A reassessment of the importance of "low-count" bacteriuria in young women with acute urinary symptoms. Ann Intern Med 1993; 119(6):454–60.

25. Fenwick EA, Briggs AH, Hawke CI. Management of urinary tract infection in general practice: a cost-effectiveness analysis. Br J Gen Pract 2000;50(457):635–9.

26. Saint S, Scholes D, Fihn SD, et al. The effectiveness of a clinical practice guideline for the management of presumed uncomplicated urinary tract infection in women. Am J Med 1999;106(6):636–41.

27. O'Connor PJ, Solberg LI, Christianson J, et al. Mechanism of action and impact of a cystitis clinical practice guideline on outcomes and costs of care in an HMO. Jt Comm J Qual Improv 1996;22(10):673–82.

28. Little P, Moore MV, Turner S, et al. Effectiveness of five different approaches in management of urinary tract infection: randomised controlled trial. BMJ 2010; 340:c199.

29. Vellinga A, Murphy AW, Hanahoe B, et al. A multilevel analysis of trimethoprim and ciprofloxacin prescribing and resistance of uropathogenic Escherichia coli in general practice. J Antimicrob Chemother 2010;65(7):1514–20.

30. Zhanel GG, Hisanaga TL, Laing NM, et al. Antibiotic resistance in Escherichia coli outpatient urinary isolates: final results from the North American Urinary Tract Infection Collaborative Alliance (NAUTICA). Int J Antimicrob Agents 2006;27(6):468–75.

31. Colgan R, Johnson JR, Kuskowski M, et al. Risk factors for trimethoprim-sulfamethoxazole resistance in patients with acute uncomplicated cystitis. Antimicrobial Agents Chemother 2008;52(3):846–51.

32. Vellinga A, Tansey S, Hanahoe B, et al. Trimethoprim and ciprofloxacin resistance and prescribing in urinary tract infection associated with Escherichia coli: a multilevel model. J Antimicrob Chemother 2012;67(10):2523–30.

33. Brumfitt W, Hamilton-Miller JM. Efficacy and safety profile of long-term nitrofurantoin in urinary infections: 18 years' experience. J Antimicrob Chemother 1998;42(3):363–71.

34. MACROBID (nitrofurantoin monohydrate and nitrofurantoin, macrocrystalline) capsule [Procter and Gamble Pharmaceuticals, Inc.]. Daily Med Current Medication Information. Available at: http://dailymed.nlm.nih.gov/dailymed/lookup.cfm?setid=1971e893-5fdb-41e3-a1e9-5e52deed03d1. Accessed December 5, 2012.

35. Petri W. Goodman & Gilman's the pharmacological basis of therapeutics. 12th edition. New York: McGraw-Hill; 2011.

36. Penn RG, Griffin JP. Adverse reactions to nitrofurantoin in the United Kingdom, Sweden, and Holland. Br Med J (Clin Res Ed) 1982;284(6327):1440–2.

37. Mendez JL, Nadrous HF, Hartman TE, et al. Chronic nitrofurantoin-induced lung disease. Mayo Clin Proc 2005;80(10):1298–302.

38. ACOG Committee Opinion No. 494. Sulfonamides, nitrofurantoin, and risk of birth defects. Obstet Gynecol 2011;117(6):1484–5.

39. LactMed. Drugs and lactation database. 2010. Available at: http://toxnet.nlm.nih.gov/cgi-bin/sis/search/f?./temp/~v5mwMX:1. Accessed December 5, 2012.

40. Linnebur SA, Parnes BL. Pulmonary and hepatic toxicity due to nitrofurantoin and fluconazole treatment. Ann Pharmacother 2004;38(4):612–6.

41. Iravani A, Klimberg I, Briefer C, et al. A trial comparing low-dose, short-course ciprofloxacin and standard 7 day therapy with co-trimoxazole or nitrofurantoin in the treatment of uncomplicated urinary tract infection. J Antimicrob Chemother 1999;43(Suppl A):67–75.

42. Gupta K, Hooton TM, Roberts PL, et al. Short-course nitrofurantoin for the treatment of acute uncomplicated cystitis in women. Arch Intern Med 2007;167(20):2207–12.

43. Ho JM, Juurlink DN. Considerations when prescribing trimethoprim-sulfamethoxazole. CMAJ 2011;183(16):1851–8.

44. Alappan R, Perazella MA, Buller GK. Hyperkalemia in hospitalized patients treated with trimethoprim-sulfamethoxazole. Ann Intern Med 1996;124(3):316–20.

45. Alappan R, Buller GK, Perazella MA. Trimethoprim-sulfamethoxazole therapy in outpatients: is hyperkalemia a significant problem? Am J Nephrol 1999;19(3):389–94.

46. Fischer HD, Juurlink DN, Mamdani MM, et al. Hemorrhage during warfarin therapy associated with cotrimoxazole and other urinary tract anti-infective agents: a population-based study. Arch Intern Med 2010;170(7):617–21.

47. Ressel G. AAP updates statement for transfer of drugs and other chemicals into breast milk. American Academy of Pediatrics. Am Fam Physician 2002;65(5):979–80.

48. Minassian MA, Lewis DA, Chattopadhyay D, et al. A comparison between single-dose fosfomycin trometamol (Monuril) and a 5-day course of trimethoprim in the treatment of uncomplicated lower urinary tract infection in women. Int J Antimicrob Agents 1998;10(1):39–47.

49. Deck D, Winston L. Beta-Lactam and other cell wall- and membrane-active antibiotics. In: Basic & clinical pharmacology. 12th edition. New York: McGraw-Hill; 2012.

50. Trevor A, Katzunk B, Masters S. Beta-Lactam antibiotics and other cell wall synthesis inhibitors. In: Pharmacology: examination and board review. 9th edition. New York: McGraw-Hill; 2010.

51. Patel SS, Balfour JA, Bryson HM. Fosfomycin tromethamine. A review of its antibacterial activity, pharmacokinetic properties and therapeutic efficacy as a single-dose oral treatment for acute uncomplicated lower urinary tract infections. Drugs 1997;53(4):637–56.

52. Michalopoulos AS, Livaditis IG, Gougoutas V. The revival of fosfomycin. Int J Infect Dis 2011;15(11):e732–9.

53. Naber KG. Fosfomycin trometamol in treatment of uncomplicated lower urinary tract infections in adult women–an overview. Infection 1992;20(Suppl 4):S310–2.

54. Reeves DS. Fosfomycin trometamol. J Antimicrob Chemother 1994;34(6):853–8.

55. Falagas ME, Kastoris AC, Kapaskelis AM, et al. Fosfomycin for the treatment of multidrug-resistant, including extended-spectrum beta-lactamase producing, Enterobacteriaceae infections: a systematic review. Lancet Infect Dis 2010;10(1):43–50.

56. Stein GE. Comparison of single-dose fosfomycin and a 7-day course of nitrofurantoin in female patients with uncomplicated urinary tract infection. Clin Ther 1999;21(11):1864–72.

57. Henry DC Jr, Bettis RB, Riffer E, et al. Comparison of once-daily extended-release ciprofloxacin and conventional twice-daily ciprofloxacin for the treatment of uncomplicated urinary tract infection in women. Clin Ther 2002;24(12):2088–104.

58. Van der Linden PD, Sturkenboom MC, Herings RM, et al. Fluoroquinolones and risk of Achilles tendon disorders: case-control study. BMJ 2002;324(7349): 1306–7.
59. Deck D, Winston L. Sulfonamides, trimethoprim, quinolones. In: Basic and clinical pharmacology. 12th edition. New York: McGraw-Hill; 2012.
60. Hooton TM, Roberts PL, Stapleton AE. Cefpodoxime vs ciprofloxacin for short-course treatment of acute uncomplicated cystitis: a randomized trial. JAMA 2012;307(6):583–9.
61. Kavatha D, Giamarellou H, Alexiou Z, et al. Cefpodoxime-proxetil versus trimethoprim-sulfamethoxazole for short-term therapy of uncomplicated acute cystitis in women. Antimicrobial Agents Chemother 2003;47(3):897–900.
62. Horn J, Hansten P. Drug interactions: absence of proof is not proof of absence. Pharmacy Times 2010;46.
63. Dickinson B, Altman R, Nielsen N, et al. Drug interactions between oral contraceptives and antibiotics. Obstet Gynecol 2001;98(5 Pt 1):853–60.
64. Foxman B. Recurring urinary tract infection: incidence and risk factors. Am J Public Health 1990;80(3):331–3.
65. Stamm WE, McKevitt M, Roberts PL, et al. Natural history of recurrent urinary tract infections in women. Rev Infect Dis 1991;13(1):77–84.
66. Foxman B, Gillespie B, Koopman J, et al. Risk factors for second urinary tract infection among college women. Am J Epidemiol 2000;151(12):1194–205.
67. Scholes D, Hooton TM, Roberts PL, et al. Risk factors for recurrent urinary tract infection in young women. J Infect Dis 2000;182(4):1177–82.
68. Hooton TM, Scholes D, Hughes JP, et al. A prospective study of risk factors for symptomatic urinary tract infection in young women. N Engl J Med 1996;335(7): 468–74.
69. Fihn SD, Latham RH, Roberts P, et al. Association between diaphragm use and urinary tract infection. JAMA 1985;254(2):240–5.
70. Scholes D, Hawn TR, Roberts PL, et al. Family history and risk of recurrent cystitis and pyelonephritis in women. J Urol 2010;184(2):564–9.
71. Ikäheimo R, Siitonen A, Heiskanen T, et al. Recurrence of urinary tract infection in a primary care setting: analysis of a 1-year follow-up of 179 women. Clin Infect Dis 1996;22(1):91–9.
72. Hooton TM, Stapleton AE, Roberts PL, et al. Perineal anatomy and urine-voiding characteristics of young women with and without recurrent urinary tract infections. Clin Infect Dis 1999;29(6):1600–1.
73. Sheinfeld J, Schaeffer AJ, Cordon-Cardo C, et al. Association of the Lewis blood-group phenotype with recurrent urinary tract infections in women. N Engl J Med 1989;320(12):773–7.
74. Hawn TR, Scholes D, Li SS, et al. Toll-like receptor polymorphisms and susceptibility to urinary tract infections in adult women. PLoS One 2009;4(6): e5990.
75. Foxman B, Marsh J, Gillespie B, et al. Condom use and first-time urinary tract infection. Epidemiology 1997;8(6):637–41.
76. Stamatiou C, Bovis C, Panagopoulos P, et al. Sex-induced cystitis–patient burden and other epidemiological features. Clin Exp Obstet Gynecol 2005; 32(3):180–2.
77. McGroarty JA, Tomeczek L, Pond DG, et al. Hydrogen peroxide production by *Lactobacillus* species: correlation with susceptibility to the spermicidal compound nonoxynol-9. J Infect Dis 1992;165(6):1142–4.

78. Hooton TM, Fennell CL, Clark AM, et al. Nonoxynol-9: differential antibacterial activity and enhancement of bacterial adherence to vaginal epithelial cells. J Infect Dis 1991;164(6):1216–9.

79. Klebanoff SJ. Effects of the spermicidal agent nonoxynol-9 on vaginal microbial flora. J Infect Dis 1992;165(1):19–25.

80. US Food and Drug Administration. Drug approvals and databases. Available at: http://www.fda.gov/Drugs/InformationOnDrugs/default.htm. Accessed November 9, 2012.

81. Falagas ME, Betsi GI, Tokas T, et al. Probiotics for prevention of recurrent urinary tract infections in women: a review of the evidence from microbiological and clinical studies. Drugs 2006;66(9):1253–61.

82. Karlsson M, Scherbak N, Khalaf H, et al. Substances released from probiotic *Lactobacillus rhamnosus* GR-1 potentiate NF-κB activity in *Escherichia coli*-stimulated urinary bladder cells. FEMS Immunol Med Microbiol 2012;66(2): 147–56.

83. Gupta K, Stapleton AE, Hooton TM, et al. Inverse association of H2O2-producing lactobacilli and vaginal *Escherichia coli* colonization in women with recurrent urinary tract infections. J Infect Dis 1998;178(2):446–50.

84. Barrons R, Tassone D. Use of *Lactobacillus* probiotics for bacterial genitourinary infections in women: a review. Clin Ther 2008;30(3):453–68.

85. Stapleton AE, Au-Yeung M, Hooton TM, et al. Randomized, placebo-controlled phase 2 trial of a *Lactobacillus crispatus* probiotic given intravaginally for prevention of recurrent urinary tract infection. Clin Infect Dis 2011;52(10):1212–7.

86. Beerepoot MA, Ter Riet G, Nys S, et al. Lactobacilli vs antibiotics to prevent urinary tract infections: a randomized, double-blind, noninferiority trial in postmenopausal women. Arch Intern Med 2012;172(9):704–12.

87. Tempera G, Corsello S, Genovese C, et al. Inhibitory activity of cranberry extract on the bacterial adhesiveness in the urine of women: an ex-vivo study. Int J Immunopathol Pharmacol 2010;23(2):611–8.

88. Wang CH, Fang CC, Chen NC, et al. Cranberry-containing products for prevention of urinary tract infections in susceptible populations: a systematic review and meta-analysis of randomized controlled trials. Arch Intern Med 2012; 172(13):988–96.

89. Stapleton AE, Dziura J, Hooton TM, et al. Recurrent urinary tract infection and urinary *Escherichia coli* in women ingesting cranberry juice daily: a randomized controlled trial. Mayo Clin Proc 2012;87(2):143–50.

90. Beerepoot MA, Ter Riet G, Nys S, et al. Cranberries vs antibiotics to prevent urinary tract infections: a randomized double-blind noninferiority trial in premenopausal women. Arch Intern Med 2011;171(14):1270–8.

91. Lee BS, Bhuta T, Simpson JM, et al. Methenamine hippurate for preventing urinary tract infections. Cochrane Database Syst Rev 2012;(10):CD003265.

92. Suckling J, Lethaby A, Kennedy R. Local oestrogen for vaginal atrophy in postmenopausal women. Cochrane Database Syst Rev 2006;(4):CD001500.

93. Pabich WL, Fihn SD, Stamm WE, et al. Prevalence and determinants of vaginal flora alterations in postmenopausal women. J Infect Dis 2003;188(7):1054–8.

94. Perrotta C, Aznar M, Mejia R, et al. Oestrogens for preventing recurrent urinary tract infection in postmenopausal women. Cochrane Database Syst Rev 2008;(2):CD005131.

95. Engel JD, Schaeffer AJ. Evaluation of and antimicrobial therapy for recurrent urinary tract infections in women. Urol Clin North Am 1998;25(4):685–701, x.

96. Johansen TE. The role of imaging in urinary tract infections. World J Urol 2004; 22(5):392–8.

97. Van Haarst EP, Van Andel G, Heldeweg EA, et al. Evaluation of the diagnostic workup in young women referred for recurrent lower urinary tract infections. Urology 2001;57(6):1068–72.

98. Lawrentschuk N, Ooi J, Pang A, et al. Cystoscopy in women with recurrent urinary tract infection. Int J Urol 2006;13(4):350–3.

99. Albert X, Huertas I, Pereiró II, et al. Antibiotics for preventing recurrent urinary tract infection in non-pregnant women. Cochrane Database Syst Rev 2004;(3):CD001209.

100. Stapleton A, Latham RH, Johnson C, et al. Postcoital antimicrobial prophylaxis for recurrent urinary tract infection. A randomized, double-blind, placebo-controlled trial. JAMA 1990;264(6):703–6.

101. Melekos MD, Asbach HW, Gerharz E, et al. Post-intercourse versus daily ciprofloxacin prophylaxis for recurrent urinary tract infections in premenopausal women. J Urol 1997;157(3):935–9.

102. Zhong YH, Fang Y, Zhou JZ, et al. Effectiveness and safety of patient initiated single-dose versus continuous low-dose antibiotic prophylaxis for recurrent urinary tract infections in postmenopausal women: a randomized controlled study. J Int Med Res 2011;39(6):2335–43.

Index

Note: Page numbers of article titles are in **boldface** type.

A

Abdominal infections, streptococci group A, 724
Abscesses, MRSA, 605–607, 609–610
Acute retinal necrosis, in herpes zoster, 508
Acyclovir, for herpes zoster, 513–514
Adamantanes, for influenza, 630
Adenylate cyclase toxin, *Bordetella pertussis,* 539
African tick bite fever, in returning travelers, 713
Agranulocytosis, drug-induced, 668
Albendazole, for cutaneous larva migrans, 705
Albumin replacement, for streptococcal group A infections, 728
Allergic interstitial nephritis, drug-induced, 670
Allopurinol, complications of, 672
Amikacin
    for multidrug-resistant tuberculosis, 563
    resistance to, 562
Aminoglycosides, complications of, 670–671
Amitriptyline, for post-herpetic neuralgia, 512
Amoxicillin, complications of, 669
Amoxicillin/clavulanate
    complications of, 670
    for *Streptococcus pneumoniae* infections, 656
Amphotericin
    complications of, 670
    for leishmaniasis, 706
Ampicillin, complications of, 673
Anemia, hemolytic. *See* Hemolytic anemia.
Animal exposure, by travelers, 702
Antibiotics. *See also specific antibiotics.*
    Clostridium difficile infections due to, 524, 527
    complications of, **667–679**
        by agent, 674
        by system, 667–674
        drug-drug interactions, 674–676
    resistance to. *See* Drug resistance.
Antidepressants, for post-herpetic neuralgia, 512
Antigenic changes, in influenza virus, 622–623
Antimonials, for leishmaniasis, 706
Aplastic anemia, drug-induced, 668
Artemether-lumefantrine, for malaria, 710–711
Arthritis, streptococci group A, 724–725, 730
Asplenia, traveler's infections with, 715

Med Clin N Am 97 (2013) 759–774
http://dx.doi.org/10.1016/S0025-7125(13)00080-1
0025-7125/13/$ – see front matter © 2013 Elsevier Inc. All rights reserved.

medical.theclinics.com

Atovaquone-proguanil, for malaria, 701, 710–711
Avian influenza, 622–624
Azathioprine, immunodeficiency from, traveler's infections with, 715
Azithromycin
    complications of, 668
    drug interactions with, 675
    for enteric fever, 714
    for pertussis, 546
    for streptococcal group A infections, 730
    for *Streptococcus pneumoniae* infections, 651
    for traveler's diarrhea, 700

B

BACTEC460 radiometric test, for multidrug-resistant tuberculosis, 559–561
Bacteremia
    MRSA, 610–612
    streptococci group A, 724–725
    Streptococcus pneumoniae, 650–651
Berdaquiline, multidrug-resistant tuberculosis in, 565–566
Bismuth, for traveler's diarrhea, 703
Blood smear, for malaria detection, 709
Bordetella parapertussis infections, 538
Bordetella pertussis infections. *See* Pertussis.
Botfly bites, myiasis in, 706–707
Bronchitis, in returning travelers, 715

C

Candidiasis, vulvovaginal, drug-induced, 671
Capreomycin
    complications of, 671
    for multidrug-resistant tuberculosis, 563
    resistance to, 562
Capsaicin, for post-herpetic neuralgia, 512
Capsule, *Streptococcus pneumoniae,* 649
Cardiac complications, drug-induced, 668–669
Cefotaxime, for *Streptococcus pneumoniae* infections, 653–657
Cefpodoxime, for urinary tract infections, 747
Ceftaroline, for MRSA infections, 613–614
Ceftriaxone
    complications of, 670
    for streptococcal group A infections, 730
    for *Streptococcus pneumoniae* infections, 656
Cellulitis
    in herpes zoster, 509–510
    streptococci group A, 725
Cephalosporins
    complications of, 668, 670, 673
    for enteric fever, 714
    for MRSA infections, 613–614

Chemoprophylaxis, for influenza, 635–636
Chemotherapy, immunodeficiency from, traveler's infections with, 715
Chicken pox, herpes zoster after. *See* Herpes zoster.
Chills, in enteric fever, 714
Chloroquine, for malaria, 701, 710–711
Ciprofloxacin
    complications of, 670, 673, 746
    for *Streptoco ccus pneumoniae* infections, 656–657
    for traveler's diarrhea, 700
    for urinary tract infections, 743, 746–747
Clarithromycin
    complications of, 668
    drug interactions with, 675–676
    for pertussis, 546
Clindamycin
    for malaria, 710–711
    for MRSA infections, 606–608
    for streptococcal group A infections, 727, 729, 731
    for *Streptococcus pneumoniae* infections, 656
Clostridium difficile infections, **523–536**
    clinical manifestations of, 525–527
    diagnosis of, 525–527
    epidemiology of, 524–525
    microbiology of, 523–524
    prevention of, 527–528
    recurrence of, 531–532
    risk factors for, 524–525
    severity of, 525
    surveillance for, 526–527
    treatment of, 528–532
Colistin, complications of, 670
Colitis, pseudomembranous, in *Clostridium difficile* infections, 525
Colonization, by MRSA, 604–605, 610–611
Computed tomography, for *Clostridium difficile* infections, 526
Contraceptive methods, urinary tract infections and, 748
Corticosteroids
    for herpes zoster, 512
    for *Streptococcus pneumoniae* meningitis, 652
    immunodeficiency from, traveler's infections with, 715
Cough
    in influenza, 625–626
    in pertussis, 541–543, 547
    in tuberculosis, 558
Cranberries, for urinary tract infection prevention, 748–749
Croupous colitis, 650
Cryptosporidiosis, in solid organ transplant patients, 590–592
Culture
    for *Bordetella pertussis,* 544
    for enteric fever, 714
    for enterohemorrhagic *Escherichia coli,* 686
    for influenza, 626–627

Culture (*continued*)
>   for multidrug-resistant tuberculosis, 559–560
>   for urinary tract infections, 740–742
Cutaneous larva migrans, 704–705
Cyclophosphamide, immunodeficiency from, traveler's infections with, 715
Cycloserine, for multidrug-resistant tuberculosis, 555, 563
Cystitis
>   antibiotic-resistant. *See* Urinary tract infections.
>   in solid organ transplant patients, 592–594
Cystoscopy, for urinary tract infections, 750–751

D

Dapsone, complications of, 668, 672–673
Debridement, for necrotizing fasciitis, 727
Decolonization, for MRSA infections, 610–611
DEET, for insect protection, 700
Delamanid, for multidrug-resistant tuberculosis, 564–565
Delirium, drug-induced, 673
Dengue fever, 710, 712
Dermatologic complications, drug-induced, 672–673
Dermatomes, herpes zoster manifestations in, 505–507
Desipramine, for post-herpetic neuralgia, 512
Diarrhea
>   drug-induced, 669–670
>   in *Clostridium difficile* infections, 525
>   in enterohemorrhagic *Escherichia coli* infections, **681–695**
>   in solid organ transplant patients, 590–592
>   traveler's, 699–700, 702–703
Diphtheria vaccine, for solid organ transplant patients, 595
Dipstick analysis, for urinary tract infections, 740–742
Direct fluorescent antibody test
>   for *Bordetella pertussis,* 545
>   for herpes zoster, 510
Directly Observed Therapy-Short Course treatment, for tuberculosis, 556, 562
Doxycycline
>   complications of, 670, 673
>   for malaria, 701
>   for MRSA infections, 606, 608
>   for rickettsial infections, 713
>   for *Streptococcus pneumoniae* infections, 651
Drainage, of MRSA abscess, 605–606
DRESS (Drug Rash with Eosinophilia and Systemic Systems), 672
Drug fever, 673
Drug resistance
>   in urinary tract infections, **737–757**
>   *Mycobacterium tuberculosis. See* Multidrug-resistant tuberculosis.
>   *Staphylococcus aureus,* **601–619**
>   *Streptococcus pneumoniae,* 652–658
Drug-induced liver injury, 670

E

Ear, herpes zoster of, 509

Eculizumab, for enterohemorrhagic *Escherichia coli* infections, 689

Elderly persons, influenza in, 626, 632, 634

Electrolyte abnormalities, drug-induced, 670–671

Empyema, in streptococcal group A infections, 730

Endocarditis

   MRSA, 613

   streptococci group A, 724, 731

Enteric fever, in returning travelers, 714

Enteric infections

   in returning travelers, 714

   in solid organ transplant patients, 590–592

Enterobacteriaceae infections, urinary tract, 739

Enterohemorrhagic *Escherichia coli* infections and hemolytic-uremic syndrome, **681–695**

   clinical presentation of, 685–687

   diagnosis of, 686, 688

   epidemiology of, 682–684

   pathogenesis of, 684–685

   prevention of, 690

   prognosis for, 689–690

   transmission of, 682–684

   treatment of, 688–689

Enzyme immunoassay, for *Clostridium difficile,* 526

Eosinophilia, drug-induced, 673

Eosinophiluria, drug-induced, 670

Epsilometer test, for multidrug-resistant tuberculosis, 559–560

Erythromycin

   complications of, 668–670

   for pertussis, 546

   for *Streptococcus pneumoniae* infections, 653–657

Escherichia coli infections

   enterohemorrhagic, hemolytic-uremic syndrome and, **681–695**

   nomenclature of, 684

   urinary tract, 738

Esophagitis, pill, 670

Estrogen, for urinary tract infection prevention, 749

Ethambutol, for multidrug-resistant tuberculosis, 555

Ethionamide, for multidrug-resistant tuberculosis, 563–564

Exanthem, drug-induced, 672

Exotoxins, of streptococci group A, 722–723

Extended spectrum beta-lactamases, in resistance development, 738–739

Eye, herpes zoster of, 507–509, 513–514

F

Facial nerve, herpes zoster of, 509

Famciclovir, for herpes zoster, 514

Fecal microbiota transplantation, for *Clostridium difficile* infections, 532

Fever
    drug, 673
    in returning travelers, 707–714
        dengue, 710, 712
        diagnosis of, 708
        epidemiology of, 707–708
        malaria, 708–711
Fidaxomicin, for *Clostridium difficile* infections, 529
Fixed drug eruptions, 672–673
Fluid therapy
    for enterohemorrhagic *Escherichia coli* infections, 688–689
    for streptococcal group A infections, 727
    for traveler's diarrhea, 703
Fluorometric assay, for multidrug-resistant tuberculosis, 559–560
Fluoroquinolones. *See also specific drugs.*
    complications of, 674
Folliculitis, MRSA, 605–606
Food, traveler's diarrhea related to, 699–700
FoodNet report, on enterohemorrhagic *Escherichia coli* infections, 682
Fosfomycin, for urinary tract infections, 743, 746–747

G

Gabapentin, for post-herpetic neuralgia, 512
Gastric acid suppression, *Clostridium difficile* infections in, 525
Gastroenteric infections, in returning travelers, 714
Gastrointestinal complications, drug-induced, 669–670
Gatifloxacin
    complications of, 668
    for multidrug-resistant tuberculosis, 564
Gemifloxacin, for *Streptococcus pneumoniae* infections, 651, 657
Genetics, of influenza virus, 622–623
GeneXpert MTB/RIF assay, for multidrug-resistant tuberculosis, 561
Genitourinary complications, drug-induced, 671
Genotypic tests, for multidrug-resistant tuberculosis, 560–561
Gentamicin, for MRSA infections, 610, 612
GeoSentinel network, for traveler's infections, 704
Global Alliance for TB Drug Development, 566
Glucose-6-phosphate deficiency, hemolytic anemia in, 668

H

Hemagglutinin, influenza virus, 622–626
Hematologic complications, drug-induced, 667–668
Hemolysis, in streptococcal group A infections, 728–729
Hemolytic anemia
    immune, 667–668
    in enterohemorrhagic *Escherichia coli* infections, **681–695**
Hemolytic-uremic syndrome and enterohemorrhagic *Escherichia coli* infections, **681–695**
Hepatobiliary complications, drug-induced, 670

Herpes zoster, **503–522**
    clinical presentation of, 505–507
    complications of, 507–509
    contagiousness of, 511
    diagnosis of, 510–511
    differential diagnosis of, 509–510
    disseminated, 505
    epidemiology of, 503–505
    in pregnancy, 513
    pathogenesis of, 505
    prodrome of, 506–507
    recurrence of, 507
    treatment of, 511–514
    vaccine for, 514–517
Herpes zoster ophthalmicus, 507–509, 513–514
Herpes zoster oticus, 509
Hives, drug-induced, 672
Human immunodeficiency virus infection, 513
    herpes zoster in, 506, 508
    influenza vaccine for, 635
    multidrug-resistant tuberculosis in, 558, 564–565
    Streptococcus pneumoniae infections in, 648–649
    traveler's infections with, 715
Human papilloma virus vaccine, for solid organ transplant patients, 596–597
Hutchinson sign, 507–508, 513–514
Hyperkalemia, drug-induced, 670–671
Hypersensitivity, drug-induced, 672
Hypokalemia, drug-induced, 671

I

Imipenem, complications of, 673
Immunization. *See* Vaccines and vaccination.
Immunodeficiency
    herpes zoster in, 504–507, 515–517
    influenza vaccine for, 635
    Streptococcus pneumoniae infections in, 648–649
    traveler's infections with, 715–716
Immunofluoresence test, for influenza, 626–627
Immunoglobulin G, intravenous, for streptococcal group A infections, 729
Immunosuppressive therapy, for solid organ transplantation, infections due to, **581–600**
Infection control
    for *Clostridium difficile,* 527
    for enterohemorrhagic *Escherichia coli* infections, 690
    for influenza, 636
    in animal exposure, 702
Inflammatory bowel disease, *Clostridium difficile* infections with, 525
Influenza, **621–645**
    B type, 622
    biology of, 622–623

Influenza (*continued*)
    C type, 622
    complications of, 636–637
    diagnosis of, 625–628
    genetics of, 622–623
    history of, 623–625
    H1N1 (1918), 622
    H1N1 (2009), 624–625, 632–633
    H2N2 (1957), 623–624
    H3N2, 623–624
    H5N1, 623–624
    in elderly persons, 626, 632, 634
    in returning travelers, 715
    in solid organ transplant patients, 585–587
    prevention of, 633–636
    transmission of, 633–634
    treatment of, 628–633
    vaccines for, 595, 634–635
Insect-borne diseases, in travelers, 700
Insurance, for travelers, 698
International Health Regulations, vaccine requirements of, 699
Isoniazid
    complications of, 671, 673
    for multidrug-resistant tuberculosis, 555
Ivermectin, for cutaneous larva migrans, 705

K

Kanamycin
    for multidrug-resistant tuberculosis, 563
    resistance to, 562
Kidney injury
    drug-induced, 670
    in enterohemorrhagic *Escherichia coli* infections, **681–695**
    in streptococcal group A infections, 728
Klebsiella pneumoniae infections, urinary tract, 738–739

L

Larva migrans, cutaneous, 704–705
Leishmaniasis, 705–706
Leukocytosis, in *Clostridium difficile* infections, 525
Leukopenia, in dengue fever, 712
Levofloxacin
    drug interactions with, 675
    for multidrug-resistant tuberculosis, 563
    for *Streptococcus pneumoniae* infections, 651, 653–657
    for urinary tract infections, 746–747
Lidocaine, for post-herpetic neuralgia, 512–513
Line probe assay, for multidrug-resistant tuberculosis, 560–561

Linezolid
    complications of, 668, 675
    for MRSA infections, 606, 608, 613
    for multidrug-resistant tuberculosis, 564
Liver, drug-induced toxicity to, 670
Loperamide, for traveler's diarrhea, 703
Lung
    drug-induced toxicity to, 669
    surgery on, for multidrug-resistant tuberculosis, 566
Lupus, drug-induced, 671

M

M protein, of streptococci group A, 722, 732
Malaria, in travelers, 700, 708–711
Management of Adolescent and Adult Illness Project, for tuberculosis treatment, 562
Mediterranean spotted fever, in returning travelers, 713
Mefloquine, for malaria, 701, 710–711
Meningitis
    streptococcal group A, 724, 731
    Streptococcus pneumoniae, 652, 655
Methenamine salts, for urinary tract infection prevention, 749
Methicillin-resistant *Staphylococcus aureus* infections. *See* MRSA (methicillin-resistant *Staphylococcus aureus*) infections.
Methotrexate, immunodeficiency from, traveler's infections with, 715
Metronidazole
    complications of, 669, 673
    drug interactions with, 676
    for *Clostridium difficile* infections, 528–532
Microscopic-observation drug susceptibility test, for multidrug-resistant tuberculosis, 559
Microscopy, for malaria detection, 709
Minocycline
    complications of, 670–673
    for MRSA infections, 606, 608
Molecular tests, for multidrug-resistant tuberculosis, 560–561
Moxifloxacin
    complications of, 668
    for multidrug-resistant tuberculosis, 563, 566
    for *Streptococcus pneumoniae* infections, 651, 657
MRSA (methicillin-resistant *Staphylococcus aureus*) infections, **601–619**
    abscesses, 605–607, 609–610
    bacteremia, 610–612
    ceftaroline for, 613–614
    colonization by, 604–605, 610–611
    community-acquired, 603–604
    consultation in, 614
    decolonization in, 610–611
    future of, 614–615
    hospital-acquired, 603–604
    information resources for, 615

MRSA (*continued*)
origin of, 602–603
pneumonia, 613–614
systemic, 607–609
urinary tract, 612–613
vaccine for, 615
versus methicillin-sensitive *Staphylococcus aureus,* 603–604
worries about, 604–605
MTBDR*plus* assay, for multidrug-resistant tuberculosis, 560–561
MTBDRs/ assay, for multidrug-resistant tuberculosis, 562
MTB/RIF test, 561
Multidrug-resistant tuberculosis, **553–579**
diagnosis of, 558–562
epidemiology of, 556–558
extrapulmonary, 558
extreme, 562–564, 568
historical perspective of, 554–556
infection control for, 567–569
totally, 567
treatment of, 562–567
Murine typhus, in returning travelers, 713
Myalgia, in influenza, 625–626
Mycobacterium tuberculosis infections, multidrug-resistant. *See* Multidrug-resistant
tuberculosis.
Myiasis, 706–707
Myocarditis, in influenza, 636

N

Nasociliary nerve, herpes zoster of, 508–509
National Antimicrobial Resistance Monitoring System, 739
Nausea, drug-induced, 669–670
Necrotizing pneumonitis, in streptococcal group A infections, 730
Necrotizing soft tissue infections, streptococci group A, 723–727, 731
Nephritis, allergic interstitial, 670
Nephrotoxicity, of antibiotics, 670
Neuralgia, post-herpetic, 504, 507–508, 511–514
Neuraminidase, influenza virus, 622–626
Neurologic disorders
drug-induced, 673, 675
in herpes zoster, 509
in influenza, 636–637
Nikolsky's sign, 672
Nitrate reductase assay, for multidrug-resistant tuberculosis, 559
Nitrofurantoin
complications of, 668–671, 673, 744
for urinary tract infections, 742–744, 746
Nortriptyline, for post-herpetic neuralgia, 512
Nucleic acid amplification tests
for *Clostridium difficile,* 526
for multidrug-resistant tuberculosis, 561

O

Obesity, influenza in, 624
Oncologic medications, immunodeficiency from, traveler's infections with, 715
Opioids, for post-herpetic neuralgia, 513
Oral contraceptives, drug interactions with, 676, 747
Oral rehydration solution, for traveler's diarrhea, 703
Oseltamivir, for influenza, 628–632, 636–637
Osteomyelitis, streptococci group A, 724
Otitis media, *Streptococcus pneumoniae,* 652

P

PA-824, for multidrug-resistant tuberculosis, 566
Pain
    in enteric fever, 714
    in enterohemorrhagic *Escherichia coli* infections, 686
    in herpes zoster, 506
    in necrotizing fasciitis, 724
    post-herpetic, 504, 507–508, 515–517
Para-amino salicylic acid, for multidrug-resistant tuberculosis, 555, 563
Paratyphoid fever, in returning travelers, 714
Partners in Health, for tuberculosis treatment, 562
Penicillin(s)
    complications of, 668, 671–673
    for streptococcal group A infections, 727, 731
    for *Streptococcus pneumoniae* infections, 653–657
Peripheral neuropathy, drug-induced, 673
Pertussis, **537–552**
    age-related differences in, 541–542
    classic, 541
    clinical manifestations of, 540–542
    complications of, 542
    diagnosis of, 543–545
    differential diagnosis of, 542–543
    epidemiology of, 539–540
    in pregnancy, 548–549
    laboratory findings in, 541
    microbiology of, 538
    pathogenesis of, 539
    phases of, 541
    physical examination in, 541
    radiography for, 541
    toxins of, 539
    transmission of, 538
    treatment of, 546–547
    vaccine for, 547–549, 595
Pharyngitis, in returning travelers, 714–715
Phenotypic assays, for multidrug-resistant tuberculosis, 559–560
Photosensitivity, drug-induced, 673
Pill esophagitis, 670

Plasmapheresis, for enterohemorrhagic *Escherichia coli* infections, 689
Plasmodium infections (malaria), 708–711
Pneumococcal infections. *See Streptococcus pneumoniae* infections.
Pneumococcal urinary antigen, 650
Pneumococcal vaccine, for solid organ transplant patients, 595
Pneumolysin, 649
Pneumonia
    in influenza, 632–633
    in pertussis, 542
    in returning travelers, 715
    in solid organ transplant patients, 588–590
    MRSA, 613–614
    streptococci group A, 724–725, 729–731
    Streptococcus pneumoniae, 649–650
Polymerase chain reaction
    for herpes zoster, 510
    for influenza, 626–627
    for malaria, 709
    for multidrug-resistant tuberculosis, 560
    for pertussis, 544
Post-herpetic neuralgia, 504, 507–508, 511–514
Pregabalin, for post-herpetic neuralgia, 512
Pregnancy
    herpes zoster in, 513
    influenza in, 624, 631–632
    pertussis in, 548–549
Primaquine, for malaria, 710–711
Probiotics
    for *Clostridium difficile* infection prevention, 527–528, 532
    for urinary tract infections, 748
    for vulvovaginal candidiasis, 671
Pruritus, drug-induced, 672
Pseudomembranous colitis, in *Clostridium difficile* infections, 525
Pseudomonas aeruginosa infections, urinary tract, 739
Puerperal sepsis, streptococci group A, 724, 730
Pyelonephritis
    antibiotic-resistant. *See* Urinary tract infections.
    in solid organ transplant patients, 592–594
Pyomyositis, streptococci group A, 724, 731
Pyrazinamide
    for multidrug-resistant tuberculosis, 555, 563–564, 566
    resistance to, 561
Pyridoxine, for multidrug-resistant tuberculosis, 563

Q

QT prolongation, drug-induced, 668–669
Quinidine, for malaria, 710–711
Quinine, for malaria, 710–711
Quinolones, for enteric fever, 714

R

Rabies, in travelers, 702
Radiography
    for pertussis, 541
    for *Streptococcus pneumoniae* infections, 650
Ramsay Hunt syndrome, 509
Rapid tests, for influenza, 626–627
Rash
    differential diagnosis of, 509–510
    drug, 672
    in cutaneous larva migrans, 704–705
    in dengue fever, 712
    in herpes zoster, 505–510
Respiratory disorders
    drug-induced, 669
    in returning travelers, 714–715
Retinal detachment, drug-induced, 675
Retinal necrosis, in herpes zoster, 508
Rheumatologic complications, drug-induced, 671
Ribavirin, for influenza, 630
Rickettsial infections, in returning travelers, 713
Rifampin
    drug interactions with, 676
    for MRSA infections, 608
    for multidrug-resistant tuberculosis, 555
    resistance to, 561
Rifaxamin, for traveler's diarrhea, 700
Rocky Mountain spotted fever, in returning travelers, 713

S

Salmonella infections
    from animal exposure, 702
    in returning travelers, 714
Sand flea bites, tungiasis in, 707
Scrub typhus, in returning travelers, 713
Seizures, drug-induced, 673
SENTRY Antimicrobial Surveillance Program, 653–654
Septic arthritis, streptococci group A, 724–725, 730
Septic shock, in *Streptococcus pneumoniae* infections, 651
Serologic tests, for *Bordetella pertussis,* 545
Serotonin syndrome, 675
Sexual activity, in travelers, protection in, 701–702
Shiga toxin, *Escherichia coli,* 684–686
Shingles. *See* Herpes zoster.
Shingles Prevention Study, 514
Skin lesions
    drug-induced, 672–673
    in travelers, 703–707
Spermicide use, urinary tract infections and, 748

Splenectomy, traveler's infections after, 715
Spotted fever, in returning travelers, 713
Sputum collection, for *Streptococcus pneumoniae* infections, 650
Staphylococcus aureus infections, methicillin-resistant. *See* MRSA (methicillin-resistant *Staphylococcus aureus*) infections.
Staphylococcus saprophyticus infections, 738
Stevens-Johnson syndrome, 672
Streptococcal group A infections, **721–736**
    clinical presentation of, 723–731
    epidemiology of, 723
    incidence of, 722
    microbiology of, 722–723
    pathophysiology of, 722–723
    prevention of, 732
    spectrum of, 721
    treatment of, 731–732
Streptococcal infections, pyogenic, 605–606
Streptococcus pneumoniae infections, **647–666**
    antimicrobial resistance in, 652–658
    bacteremia, 650–651
    bacterial structure and, 649
    colonization and, 649
    epidemiology of, 648
    invasive, 648
    meningitis, 652
    otitis media, 652
    pathogenesis of, 649
    pneumonia, 649–650
    risk factors for, 648–649
    vaccines for, 658–660
Streptococcus pyogenes infections. *See* Streptococcal group A infections.
Streptomycin, for multidrug-resistant tuberculosis, 563
Sulfonamides, complications of, 668, 670, 672–673
Swelling, in necrotizing fasciitis, 724
Swine influenza, 622–624
Systemic lupus erythematosus, drug-induced, 671

T

Tendinopathy, drug-induced, 675
Tetanus vaccine, for solid organ transplant patients, 595
Tetracyclines
    complications of, 673
    for malaria, 710–711
    for MRSA infections, 608
    for *Streptococcus pneumoniae* infections, 653–657
Thin-layer agar assay, for multidrug-resistant tuberculosis, 559
Thrombocytopenia
    drug-induced, 668
    in dengue fever, 712
Thrombotic microangiopathy, in enterohemorrhagic *Escherichia coli* infections, 685

Tonsillitis, in returning travelers, 714–715

Torsades de pointes, drug-induced, 668

Totally drug-resistant tuberculosis, 567

Toxic epidermal necrolysis, drug-induced, 672

Toxic shock syndrome, streptococci group A, 724–725, 727–729, 731

Toxins
    Bordetella pertussis, 539
    Clostridium difficile, 523–524, 526
    streptococci group A, 722–723

Tracheal cytotoxin, *Bordetella pertussis,* 539

Transaminitis, drug-induced, 673

Transplantation
    fecal microbiota, for *Clostridium difficile* infections, 532
    solid organ
        infections in, **581–600**
            case studies of, 585–597
            herpes zoster, 506
            practical issues in, 582–585
            statistics on, 581–582
            timeline of susceptibility in, 584
            vaccines for, 635
        traveler's infections with, 715–716

Traveler's infections, **697–720**
    after return from trip, 702–716
        diarrhea, 702–703
        enteric, 714
        fever, 707–712
        respiratory disorders, 714–715
        rickettsial, 713
        skin lesions, 703–707
    counseling on, 699–702
    in immunodeficiency, 715–716
    preetravel visit for, 698–699

Trigeminal ganglion, herpes zoster in, 513–514

Trimethoprim-sulfamethoxazole
    complications of, 668–672, 675, 745
    drug interactions with, 675, 745
    for MRSA infections, 606, 608
    for pertussis, 546
    for *Streptococcus pneumoniae* infections, 653–657
    for urinary tract infections, 743–745, 751

Tuberculosis, multidrug-resistant. *See* Multidrug-resistant tuberculosis.

Tumor necrosis inhibitor therapy, immunodeficiency from, traveler's infections with, 715

Tungiasis, 707

Typhoid fever, in returning travelers, 714

Typhus, in returning travelers, 713

U

Ulcerative colitis, *Clostridium difficile* infections with, 525

Ultrasonography, for urinary tract infections, 750

Urinary tract infections
    antibiotic-resistant, **737–757**
        evaluation of, 740–742
        impact of, 738
        incidence of, 738
        microbiology of, 738–740
        prevention of, 747–751
        recurrent, 747–751
        resistance mechanisms in, 738–740
        risk factors for, 738–740, 742
        treatment of, 742–747
    in solid organ transplant patients, 592–595
    MRSA, 612–613
Urticaria, drug-induced, 672

V

Vaccines and vaccination
    for solid organ transplant patients, 594–597
    for travelers, 698–699
    herpes zoster, 514–517
    influenza, 595, 634–635
    MRSA, 615
    streptococcal group A infections, 732
    Streptococcus pneumoniae, 658–660
    typhoid fever, 714
Valacyclovir, for herpes zoster, 514
Vancomycin
    complications of, 670, 672
    for *Clostridium difficile* infections, 528–532
    for MRSA infections, 607–609, 612–613
    for *Streptococcus pneumoniae* infections, 653–658
Varicella zoster virus infections, herpes zoster in. *See* Herpes zoster.
Verotoxin, *Escherichia coli,* 684–686
Vision loss, in herpes zoster, 507–508
Voiding habits, urinary tract infections and, 748
Vomiting, in pertussis, 541–543
Vulvovaginal candidiasis, drug-induced, 671

W

Warfarin, drug interactions with, 674–675
Water, traveler's diarrhea related to, 699–700
Whooping cough. *See* Pertussis.
World Health Organization, multidrug-resistant tuberculosis involvement by, 554–556

Z

Zanamavir, for influenza, 628–630
Zoster. *See* Herpes zoster.
Zoster sine herpete, 507

Moving?

Make sure your subscription moves with you!

To notify us of your new address, find your **Clinics Account Number** (located on your mailing label above your name), and contact customer service at:

Email: journalscustomerservice-usa@elsevier.com

800-654-2452 (subscribers in the U.S. & Canada)
314-447-8871 (subscribers outside of the U.S. & Canada)

Fax number: 314-447-8029

Elsevier Health Sciences Division
Subscription Customer Service
3251 Riverport Lane
Maryland Heights, MO 63043

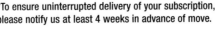

*To ensure uninterrupted delivery of your subscription,
please notify us at least 4 weeks in advance of move.